AF335612

SCOPE 41
IPCS JOINT SYMPOSIA 8

SGOMSEC 4

Short-term Toxicity Tests for Non-genotoxic Effects

Scientific Committee on Problems of the Environment
SCOPE
Executive Committee, elected 10 June 1988

Officers

President: Professor F. di Castri, CNRS, Centre L. Emberger. Route de Mende, BP 5051, 34033 Montpellier Cedex, France

Vice-President: Academician M.V. Ivanov, Institute of Microbiology, USSR Academy of Sciences, GSP-7 Prospekt 60 letija Oktjabrja 7-2, 117811, Moscow, USSR

Vice-President: Professor C.R. Krishna Murti, Scientific Commission for Continuing Studies on Effects of Bhopal Gas Leakage on Life Systems, Cabinet Secretariat, 2nd Floor, Sardar Patel Bhavan, New Delhi 110001, India

Treasurer: Dr T.E. Lovejoy, Smithsonian Institution, Washington, DC, 20560, USA

Secretary-General: Professor J.W.B. Stewart, Saskatchewan Institute of Pedology, University of Saskatchewan, Saskatoon, Saskatchewan, S7N 0W0, Canada

Members

Professor M.O. Andreae (I.U.G.G. representative), Max-Planck-Institut für Chemie, Postfach 3060, D-6500 Mainz, FRG

Professor M.A. Ayyad, Faculty of Science, Alexandria University, Moharram Bey, Alexandria, Egypt

Professor R. Herrera (I.U.B.S. representative), Centro de Ecologia y Ciencias Ambientales (IVIC), Carretera Panamericana km. 11, Apartado 21827, Caracas, Venezuela

Professor M. Kecskés, Department of Microbiology, University of Agricultural Sciences, Pater K. utca 1, 2103 Gödöllö, Hungary

Professor R.O. Slatyer, Chief Scientist, Office of the Prime Minister and Cabinet, 3–5 National Circuit, Barton, ACT 2600, Australia.

Editor-in-Chief

Professor R.E. Munn, Institute of Environmental Studies, University of Toronto, Toronto, Ontario M5S 1A4, Canada

SCOPE 41
IPCS JOINT SYMPOSIA 8

SGOMSEC 4

Short-term Toxicity Tests for Non-genotoxic Effects

Edited by

Philippe Bourdeau
Commission of the European Communities, Brussels, Belgium

Emmanuel Somers
Health and Welfare Canada, Ottawa, Canada

G. Mark Richardson
Health and Welfare Canada, Ottawa, Canada

and

J.R. Hickman
Health and Welfare Canada, Ottawa, Canada

Prepared by
Scientific Group on Methodologies for the
Safety Evaluation of Chemicals
(SGOMSEC)

Published on behalf of the
Scientific Committee on Problems of the Environment (SCOPE)
of the International Council of Scientific Unions (ICSU),
and the International Programme on Chemical Safety (IPCS)
of the World Health Organization (WHO),
the United Nations Environment Programme (UNEP)
and the International Labour Organization (ILO)

by

JOHN WILEY & SONS
Chichester · New York · Brisbane · Toronto · Singapore

Other Wiley Editorial Offices

John Wiley & Sons, Inc., 605 Third Avenue,
New York, NY 10158-0012, USA

Jacaranda Wiley Ltd, G.P.O. Box 859, Brisbane,
Queensland 4001, Australia

John Wiley & Sons (Canada) Ltd, 22 Worcester Road,
Rexdale, Ontario M9W 1L1, Canada

John Wiley & Sons (SEA) Pte Ltd, 37 Jalan Pemimpin 05-04,
Block B, Union Industrial Building, Singapore 2057

Library of Congress Cataloging-in-Publication Data

Short-term toxicity tests for non-genotoxic effects   /   edited by
   Philippe Bourdeau . . . [et al.].
      p.   cm. — (SCOPE   ;   41)   (IPCS joint symposium   ;   8)   (SGOMSEC)
      ;   4)
      "Published on behalf of the Scientific Committee on Problems of
the Environment (SCOPE) of the International Council of Scientific
Unions (ICSU) . . . [et al]."
   Includes bibliographical references.
   ISBN 0 471 92506 3
   1.   Acute toxicity testing.   I.   Bourdeau, Philippe.
II.   International Council of Scientific Unions.   Scientific
Committee on Problems of the Environment.   III.   Series.   IV.   Series:
SCOPE report   ;   41.   V.   Series: SGOMSEC (Series)   ;   4.
RA1199.4.A38S56   1990
615.9'07—dc20   89-22693
                                                                                    CIP

British Library Cataloguing in Publication Data

Short-term toxicity tests for non-genotoxic effects.
   1. Man.   Toxic effects of chemicals.   Research.   Use of laboratory animals
I.   Bourdeau, Philippe   II.   Series   III.   Series   IIII.
Series
615.9'00724

ISBN 0 471 92506 3

Typeset by Inforum Typesetting, Portsmouth
Printed in Great Britain by Biddles Ltd., Guildford, Surrey

SCOPE 1: Global Environmental Monitoring 1971, 68 pp (out of print)
SCOPE 2: Man-Made Lakes as Modified Ecosystems, 1972, 76 pp (out of print)
SCOPE 3: Global Environmental Monitoring Systems (GEMS): Action Plan for Phase 1, 1973, 132 pp (out of print)
SCOPE 4: Environmental Sciences in Developing Countries, 1974, 72 pp (out of print)
Environment and Development, proceedings of SCOPE/UNEP Symposium on Environmental Sciences in Developing Countries, Nairobi, February 11–23, 1974, 418 pp (out of print)
SCOPE 5: Environmental Impact Assessment: Principles and Procedures, Second Edition, 1979, 208 pp
SCOPE 6: Environmental Pollutants: Selected Analytical Methods, 1975, 277 pp (out of print)
SCOPE 7: Nitrogen, Phosphorus and Sulphur: Global Cycles, 1975, 129 pp (out of print)
SCOPE 8: Risk Assessment of Environmental Hazard, 1978, 132 pp (out of print)
SCOPE 9: Simulation Modelling of Environmental Problems, 1978, 128 pp (out of print)
SCOPE 10: Environmental Issues, 1977, 242 pp (out of print)
SCOPE 11: Shelter Provision in Developing Countries, 1978, 112 pp (out of print)
SCOPE 12: Principles of Ecotoxicology, 1978, 372 pp (out of print)
SCOPE 13: The Global Carbon Cycle, 1979, 491 pp (out of print)
SCOPE 14: Saharan Dust: Mobilization, Transport, Deposition, 1979, 320 pp (out of print)
SCOPE 15: Environmental Risk Assessment, 1980, 176 pp (out of print)
SCOPE 16: Carbon Cycle Modelling, 1981, 404 pp (out of print)
SCOPE 17: Some Perspectives of the Major Biogeochemical Cycles, 1981, 175 pp (out of print)
SCOPE 18: The Role of Fire in Northern Circumpolar Ecosystems, 1983, 344 pp
SCOPE 19: The Global Biogeochemical Sulphur Cycle, 1983, 495 pp
SCOPE 20: Methods for Assessing the Effects of Chemicals on Reproductive Functions, 1983, 568 pp
SCOPE 21: The Major Biogeochemical Cycles and Their Interactions, 1983, 554 pp (out of print)
SCOPE 22: Effects of Pollutants at the Ecosystem Level, 1984, 460 pp
SCOPE 23: The Role of Terrestrial Vegetation in the Global Carbon Cycle: Measurement by Remote Sensing, 1984, 272 pp
SCOPE 24: Noise Pollution, 1986, 466 pp
SCOPE 25: Appraisal of Tests to Predict the Environmental Behaviour of Chemicals, 1985, 400 pp
SCOPE 26: Methods for Estimating Risks of Chemical Injury: Human and Non-Human Biota and Ecosystems, 1985, 712 pp
SCOPE 27: Climate Impact Assessment: Studies of the Interaction of Climate and Society, 1985, 650 pp

Funds to meet SCOPE expenses are provided by contributions from SCOPE Committees, an annual subvention from ICSU (and through ICSU, from UNESCO), an annual subvention from the French Ministère de l'Environnement, contracts with UN Bodies, particularly UNEP, and grants from Foundations and industrial enterprises.

International Council of Scientific Unions (ICSU)
Scientific Committee on Problems of the Environment (SCOPE)

SCOPE is one of a number of committees established by a non-governmental group of scientific organizations, the International Council of Scientific Unions (ICSU). The membership of ICSU includes representatives from 74 National Academies of Science, 20 International Unions and 26 other bodies called Scientific Associates. To cover multidisciplinary activities which include the interests of several unions, ICSU has established 10 scientific committees, of which SCOPE is one. Currently, representatives of 35 member countries and 20 international scientific bodies participate in the work of SCOPE, which directs particular attention to the needs of developing countries. SCOPE was established in 1969 in response to the environmental concerns emerging at that time; ICSU recognized that many of these concerns required scientific inputs spanning several disciplines and ICSU Unions. SCOPE's first task was to prepare a report on Global Environmental Monitoring (SCOPE 1, 1971) for the UN Stockholm Conference on the Human Environment.

The mandate of SCOPE is to assemble, review, and assess the information available on man-made environmental changes and the effects of these changes on man; to assess and evaluate the methodologies of measurement of environmental parameters; to provide an intelligence service on current research; and by the recruitment of the best available scientific information and constructive thinking to establish itself as a corpus of informed advice for the benefit of centres of fundamental research and of organizations and agencies operationally engaged in studies of the environment.

SCOPE is governed by a General Assembly, which meets every three years. Between such meetings its activities are directed by the Executive Committee.

R.E. Munn
Editor-in-Chief
SCOPE Publications

Executive Secretary: V. Plocq

Secretariat: 51 Bld de Montmorency
           75016 PARIS

Contents

PART A   JOINT REPORT

Chapter 13   Short-term Tests for Neurotoxicity ... 193

Silvio Garattini

Chapter 14   Methods for Assessing the Effects of Chemicals on the Endocrine System ... 221

J. H. Clark and F. X. R. van Leeuwen

Foreword

While SCOPE is primarily an organization devoted to scientific inquiry, it is, of course, highly sensitive to societal priorities and, hence, also has a keen interest in mechanisms that quickly deliver scientific results to decision-makers and organizations in a position to apply these results in practice.

One such mechanism is provided by the Scientific Group on Methodologies for the Safety Evaluation of Chemicals (SGOMSEC). This group was set up in 1978 and is supported by SCOPE as well as the World Health Organization (WHO), the United Nations Environment Programme (UNEP) and the International Labour Organization (ILO) with the framework of the International Programme on Chemical Safety (IPCS).

The present study is the fourth book produced by this successful group and deals with an important, practical and very specific topic within its wide mandate: reliable *in vitro* tests for toxicity which are a cornerstone in the development of environmentally acceptable chemicals as they have a direct impact on the costs of R & D for new chemicals. In this sense SGOMSEC has been working in this study, as it should, at the cutting edge between science and society.

J.W.W. LaRivière
President, SCOPE (1984)

Foreword

Toxicity testing of chemicals in experimental animals to detect potential hazards to human health and the environment for decades has been the cornerstone of national and international programmes on chemical safety. Over the last several years, major advances in the biological and medical sciences have led to the development of new short-term tests for non-genotoxic end-points. Although many of these tests hold great promise for improving the risk assessment process, as well as for decreasing the use of experimental animals in toxicology, the relevance to the intact animal of the scientific data obtained from such short-term tests have yet to be evaluated. The fourth workshop of the Scientific Group on Methodologies for the Safety Evaluation of Chemicals (SGOMSEC) was organized to address such important scientific issues, providing assistance to the scientific community to develop new and improved methods for assessing risks from chemical exposures.

It is hoped that the personal views and opinions expressed by the individual experts in their Contributed Papers will lead to in-depth scientific discussions followed by the research needed to develop new short-term tests well supported by scientific data, perhaps, even more relevant to the intact animal than that obtained from those tests presently available. The Joint Workshop Report, in turn, should provide scientists and decision makers with a summary of the potential uses of presently available methodologies and the research needed to validate these short term tests, leading to their more widespread use.

Both of these results will be of great assistance to the IPCS as we attempt to promote the development, improvement, validation, and use of methods (laboratory, epidemiological and ecological) suitable for the evaluation of health and environmental risks and hazards from chemicals in an effort to provide scientific guidance to national chemical safety programmes.

MICHEL J. MERCIER
Manager
International Programme on Chemical Safety

Preface

This study was undertaken by the Scientific Group on Methodologies for the Safety Evaluation of Chemicals (SGOMSEC), an international group which examines difficult issues relating to safety evaluation. In doing so, it attempts to identify those methods that may be adequate and useful at this time, those which need improvement, and to suggest research that may improve them.

SGOMSEC operates under the sponsorship of the International Programme on Chemical Safety (IPCS) within the World Health Organization (WHO), which has the joint input of the United Nations Environment Program (UNEP) and the International Labour Organization (ILO). A second sponsor is the Scientific Committee on Problems of the Environment (SCOPE), which operates under the International Council of Scientific Unions (ICSU).

This project was held in Ottawa, Canada, 13–16 August 1984. It was undertaken with the view that something less than full scale *in vivo* studies may have useful predictive value in characterizing the toxicity of chemicals of public health and ecological importance. It was not anticipated that this exploratory study would necessarily reveal techniques ready at this time to serve as substitutes for classical toxicological and environmental assessments. However, in some instances, it has been possible to identify experimental approaches to the resolution of specific questions relating to the adverse effects of chemicals and thus supplement classical *in vivo* approaches. Not surprisingly, in some cases, there were substantial limitations in the information that could be secured in simplified systems.

The issue was dealt with through a series of inquiries: cell cultures involving primarily undifferentiated cells; a systematic examination of short-term tests of the functional ability of organs or components thereof; and a series of systems—haematopoietic, immunologic, reproductive, and so forth—were also examined.

In each such instance, experts in the respective fields undertook the preparation of background papers exploring the presently available information. At the Workshop, these contributors, together with other experts, prepared a Joint Report by collectively examining each of the various topics.

The Joint Report is published together with the contributed papers; we thus have in this volume an examination of the ability of short-term tests to provide useful supplementary information for the evaluation of the effects of chemicals in mammalian systems and in non-human biota.

This is the fourth volume in the SGOMSEC series. This activity was guided by the co-chairpersons, Dr Emmanuel Somers of the Department of National Health and Welfare, Canada, and Dr Philippe Bourdeau, Director of Environmental Research, Commission of the European Communities. The participants who contributed papers and who participated in the preparation of the Joint Report are included in the list of *Participants of the Workshop*.

The entire volume has been edited by and prepared under the supervision of Mr J.R. Hickman of the Department of National Health and Welfare, Canada, to whom we owe much for his skill and discernment.

It is hoped that this survey will provide a useful starting point for further exploration in an endeavour to improve the efficiency of safety evaluation of chemicals and thus aid in providing needed information more quickly and more economically. Obviously, much additional work in nearly every area will be required before major gains can be secured in these objectives.

SGOMSEC is indebted for encouragement or financial support to a number of sponsors, including the Scientific Committee on Problems of the Environment, the International Programme on Chemical Safety, the Canadian Department of National Health and Welfare, the National Research Council of Canada, the Commission of European Communities, the US National Institute of Environmental Health Sciences, the US Environmental Protection Agency, and to many other organizations and individuals.

Co-operation in Ottawa included many services and facilities, which are most gratefully acknowledged. This came from the National Research Council of Canada, where the Workshop was held, and the Environmental Health Directorate of the Canadian Department of National Health and Welfare. We owe much to the secretarial services of Ms Anita Redfern (Mr Hickman's secretary), and Mrs Jane Calvin of New York University, who was of indispensable aid to the Chairman of SGOMSEC in the guiding and control of the manuscripts as they were completed.

NORTON NELSON
Chairman
Scientific Group on Methodologies for the
Safety Evaluation of Chemicals

Scientific Group on Methodologies for the Safety Evaluation of Chemicals

***Philippe Bourdeau,**   *Director of Environmental Research, Commission of the European Communities, Rue de la Loi 200, B-1049, Brussels, Belgium*

N.P. Bockov,   *Director, Institute of Medical Genetics, Kasirskoe sosse 6A, Moscow 115478, USSR*

***Gordon C. Butler,**   *Director, Division of Biological Sciences, National Research Council of Canada, 100 Sussex Drive, Ottawa, Canada K1A 0R6*

***J.R. Hickman,**   *Director General, Environmental Health Directorate, Health Protection Branch, Health and Welfare Canada, Ottawa, Ontario, Canada K1A 0L2*

C.R. Krishna Murti,   *SWATI, 27, Dr. Radhakrishnan Salai, Mylapore, Madras 600 004, India*

V. Landa,   *Czechoslovak Academy of Sciences, Institute of Entomology, Vinicna 7, Prague 2, Czechoslovakia*

Aly Massoud,   *Professor and Chairman, Departments of Community, Environmental and Occupational Medicine, Ein Shams University, PO Box 38, Abbassia, Cairo, Egypt*

***Norton Nelson,**   *Institute for Environmental Medicine, New York University Medical Center, 550 First Avenue, New York, New York, USA 10016 (Chairman)*

Blanca Ordonez,   *Environmental Advisory of the Minister of Health, Lopez Cotilla 739, Col del. Valle 03100 D.V., Mexico*

Jiri Parizek,   *International Programme on Chemical Safety, Division of Environmental Health, World Health Organization, 1211 Geneva 27, Switzerland*

David Peakall,   *Head, Toxicology Section, National Wildlife Research Centre, Canadian Wildlife Service, Ottawa, Ontario, Canada K1A 0E7*

Patrick Sheehan,   *Division of Biological Sciences, National Research Council of Canada, Ottawa, Ontario, Canada K1A 0R6*

***Emmanuel Somers,**   *Director General, Drugs Directorate, Health Protection Branch, Health and Welfare Canada, Health Protection Building, Tunney's Pasture, Ottawa, Ontario, Canada K1A 0L2*

R. Truhaut,   *Laboratoire de Toxicologie et d'Hygiene Industrielle, Faculté des Sciences, Pharmaceutiques et Biologiques de Paris, Université René Descartes, 4 avenue de l'Observatoire, 75006 Paris, France*

*Member of the Executive Committee.

Participants of the Workshop on Short-term Toxicity Tests for Non-genotoxic Effects

D.K. Agarwal,   *National Institute of Environmental Health Sciences, PO Box 12233, Research Triangle Park, Raleigh, North Carolina 27709, USA*

***Bernard Astill,**   *Health, Safety and Human Factors Laboratory, Eastman Kodak Company, 1669 Lake Avenue, Rochester, New York 14650, USA*

Donald Barltrop,   *Department of Child Health, Westminster Medical School, University of London, Vincent Square, London SW1P 2NS, UK*

G.C. Becking,   *Interregional Research Unit, International Programme on Chemical Safety (IPCS), National Institute of Environmental Health Science, PO Box 12233, Research Triangle Park, Raleigh, North Carolina 27709, USA*

A. Berlin,   *Health and Safety Directorate, Commission of European Communities, Plateau DE, Kirchberg L-2920, Luxemburg, OMEA*

Philippe Bourdeau,   *Director of Environmental Research, Commission of the European Communities, Rue de la Loi 200, B-1049, Brussels, Belgium (Co-Chairman)*

J.W. Bridges,   *Professor of Toxicology, Department of Biochemistry, University of Surrey, Guildford, Surrey GU2 5XH, UK*

Martin Brueton,   *Assistant Director, Department of Child Health, Westminster Medical School, University of London, Vincent Square, London SW1P 2NS, UK*

Gordon C. Butler,   *Director, Division of Biological Sciences, National Research Council of Canada, 100 Sussex Drive, Ottawa, Canada K1A 0R6*

Davide Calamari, *Faculty of Agriculture, University of Milan, Via Celoria 2, 20133 Milan, Italy*

Neil Chernoff, *Director, Division of Reproductive and Developmental Toxicology, Health Effects Laboratory, MD-67, U.S. Environmental Protection Agency, Research Triangle Park, North Carolina 27709, USA*

James Clark, *Department of Cell Biology, Baylor College of Medicine, Houston, Texas 77003, USA*

Jack H. Dean, *Head, Immunobiology Program and Immunotoxicology/Cell Biology Section, Chemical Industry Institute of Toxicology, PO Box 12137, Research Triangle Park, North Carolina 27709, USA*

Robert L. Dixon, *Sterling-Winthrop Research Institute, Rensellaer, New York, USA*

B. Ekwall, *Toxicology Laboratory, National Food Administration, Uppsala, Sweden*

Nilda Fernicola, *Pan American Center for Human Ecology and Health, Apartado Postal 249, Toluca, Mexico*

Theodor Fliedner, *Rector, University of Ulm, D 79 Ulm, Federal Republic of Germany*

J. Friedrich, *Lehrstuhl für Organische Chemie, T.U., Lichtenbergstr 4, 8046 Garching, Federal Republic of Germany*

Silvio Garattini, *Direttore, Istituto di Ricerche Pharmacologiche, Mario Negri, Via Eritrea 62, Milan, Italy*

James W. Gillett, *114 Fernow Hall, Cornell University, Department of Natural Resources, Ithaca, New York 14853–0188, USA*

Alan Goldberg, *Department of Environmental Health Sciences, Johns Hopkins School of Hygiene, 615 N. Wolfe Street, Baltimore, Maryland 21205, USA*

M.I. Gounar, *International Programme on Chemical Safety (IPCS), Division of Environmental Health, World Health Organization, 1211 Geneva 27, Switzerland*

H. Heit, *University of Ulm, D 79 Ulm, Federal Republic of Germany*

J.R. Hickman, *Director General, Environmental Health Directorate, Health Protection Branch, Health and Welfare Canada, Ottawa, Ontario, Canada K1A 0L2*

Fina Kalayanova,	*Director, Institute of Hygiene and Occupational Health, Academy of Medicine, Boul. D. Nestorov 15, Sofia 1431, Bulgaria*
K. Khera,	*General Toxicology Section, Food Directorate, Health Protection Branch, Health and Welfare Canada, Ottawa, Ontario, Canada K1A 0L2*
C.R. Krishna Murti,	*SWATI, 27, Dr. Radhakrishnan Salai, Mylapore, Madras 600 004, India*
Ralf Krowke,	*Institute für Toxikologie und Embryopharmakologie, Freie Universität Berlin, Garystr. 5, 1000 Berlin 33, Federal Republic of Germany*
V. Landa,	*Czechoslovak Academy of Sciences, Institute of Entomology, Vinicna 7, Prague 2, Czechoslovakia*
B.V. Leonov,	*Head, Laboratories for Experimental Embryology, All Union Research Institute of OBS/GYN, Elansky Street, Moscow 119435, USSR*
Carlton Nadolney,	*U.S. Environmental Protection Agency, Mail Drop RE 683, 401 M Street S.W., Washington, D.C. 20460, USA*
Norton Nelson,	*Institute for Environmental Medicine, New York University Medical Center, 550 First Avenue, New York, New York 10016, USA*
***D. Neubert,**	*Institut für Toxikologie und Embryopharmakologie der Freien Universität Berlin, Garysterasse 9, D-1000, Berlin 33, Federal Republic of Germany*
B. Ordonez,	*Environmental Advisory of the Minister of Health, Lopez Cotilla 739, COL del. Valle 03100 D.V., Mexico*
G. Pabst,	*University of Ulm, D 79 Ulm, Federal Republic of Germany*
Jiri Parizek,	*International Programme on Chemical Safety, Division of Environmental Health, World Health Organization, 1211 Geneva 27, Switzerland*
D. Peakall,	*Head, Toxicology Section, National Wildlife Research Centre, Canadian Wildlife Service, Ottawa, Ontario, Canada K1A 0E7*
G. Persoone,	*Director, Laboratory for Biological Research in Environmental Pollution, State University of Ghent, J. Plateaustraat 22, B-9000, Ghent, Belgium*
Andrew Rowan,	*Assistant Dean, Tufts School of Veterinary Medicine, 203 Harrison Avenue, Boston, Massachusetts 02111, USA*

I.V. Sanockij, *Institute of Industrial Hygiene and Occupational Diseases, Academy of Medical Science of USSR, PROSP Budennoga 31, Moscow 105275, USSR*

Lauri Saxén, *University of Helsinki, Haartmaninkatu 3, 00290 Helsinki 29, Finland*

P. Sheehan, *Division of Biological Sciences, National Research Council of Canada, Ottawa, Ontario, Canada K1A 0R6*

***Vittorio Silano,** *Istituto Superiore di Sanità, Viale Regina Elena 299, 00161 Rome, Italy*

Emmanuel Somers, *Director General, Drugs Directorate, Health Protection Branch, Health and Welfare Canada, Health Protection Building, Tunney's Pasture, Ottawa, Ontario, Canada K1A 0L2 (Co-chairman)*

A.L. Stammati, *Istituto Superiore di Sanità, Viale Regina Elena 299, 00161 Rome, Italy*

Raymond Suskind, *University of Cincinnati Medical Center, Institute of Environmental Health, Kettering Laboratory (#56), 3223 Eden Avenue, Cincinnati, Ohio 45267, USA*

Sonia Tabakova, *Institute of Hygiene and Occupational Health, Academy of Medicine, Boul. D. Nestorov 15, Sofia 1431, Bulgaria*

R. Truhaut, *Laboratoire de Toxicologie et d'Hygiene Industrielle, Faculté des Sciences, Pharmaceutiques et Biologiques de Paris, Université René Descartes, 4 avenue de l'Observatoire, 75006 Paris, France*

***Ivar Ugi,** *Lehrstuhl für Organische Chemie, T.U., Lichtenbergstr 4, 8046 Garching, Federal Republic of Germany*

F.X.R. van Leeuwen, *National Institute of Public Health, PO Box 1, Bilthoven, The Netherlands*

J.G. Vos, *National Institute of Public Health and Environmental Protection, PO Box 1, Bilthoven, The Netherlands*

Peter Wells, *Toxic Chemicals Management Center, Environment Canada, Place Vincent Massey, 351 St. Joseph Boulevard, Hull, Quebec, Canada K1A 1C8*

F. Zucco, *Istituto di Tecnologie Biomediche, C.N.R., Rome, Italy*

*Did not attend Workshop.

PART A

JOINT REPORT

Short-term Toxicity Tests for Non-genotoxic Effects
Edited by P. Bourdeau *et al.*
© 1990 SCOPE. Published by John Wiley & Sons Ltd

CHAPTER 1

*Introduction, General Conclusions and Recommendations**

1.1 INTRODUCTION

The safety evaluation of chemicals depends heavily on the use of animal tests from which inferences are drawn about the degree of risk to human health and the environment. There is now general agreement on the principles and methods for testing and evaluating chemicals (World Health Organization, 1978, 1984; Vouk and Sheehan, 1983; OECD, 1981; IARC, 1980). However, the methods involved are costly, require skilled manpower and specialized facilities, and take several years to complete. Furthermore, there is a growing number of examples of chemical toxicity in man that were not predicted by routine toxicity tests involving lifetime rodent bioassays. This is particularly the case for chemical agents that cause direct toxic effects on the endocrine, immune and nervous systems and on the developing organism.

It is also difficult to detect, by established, routine methods, subtle damage to organs and systems that have a large functional reserve or which display tolerance to toxic insults. Examples include effects on the liver and kidney, on the intestinal tract and on haematopoietic and immune response processes.

For these reasons, there is a continuing and justifiable interest in new approaches that may be able to provide more specific information concerning the effects of chemicals on particular organs or biological systems. Recent advances in biology and chemistry have opened up the possibility to study the effects of chemicals on living matter at the cellular and subcellular level. Better knowledge of the relationship between chemical and physical characteristics of toxic substances and their biological activity has opened up possibilities for predicting toxicity based on a study of these relationships. In consequence, new procedures and techniques have been developed that provide much useful information about the mechanisms whereby chemicals exert their toxic actions. Some of these appear to have potential as bioassay techniques that yield results more rapidly than the traditional methods now

*This chapter was prepared by a Workgroup chaired by A. N. Rowan. Other members were A. Berlin (rapporteur), G. C. Becking, B. Ekwall, N. Fernicola, J. Friedrich, M. I. Gounar, F. Kaloyanova, C. R. Krishna Murti, B. Ordonez, I. V. Sanockij, and A. L. Stammati.

used in toxicology. Accordingly, tests of this type are often referred to as 'short-term tests'.

Best known and most widely applied of the short-term tests are those that serve as indicators of mutagenic activity and are predictive of carcinogenic potential. The Workshop excluded these short-term tests for genotoxic effects from its cosideration since this group of tests has been recently reviewed and evaluated elsewhere (International Agency for Research on Cancer, 1980; International Life Sciences Institute, 1984). This report reviews current short-term tests other than those based on genotoxicity, with a view to describing their potential as predictive methods for toxicity and ecotoxicity and their current limitations.

The choice of this subject for study by a SGOMSEC workshop arises from a need for rapid and inexpensive methods that can be used to set priorities for testing a large number of substances present in our environment, to make it possible to rapidly screen new products in order to concentrate industrial research and development efforts on those with the least potential for toxicity, and to enable preliminary, but important, decisions to be made about chemicals in order to institute control procedures without the delay that would be required for complete toxicological assessment.

The Workshop concentrated on those tests, procedures and techniques that produce results within a few weeks rather than the two or three years required for traditional safety testing procedures usually applied to chemicals. It was noted that many tests of this type have the merit of low cost, and are easily manageable although it must be acknowledged that this is not always the case.

1.2   GENERAL CONCLUSIONS AND RECOMMENDATIONS

(1)   Short-term tests provide a great deal of information relevant to the evaluation of the safety of chemicals, particularly the mechanism(s) of action, but are not yet developed to the stage where they can replace long-term animal tests as a basis for safety judgement.

(2)   The prospects for developing *in vitro* tests for acute, local effects are encouraging. For example, recent developments indicate that it may be possible to develop an *in vitro* battery of tests to identify substances which cause acute irritation in the eye (Nardone and Bradlaw, 1983) as an alternative to the Draize test which has been used since the 1940s.

(3)   A relatively simple set of *in vitro* cytotoxicity tests will identify most substances likely to cause acute systemic toxicity; progress is being made toward quantitation of these techniques. However, the full potential of such assays will require a better understanding of the proportion of chemicals exerting an effect through general cytotoxic action compared with those affecting 'organizational aspects' of the whole organism.

(4)   Chronic effects are unlikely to be detected using currently-available *in vitro* procedures.

(5) While there are no true short-term tests for ecosystem function, two major areas show substantial promise for the shortening of time-to-decision in the ecotoxicological evaluation of chemicals: quantitative structure–activity relationships (QSAR), particularly for environmental behaviour; and multi-species test systems.

REFERENCES

International Agency for Research on Cancer (IARC) (1980). *Long-term and Short-term Screening Assays for Carcinogens: A Critical Appraisal*, IARC Monographs on the Evaluation of the Carcinogenic Risk of Chemicals to Humans, Supplement 2, IARC, Lyon.

International Life Sciences Institute (1984). *Current Issues in Toxicology*, Springer-Verlag, New York.

Nardone, R.M., and Bradlaw, J.A. (1983). Toxicity testing with *in vitro* systems: I. Occular tissue-culture. *J. Toxicol.-Cutan. Occular Toxicol.*, **2**(2–3), 81–98.

Organization for Economic Co-operation and Development (1981). *OECD Guidelines for Testing of Chemicals*, OECD, Paris.

Vouk, V.B., and P.J. Sheehan (Eds) (1983). *Methods for Assessing the Effects of Chemicals on Reproductive Functions*, SCOPE 20, John Wiley & Sons, New York.

World Health Organization (1978). *Principles and Methods for Evaluating the Toxicity of Chemicals, Part 1*, Environmental Health Criteria 6, World Health Organization, Geneva.

World Health Organization (1984). *Principles for Evaluating Health Risks to Progeny Associated with Exposure to Chemicals During Pregnancy*, Environmental Health Criteria 30, World Health Organization, Geneva.

Short-term Toxicity Tests for Non-genotoxic Effects
Edited by P. Bourdeau *et al.*
© 1990 SCOPE. Published by John Wiley & Sons Ltd

CHAPTER 2

Non-specialized Mammalian Cell Cultures for Toxicity Testing*

2.1 *IN VITRO* METHODS FOR THE ASSESSMENT OF GENERAL CELLULAR TOXICITY

These tests aim at detecting changes in common basic functions, processes and the structure of cells. These types of test have been referred to as 'general cell toxicology investigations' (Paganuzzi-Stammati *et al.*, 1981) or 'basal cytotoxicity tests' (Ekwall, 1983). Typically, they utilize cultures of undifferentiated cells (i.e. cells showing no organ-specific characteristics). These cell systems are relatively easy to culture and do not change from test to test (Ekwall, 1983). They include fibroblastic and epitheloid cell systems such as diploid human fibroblast lines and HeLa cell cultures.

Ekwall *et al.* (Chapter 7, this volume) point out that basic toxicity has often been studied in elaborate organ-specific culture systems leading to difficulties in interpretation because of confounding basic and cell-specific effects.

2.2 END-POINTS

Numerous end-points have been used by different investigators to measure toxicity. These include growth determined by protein analysis, plating efficiency, enzyme release, exclusion or inclusion of dyes or radioactive markers and metabolic alterations such as oxygen consumption and ATP levels. Most of these end-points are quantitative and can be used to plot dose–response curves. This should facilitate interlaboratory comparisons and the application of quality control methods to ensure the reliability of the results obtained. The cytotoxic concentrations of chemicals determined *in vitro* have been shown to correlate well with lethal doses in laboratory animals and man for a range of selected drugs and chemicals (Ekwall, 1983).

Morphological changes in cells exposed to chemicals, observed by light or electron microscopy, have also been used to demonstrate basic cytotoxicity. Effects

---

*This chapter was prepared by a Workgroup chaired by A. N. Rowan. Other members were A. Berlin (rapporteur), G. C. Becking, B. Ekwall, N. Fernicola, J. Friedrich, M. I. Gounar, F. Kaloyanova, C. R. Krishna Murti, B. Ordonez, I. V. Sanockij, and A. L. Stammati.

commonly observed include cytoplasmic blobs suggesting injury of the cell membrane and vacuolization (Ekwall, 1983). Although qualitative in nature, these observations may provide valuable information about the pathologic processes that occur as a consequence of exposure to a chemical substance.

2.3   CURRENT LIMITATIONS AND THE POTENTIAL FOR IMPROVED METHODS

These tests have the merit of being rapid and inexpensive to perform although a relatively high degree of skill is required to obtain reliable results. However, culture systems and conditions currently employed vary considerably from one laboratory to another. Lack of standardization in procedures has hindered inter-laboratory comparison of results that are germane to their proper validation as adequate test methods. At the present time, these tests have mainly found application as adjuncts to *in vivo* investigations, or as a screening technique.

Because basic cytotoxicity tests evaluate only the effects of a chemical on basic cellular processes, these tests have limitations in their value for predicting *in vivo* toxicity. These limitations include:

(1)   Basic cytotoxicity tests do not evaluate the capacity of highly specialized cells to carry out their organ-specific functions. Organ-specific toxicity requires testing *in vivo* or in suitable differentiated cell cultures.

(2)   Some types of toxicity involve the interactive influence of different types of cell. Toxic responses involving hormonal and nervous adjustments and immunological responses, for example, are typical of those involving organizational features characteristic of the whole organism. This type of response requires *in vivo* testing.

(3)   Many chemicals require prior biotransformation before they exert a toxic effect on cells. In such cases, tests with hepatocytes or other metabolically competent cells could be used to supplement tests on less competent cells. However, it should be noted that hepatocyte cultures undergo dedifferentiation and, as a consequence, may modify their capacity to metabolize xenobiotic chemicals (Paganuzzi-Stammati *et al.*, 1981).

(4)   *In vitro* concentrations of substances may be difficult to relate to concentrations in intact animals because of distribution phenomena (e.g. blood–brain barrier).

(5)   Most tissue culture systems involve such short incubation and observation times that they may be predictive only for acute *in vivo* effects. It is doubtful that such tests can be used to predict chronic toxicity.

2.4   CONCLUSIONS AND RECOMMENDATIONS

(1)   A number of *in vitro* methods to measure general cytoxicity based upon the

use of non-specialized cell systems have been developed but have not yet been adequately validated.

(2)   Further attention must be given to refining the choice of cell types, culture conditions and end-points as a first step toward standardization of techniques. In particular, the use of serum-free media should be encouraged.

(3)   The Workgroup noted recent developments in organizing large-scale validation studies for selected methods. Efforts in this respect are to be encouraged with particular attention focused on the reproducibility and comparability of results, comparative testing using *in vivo* and *in vitro* techniques in parallel, and by testing large series of compounds for which comprehensive animal and human toxicological data already exist.

(4)   There is a need to better determine the significance of specific end-points in all systems as they relate to *in vivo* toxicity.

REFERENCES

Ekwall, B. (1983). Screening of toxic compounds in mammalian cell cultures. *Ann. N.Y. Acad. Sci.*, **407**, 64–77.

Paganuzzi-Stammati, A., Silan, V., and Zuco, F. (1981). Toxicology investigations with cell culture systems. *Toxicol.*, **20**, 91–153.

Short-term Toxicity Tests for Non-genotoxic Effects
Edited by P. Bourdeau *et al.*
© 1990 SCOPE. Published by John Wiley & Sons Ltd

CHAPTER 3

*Methods to Detect Toxic Effects in Specific Mammalian Organs and Physiological Systems**

3.1   INTRODUCTION

Toxicity has been defined as the inherent property of a substance to cause an adverse biological effect (ECETOC, 1985). It is the result of disturbances induced by a chemical that affect complex, interrelated systems involving cells, tissues and organs and their metabolic processes. Experimental procedures to investigate toxicity may involve one or more of several levels of biological organization ranging from the molecular level to the whole animal, including tests designed to investigate effects on organelles, cellular interactions and organ-to-organ interactions in physiological systems.

Testing for toxicity at the organ or system level can be conveniently considered according to whether the investigations are designed to detect cytotoxicity, changes in metabolic processes, functional capacity or influences on differentiation and developmental processes. Biological models are available that have proved useful in the study of these various types of effect in many specific organs and organ systems. However, many of these experimental procedures require additional validation as far as reproducibility, accuracy, reliability, sensitivity and biological relevance for man are concerned.

Tables 3.1(A) to (H) list many of the tests considered by the Workgroup to be useful or potentially useful as short-term tests for chemical toxicity. These tests have been used for a variety of purposes including:

(i)   to detect and quantify organ-specific toxic effects;
(ii)   to elucidate mechanisms of toxicity;
(iii)   to provide information relevant to other organs and tissues; and
(iv)   in some instances, to permit direct experimental studies on human tissues.

---

*This chapter was prepared by a Workgroup co-chaired by J. W. Bridges and S. Garattini. Other members were D. K. Agarwal, D. Barltrop, M. J. Brueton, N. Chernoff, J. Clark, J. H. Dean, R. Dixon, T. Fliedner, L. Saxén, R. Suskind, J. G. Vos, F. X. R. Van Leeuwen, K. Khera, and S. Tabakova.

Table 3.1   Models for individual organs/systems with particular potential for assessing the adverse effects of chemicals

(A) Liver (see Bridges, Chapter 9, this volume)

Model	Purpose	End-points	Status
Microsomes	Reactive metabolite production and covalent binding/lipid peroxidation. Particularly useful for species comparisons. Often incorporated as the metabolizing system with other cell types.	Radioisotope methods, biochemical analyses	Well developed; interlaboratory standardized procedures yet to be identified
Freshly isolated hepatocytes	Xenobiotic metabolism. Initial toxic effects. Particularly employed for interspecies comparisons	Radioisotope methods, biochemical assays, morphological changes	In extensive use. Reliable methods for preparing/storing human hepatocytes particularly needed
Primary maintenance cultures of hepatocytes	Effects of chemicals on macromolecular/organelle turnover	Enzyme activity. Radioisotope incorporation	Used by many laboratories. Improved stabilization techniques for particular constituents, e.g. drug metabolizing enzymes, required
Liver perfusion	Study of short-term effects on total function	Blood flow, bile flow and composition, oxygen utilization	Reduced interpretation variability needed, needs viability period extended
Whole animal	Organ/organ interactions, particularly delayed effects. Influence of pharmacokinetic factors on the degree of toxicity	Serum chemistry. NMR	NMR still in its infancy. Serum chemistry parameters need to be adapted for each animal model used

(B) Central nervous system (see Garattini, Chapter 13, this volume)

Model	Purpose	End-points	Status
Membranes	Study of binding sites and receptors	Radioisotope methods	Well developed, relatively well reproducible but very expensive
Neuronal cultures	Study of morphological effects, cytotoxicity, biochemical activities	Radioisotope methods; biochemical assays; morphological changes	Extensive use but not for toxicological studies
Brain slices	Study of electrical activity	Voltammetry for continuous measurement or biochemical analyses of individual neurotransmitters	Extensive use, relatively well standardized but not for toxicological studies
Whole animal	Study of behaviour	Observations; behavioural measurements	Extensive use but not for toxicological studies

(C) Endocrine system (see Clark and van Leeuwen, Chapter 14, this volume)

Model	Purpose	End-points	Status
Immunocytochemical staining of endocrine glands	Determination of status of specific hormone producing cells	Appropriate staining capacity	Limited use,* reliable, well-developed
Determination of circulating hormones	Overall activity of endocrine organ function	Thyroid hormones, mineralo/glucocorticoids, etc.	Limited use, reliable, validated
Release tests *in vivo*	Test for endocrine organ function	TSH, prolactin, LH, FSH, ACTH, corticosterone, insulin in circulation	Limited use,* reliable, validated
Receptor binding	Test of inhibition of target gland function	Inhibition of TSH and ACTH binding	Not in wide use
Lipoprotein uptake by adrenal	Test for decreased adrenal function	Inhibition of uptake of lipoprotein, ^{125}I	Not in use for toxicologic evaluation
Hormone secretion by pituitary *in vitro*	Test for decreased pituitary function	Pituitary hormones in the medium	Limited use

* For several of these methods, specific antisera for the species used in the study are required.

(D) Gastrointestinal tract (see Barltrop and Brueton, Chapter 8, this volume)

Model	Purpose	End-point	Status
Whole animal and man—*in vivo*	To recognize gross damage to mucosal structure	Abnormalities seen on light and electron/microscopy, immuno-histochemimstry	Extensively used, interpretation non-specific
Whole animal and man—*in vivo*	To recognize gross damage to mucosal function	Reduction in the absorption of fat, nitrogen, carbohydrate	Extensively used, interpretation non-specific
Whole animal and man—*in vitro*	To recognize disturbances in mucosal transport	Changes in uptake kinetics in: (a) perfusion studies; (b) Ussing or Lucite chambers	Research tool; ethical considerations in man
Dissociated animal and human enterocytes in cell culture	To recognize toxic effects on cell culture systems	Changes in enzyme synthesis activity or release. Alteration of cell surface activities or metabolic pathways	Further development and validation required
Animal and human enterocyte subcellular fractions	To recognize toxic effects on subcellular function	Recognition of metabolic products; changes in enzyme synthesis, activity or release; alteration in metabolic pathways	Further development and validation required

(E) Haematological toxicity (short-term) (see Fliedner *et al.*, Chapter 12, this volume)

Haematopoietic cell renewal system	General toxicity	Blood cell counts (red cells, granulocytes, lymphocytes, platelets)	Routine haematology (species differences)
	Bone marrow impairment	Histology; EM; Cell smear; cyto/histochemistry	Routine haematology (in man and animals)
	Stem-cell pool impairment	CFU-S (mouse assay) Progenitor cell culture (CFU-GM) (CFU-GEMM)	*In vitro* cell culture (cells from man and animals)
	Cell specific functional impairment	Red cell toxicology (haemolysis); Granulocytic toxicology; Lymphocytic toxicology; platelet toxicology	*In vitro* test systems (cells from man and animals)
	Haematopoietic function impairment	^{59}Fe incorporation (erythropoiesis); ^{51}Cr blood cell survival; methaemoglobin; δ-ALA; bleeding time; granulocytic mobilization	Radionuclide methods, biochemistry of blood and urine (in man and animals)

(F) Immune system (see Vos and Dean, Chapter 15, this volume)

Model	Purpose	End-points	Status
Whole animal, *in vivo*	Initial screening for immunotoxicology	Weight and histology of thymus, spleen and lymph nodes; bone marrow cell intensity; serum immunoglobulin levels	Validated and tabulated in many laboratories
Whole animal, *in vivo*	Confirmation of altered host resistance	Resistance to infectious agents and tumour cell challenges	Validated and tabulated in many laboratories
Whole animal, *ex vivo—in vitro*	Confirmation of dysfunction of immune system	Various tests of cellular and humoral immunity, and of macrophage and natural killer cell function	Validated and tabulated in many laboratories
Whole animal, *ex vivo—in vitro*	Identification of effect on lymphoid subpopulation	Immunohistochemistry and flow cytometry using monoclonal antibodies	Under development
Lymphatic cells from rodents and man, *in vitro*	Identification of mechanism of action and development of predictive models for man	Cytotoxicity or altered functions	Under development

(G) Kidney (see Saxén, Chapter 10, this volume)

Model	Purpose	End-points	Status
Organ culture (embryonic)	Analysis of cell interactions, organogenesis, proliferation	Differentiation of the nephron at different levels	Used mainly by developmental biologists. Some toxicological applications
Chorionallantoic grafting (embryonic)	Analysis of cell interactions, organogenesis, proliferation; cell migration	Vascularization	Used mainly by developmental biologists. Some toxicological applications
In vitro perfusion (neonatal)	To examine the physiological maturation of the nephron	Ion transport, etc.	Limited use by physiologists
Culture of collecting duct epithelium (embryonic and neonatal)	Toxicity test	Viability, macromolecule synthesis	Limited use
'Biochemical end-point analysis' (embryonic)	Drug testing	Weight, protein synthesis, enzyme activity	Limited use
'Partial nephrectomy' (adult, non-differentiating)	Toxicity test	Renal histopathology; blood and urine biochemistry, metabolic disposition	Limited use

(H) Skin (see Suskind, Chapter 11, this volume)

Model	Purpose	End-points	Status
Percutaneous absorbtion *in vivo* (rodent, rabbit)	Rate of penetration from environment through epidermis to underlying tissue, blood stream and excreta	Measurement of penetrant/ metabolites	Limited use
Percutaneous absorbtion *in vitro* in static or flowing chamber models	Rate of penetration	Measurement of penetrant/ metabolites	Limited use; one processing model for assessment of biotransformation
Irritation: *in vivo*, single and repeated exposure in rodents, rabbit, man	Identify type and quantitate inflammatory response; determine threshold of irritancy	Morphologic criteria: gross and histologic	Widely used
Irritation: *in vitro*, cultured whole skin	Quantitate inflammatory response to xenobiotic	Degree of inflammation, necrosis, etc.: gross and histologic	Experimental, requires exploration
Chorioallantoic membrane of chick	Potential *in vitro* substitute for *in vivo* skin irritancy tests	Biochemical markers of injury	Experimental, requires exploration
Guinea-pigs; sensitization	Determine potential for inducing humoral antibody-associated skin reactions	Wheal-flare vascular response to elicitations; identification of humoral antibodies	Experimental
Guinea-pigs; sensitization (many models)	Determine potential for underlying cell-mediated hypersensitivity reactions	Elicitation of inflammatory response which can be quantitated grossly and histologically	Frequently used

Table 3.1 (H)   *(continued)*

Human panel; sensitization	Determine potential for underlying cell-mediated hypersensitivity reactions	Elicitation of inflammatory response which can be quantitated grossly and histologically	Frequently used
Single cell cultures, r.s.c. viral systems + UV radiation	Determine phototoxic potential	Viability of cells	No correlation with effect on man
Rodent, rabbit, hairless mouse + UV radiation; human subjects	Determine phototoxic potential	Inflammatory response	Frequently used
Guinea-pigs + UV radiation	Determine photoallergenic potential	Inflammatory response	Frequently used
In vitro tyrosinase activity, tyrosine transformation to dopa and melanin precursors	Determine change in pigment (melanin) formation	Rate of formation of dopa and precursors of melanin	Frequently used
Mouse melanoma cell culture	Determine change in melanocytes: decrease or increase in pigment	Colour and concentration of melanin granules	Frequently used
Black guinea-pigs and mice	Determine change in pigmentation	Colour and concentration of melanin granules	Frequently used

Hair strands *in vitro*	Effect on structure of keratin	Morphologic and chemical change in hair	Used by cosmetic manufacturers
Rodents with hair cycle of known duration (mice)	Effect of xenobiotic absorbed by any route on matrix cell production of hair	Rate of hair growth, hair structure, onset and persistence of hair loss; interruption of hair cycle	Occasionally used
Albino rabbit ear	Screen agent for acnegenic potential	Epidermal hyperplasia, follicular hyperkeratosis, comedones, epithelial cyst	Frequently used
Hairless mouse	Screen agent for acnegenic potential	Follicular hyperkeratosis, epidermal hyperplasia, sebaceous gland involution, keratin cyst	Research model with good potential for wider use
Human skin transplant to athymic mice	Cutaneous metabolism of xenobiotics; P450 enzyme activity	Quantitative metabolites	Experimental
Human skin transplant to athymic mice	Potential use for measuring effect on sebaceous follicles	Follicular hyperkeratosis, epidermal hyperplasia, sebaceous gland involution, keratin cyst	Experimental

The selection and development of such tests requires the application of scientific judgement and expertise if the results are to be relevant and capable of meaningful interpretation. Sections 3.2 to 3.7 of this report discuss various aspects of these tests which should be considered, as routine short-term tests methods are developed and refined.

3.2   CONSTRAINTS IN THE USE OF *IN VITRO* TESTS FOR SELECTIVE EFFECTS

Major advances in the development of cell culture systems that retain the differentiated functions and responses characteristic of the intact tissue *in vivo* have opened up possibilities for using these techniques to assess the effects of chemicals.

There are a number of considerations that relate to the use of *in vitro* test procedures. Some of the more significant ones are mentioned below.

(1)   Living organisms are characterized by homeostatic mechanisms that ensure their integrity and uniformity under differing environmental conditions. Embryo and organ cultures, cell cultures, subcellular preparations, membrane receptors and other test systems used in *in vitro* studies are more prone to artefacts because homeostatic mechanisms are considerably modified or absent.

(2)   Organs and cells cultured *in vitro* are not subject to many of the crucial influences that characterize their normal existence *in vivo*, including such influences as:

        (a)   *homeostatic* control (e.g. hormonal, nervous and immune systems);

        (b)   continuous input of nutrients and specific substances produced by other organs (e.g. liver); and

        (c)   processes which result in the elimination of catabolic products formed in organs or cells.

(3)   Exposure to chemicals, at the organ or cellular level, is the result of a dynamic situation involving absorption, distribution, metabolism and excretion processes. In contrast, exposure to chemicals *in vitro* is a static situation. In consequence, there may be differences in the response to a chemical insult *in vitro* compared to that *in vivo*. For example, a toxic effect identified *in vitro* may not occur *in vivo* because the toxicant is rapidly metabolized or excreted, or because other types of toxicity intervene at lower concentrations. Maintaining adequate concentrations of chemicals in *in vitro* systems is also a problem in some cases.

(4)   Certain tissues (e.g. brain, skin) are protected in the living organism by physiological barriers which inhibit the entry of particular chemicals. Just as access of chemicals at the tissue level may differ between the *in vitro* and *in vivo*

situations, it is conceivable that entry of a chemical into the cell and subsequent subcellular distribution may also differ.

(5) *In vitro* tests may yield misleading results for chemicals that require metabolic activation in order to exert their toxic effects. Several examples are known of chemicals that are not toxic themselves but which yield metabolites that are highly toxic (e.g. cyclophosphamide). In this context, it is worth noting that *in vivo* biotransformation of chemicals to their active metabolites may be a complex process involving large numbers of metabolites, some of which may potentiate or prolong the toxic effects and others of which may exert antagonistic actions. For example, salicylate, the major metabolite of acetylsalicylic acid, counteracts the inhibitory effect of acetylsalicylic acid on cyclo-oxygenases.

3.3 ORGAN-SPECIFIC CYTOTOXIC EFFECTS

A number of short-term tests that have found wide application in the past (e.g. the Draize tests for skin and eye irritation) depend upon the detection of cell injury or death, often by assessment of the degree of pathological sequelae such as inflammation, ulceration or immunologic responses. More recently, the possibility to culture a wide range of cell types and organs *in vitro* using relatively simple and inexpensive techniques has triggered interest in measuring adaptive changes and cell death more directly using end-points based on both cell morphology and biochemistry.

3.3.1 Skin

Topical application of chemicals to skin may result in cytotoxic effects with various sequelae depending upon the potency of the chemical and the conditions and duration of contact. These range from relatively mild, reversible effects (irritancy) to more serious effects that are irreversible such as corrosive action at the point of contact. Some chemicals require light exposure to induce a response (phototoxicity).

3.3.1.1 Primary irritation

Primary irritation is a condition in which the superficial epithelial cells of the epidermis are destroyed, provoking an inflammatory reaction. It may occur with single, short-term exposure (acute primary irritant) or only after repeated exposures. If cell injury is more severe and extensive, necrosis, ulceration and, ultimately, scarring result.

There is no single test that provides an adequate predictive model for primary irritation in humans (McCreesh and Steinberg, 1983). The most widely used methods are based on the Draize skin irritancy test (Draize *et al.*, 1944), one modification of which has been adopted as a reference method under the US Federal Hazardous Substances Act (Code of Federal Regulations, 1980) and by the Organization for

Economic Co-operation and Development (OECD, 1981). However, the Draize skin irritancy test (and modifications) suffer from a number of shortcomings, particularly in the ability of the test to predict mild or moderate irritancy. Many chemicals found to be mild irritants in rabbit or guinea-pig result in no demonstrable effects in humans (National Academy of Sciences, 1977). On the other hand, substances which elicit no irritant response (or minimal response) in rabbit are unlikely to cause a reaction in man (McCreesh and Steinberg, 1983).

In order to overcome the difficulties inherent in extrapolation of the results of irritancy testing from animal species to humans, various bioassay procedures involving human subjects have been developed (Mathias, 1983). The methods utilize the degree of erythema and oedema as indices of irritancy and are simple and convenient. Other end-points such as measurements of electrical impedance of human skin, carbon dioxide emission from skin and electrolyte flux have been used (Mathias, 1983). An in-depth review of selected issues for testing dermal toxicity has been published by the US Environmental Protection Agency (Chaube *et al.*, 1982).

No satisfactory *in vitro* methods are currently available to substitute for the Draize skin irritancy test. The potential for the development of *in vitro* methods appears promising because of improvements in culture methods for human and animal whole skin.

3.3.1.2   Changes in pigmentation

Selective melanocytotoxic action induced by chemicals results in depigmentation of the skin, a condition known clinically as 'white skin syndrome'. Animal models, using guinea-pig, mouse, cat, goldfish and rabbit, have been developed for use as *in vitro* screening techniques to detect the depigmenting action of chemicals (Gellin and Maibach, 1983). Changes in pigment, and changes in the number of melanocytes per unit area of pigmented skin of CH3 or DBA strains of mice, have been used as measures of potency.

In vitro cell systems have been used to study the effects of chemicals known to induce depigmentation. Mansur *et al.* (1978) reported studies using harvested melanocytes from the ears of black guinea-pigs. Others have used a murine melanoma strain (Dewey *et al.*, 1977). End-points include measurement of tyrosinase activity (several potent depigmenters have been shown to inhibit this enzyme) and the concentration and colour intensity of melanin granules.

3.3.1.3   Phototoxicity

Exposure to sunlight (and other sources of ultraviolet light) causes increased reactivity of many chemicals which can result in toxic skin reactions. Reactions of a non-immunologic type are usually described as phototoxic, whereas the term photoallergy has been used to describe the light-induced counterpart of contact allergy.

Phototoxicity and photoallergy testing have been primarily of interest in the cosmetic field, although light-induced reactions to drugs, industrial chemicals and environmental chemicals are of growing concern, mainly because of changing life-styles that result in increased exposure to sunlight.

Several test systems are in use to detect phototoxicity (Harber, 1981; Kornhauser *et al.*, 1983; Maibach and Marzulli, 1983) and photoallergy (Epstein, 1983) although specific tests, including *in vivo* animal tests, have not yet become standardized (Chaube *et al.*, 1982). The methods cited are all basically similar but vary in specific details such as the test species and light source to which animals are exposed to elicit a response. Rabbits, mice, guinea-pigs and miniature swine have been shown to be satisfactory models when tested with known phototoxic materials (Harber, 1981); guinea-pigs have been found suitable for photoallergy testing (Harber *et al.*, 1983). Nevertheless, because of uncertainties in the extrapolation of results obtained in laboratory animals to man, and because of the non-invasive and reversible nature of the response to most chemicals, human testing has been recommended, but only after testing in animals for both photosensitivity and systemic toxicity (Chaube *et al.*, 1982). Human testing methods for phototoxicity have been reviewed by Maibach and Marzulli (1983) and, for photoallergy, by Kaidbey (1983).

3.3.1.4 *Dermal sensitization*

Allergic reactions, or hypersensitivity, are frequently observed in response to contact with certain chemicals. Three types of injury due to the release of immunoglobulins from cells have been classified using the criteria of Coombs and Gell (1975). Briefly, these are:

(1) anaphylactic reactions involving humoral antibodies with the participation of B cells;

(2) allergic contact dermatitis in which simple chemical compounds (e.g. metal ions) are absorbed through skin, conjugate with proteins leading to recognition of the protein antigen by T lymphocytes; and

(3) cutaneous reactions to xenobiotics which involve antigen–antibody complexes forming microprecipitates in and around small blood vessels and in basement membranes.

Methods to detect the potential of chemical agents to induce various kinds of allergic response depend on short-term *in vivo* procedures reviewed by Klecak (1983) and by Chaube *et al.* (1982). The *in vivo* skin sensitization test has been standardized by the Organization for Economic Co-operation and Development (OECD, 1981).

3.3.2   Gastrointestinal tract

The gastrointestinal tract is a major portal of entry for chemical agents—a distinction shared with skin and lung. As such, it is both a major target organ for the action of ingested toxic substances, and a site for their metabolism, either during passage through the structures of the gut wall itself, or in the lumen as a result of bacterial or enzymic activity.

Toxic effects on the gastroinestinal tract structures can be identified in man by means of mucosal biopsies which are readily obtainable from the oesophagus, stomach, jejunum, sigmoid colon and rectum. A variety of cellular changes can be determined through staining, mitotic indices and the use of monoclonal antibodies. Fibre-optic endoscopy has made it possible to complement observations on biopsy material with direct observations *in situ*.

In animal models, histological and electron microscopic examination of all competent layers of the gastrointestinal tract can be carried out to determine inflammatory changes, alterations in cell types, cellular damage, ulceration, hyperplasia and changes in glandular structures and their contents. Enterocytes can be dissociated from the mucosa by chemical or mechanical means and maintained in various culture systems (Hartmann *et al.*, 1982; Gaginella *et al.*, 1977).

3.3.3   Respiratory tract

Many chemicals are known to injure the lung (Witschi, 1976) either via the airways or the bloodstream (Evans, 1982). The ciliated cells of the distal airways, the type I epithelial cells of the alveoli and the endothelial cells of the vascular system appear the most vulnerable to damage (Evans, 1982).

The pulmonary alveolar macrophages serve as an effective defence mechanism to protect the respiratory membrane against inhaled particles and micro-organisms by means of their phagocytic and lytic properties. Certain particulates are toxic to alveolar macrophages resulting in cytotoxicity. In the case of silica and asbestos, it has been postulated that macrophage injury might be the mediator of fibrosis (Brody and Davis, 1982), while macrophage dysfunction and the release of a variety of enzymes have been observed as a consequence of exposure to a number of chemical agents including oxidant gases and cigarette smoke (Brain *et al.*, 1977). In animal models, histological and electron-microscopic methods have been used to observe and quantify the degree of cellular damage. Bronchopulmonary lavage with saline solution, either in living animals or in excised lung, has been used to investigate several types of acute injury to the lung, and the inflammatory response to such an injury (Henderson *et al.*, 1979). This technique shows promise also for detecting developing chronic pulmonary conditions. It is suitable for use as a screening procedure, especially if advanced flow-cytometric instrumentation is used; this technique has been applied to toxicity studies on environmental pollutants associated with the production of synthetic fuels (Steinkamp *et al.*, 1979).

3.3.4 Haematopoietic system

In health, there is a delicate balance between the production and destruction of the cellular elements of blood (erythrocytes, leukocytes, platelets). Any chemical exerting a cytotoxic effect on the cells involved in the development of blood cells has the potential to upset this steady state equilibrium.

A large number of chemicals affect some component of the haematopoietic cell renewal system. The simplest but most effective approach to detecting this toxicity is to evaluate changes in blood cell counts in relation to the administered dosage and time. This must be done for each blood cell line independently because each of the cell types (such as erythrocytes, granulocytes, lymphocytes, monocytes and platelets) is the culmination of a renewal system with its own regulatory mechanism. However, while changes in blood counts (cells per unit volume of blood) may result from indirect action affecting precursor cells or release mechanisms, they may also result from direct effects on circulating cells (e.g. haemolysis). In many instances, disturbance of blood cell function (migration or spreading capabilities of granulocytes, monocytes or platelets, or the amount of methaemoglobin in red cells) can be detected by established methods.

Bone marrow is amenable to study either by examination of smears prepared from biopsy samples or by histological techniques applied to bone marrow sections. Bone marrow studies may provide information as to possible mechanisms of toxic action detected by systematic changes in blood counts. Specific cell types associated with cytotoxicity can be identified by appropriate staining techniques. However, it must be recognized that different animal species have specific bone marrow cytology and that the techniques involved require skill and experience.

Of particular importance for evaluating cytotoxic effects in the haematopoietic system is the study of the stem cell pool using *in vivo* or *in vitro* methods. The spleen colony assay, based on techniques developed by Till and McCulloch (1961) permits the study of chemical toxicity to pluripotent stem cells (Uyeki *et al.*, 1977). *In vitro* culture systems make it possible to study different haematopoietic progenitor cell populations (Metcalf, 1977).

3.3.5 Immune system

The potential for chemicals to alter immune response (often without causing other symptoms of overt toxicity) has been observed in both animals (for example, Goldstein *et al.*, 1976; Dean *et al.*, 1982, 1986) and man (for example, Kammuller *et al.*, 1984; Lunn *et al.*, 1967; French *et al.*, 1973). The result of such alterations is observed clinically as changes in resistance to infectious agents.

Effects on the immune system are best evaluated *in vivo* due to the complexity of the immune system. Effects can be quantified by histopathological observations on the spleen and lymph nodes which provide an indication of effects of xenobiotics on

T lymphocytes and B lymphocytes, especially when evaluated in conjunction with the weights of thymus, spleen and peripheral lymph nodes. B lymphocytes, which are primarily responsible for the production of antibodies, enter the lymphatic nodules of the spleen and are largely absent from the periarterial lymphatic sheaths; T lymphocytes, which function primarily in cellular immune response, occur mainly in the periarterial lymphatic sheaths. Atrophy of the thymus and thymus-dependent areas of the spleen and lymph nodes is indicative of immunosuppression, whereas proliferation of the high endothelial venules of thymus-dependent areas of the lymph nodes and Peyer's patches of the small intestine correlate with an enhanced immune response.

A variety of *in vitro* methods have been developed to detect or measure potential immunotoxicity (for example, Mishell and Dutton, 1967; van Furth and van Zwet, 1973; Tucker *et al.*, 1982; Graham *et al.*, 1975; Greenspan and Morrow, 1984). However, the specificity of these methods and the potential for false negative results (Kutz *et al.*, 1980) requires that they be used as part of a battery of tests (Vos and Dean, this volume). The true value of *in vitro* methods with respect to immunotoxicology is in the evaluation of modes of action of immunotoxic chemicals.

3.3.6   Liver

The liver is a biochemically diverse organ and has a wide range of important physiological functions including bile production, protein synthesis and detoxification of endogenous waste products. Despite a large functional reserve, the liver is vulnerable to effects of xenobiotics because chemicals absorbed following ingestion pass almost exclusively into the hepatic portal vein and are transported to the liver. Also, its high metabolic activity makes the liver particularly vulnerable to chemicals for which toxicity is potentiated by metabolic alteration.

A variety of accepted *in vivo* methods exist for the evaluation of cytotoxicity in the liver. These include methods for histological and histochemical assessment, and serum and tissue biochemistry (see Bridges, Chapter 9, this volume).

Liver cell lines, isolated hepatocytes and primary hepatocyte cultures have been used as *in vitro* systems to investigate general cytotoxicity, as well as liver-specific effects of xenobiotics. Hepatocytes are a particularly relevant model for evaluating the cytotoxic effects of chemicals requiring metabolic alteration to form active metabolites. Various endpoints have been monitored in these *in vitro* models including membrane damage, protein synthesis, changes in metabolic parameters, and changes in activity, growth and morphology of cell cultures.

In vitro systems lack the complexity and long-term viability to adequately assess or detect all hepatotoxic effects of chemicals. However, their use in defining mechanisms of action should be vigorously pursued, as should improvements in their preparation, maintenance and viability.

3.3.7 Kidney

Chemicals can have a variety of direct toxic or indirect effects on the kidney (Rush *et al.*, 1984; Goyer, 1983). Clinically, these effects are ultimately manifested as altered urine flow, and/or altered urine chemistry (Hayes, 1983).

A variety of kidney cell lines are available for *in vitro* assessment of chemical effects. These include baby hamster kidney fibroblasts (BHK-21), Syrian hamster kidney (HaK), monkey kidney cells (VERO), and a cell line derived from the cortex of adult pig kidney (K7) (Paganuzzi-Stammati, *et al.*, 1981). Such cell cultures can be used to assess cell specific effects, general cytotoxicity and xenobiotic metabolism. Toxic end-points include those used to investigate effects on cells of other organs (such as the liver).

Organ-specific effects are more readily investigated *in vivo* using various histological and light and electron microscopy techniques to determine the cellular pathophysiological effects of chemicals (Porter, 1982).

A practical approach to studying renal cellular effects is the *in vitro* tissue slice technique (Berndt, 1976). This technique is effective in assessing the effects of xenobiotics on renal transport processes at the cellular level, following *in vivo* chemical exposure.

3.3.8 Nervous system

Neurotoxic potential is commonly evaluated on the basis of effects on neurone and axon morphology in brain, spinal cord, and peripheral nerves. While the blood–brain barrier protects the central nervous system (CNS) against the entry of many chemicals, there are aspects of the process where the barrier is less efficient on the circumventricular organs. Systematically administered agents may affect some of these organs, such as the nucleus arcuatus of the hypothalamus, and cause selective degeneration of neurones. Cell culture systems using nervous tissue of different animal species and man can be used as test systems for effects of xenobiotics. However, due to the complexity of the CNS, it is unlikely that a few cell lines are sufficient to represent the variety of cells existing in the brain.

3.3.9 Endocrine system

Recent developments in immunocytochemistry, specifically radioimmunoassay and enzyme-linked immunosorbent assay techniques, have greatly expanded the testing possibilities for xenobiotic effects on the endocrine system. Combined with biochemical and histological observations, it is now possible to identify hormone-producing cells and quantify effects after *in vivo* chemical exposure.

In vitro, cell preparations can be used for the assessment of a variety of toxic, endocrine-specific effects including the uptake of iodide by thyroid cells, lipoprotein uptake by adrenal cells, and hormone receptor binding (see Clark and van Leeuwen, Chapter 14, this volume).

3.3.10   Reproductive system

The assessment of xenobiotic effects on cells and tissues associated with reproduction may be conducted in a wide variety of models. In animals, pre- and post-exposure models may be used and histologic, cytologic, and where appropriate, morphometric assessment of components of the male and female gonadal tissues may be carried out. Areas of investigation include aspects of maturation of gonads and accessory sex organs, ovarian cytology and ovarian growth, granulosa and thecal structure, vaginal and cervical epithelium morphology, and the quantity, quality, structure, motility, morphology, and fertility capacity of sperm. Observation of cytologic effects on reproductive processes include morphologic aspects of embryogenesis from implantation of fertilized ovum to fully developed newborn. Test models for effects on organogenesis include morphologic changes in organ cultures such as limb buds, tooth buds, liver, kidney and thyroid (see Nadolney *et al.*, Chapter 16, this volume; Saxén, Chapter 10, this volume).

3.4   METABOLIC AND BIOCHEMICAL CONSIDERATIONS

The analysis of metabolic and biochemical changes induced by xenobiotics is an important aspect of the total battery of toxicological tests. Such analyses are especially valuable in understanding mechanisms of action, and offer considerable potential for developing predictive models based on structure–function relationships. At the present time, many biochemical and metabolic tests are available; however, few of them have been used to examine toxic effects.

3.4.1   Endocrine system

The influence of endocrine secretions on metabolism is well known and it is clear that alterations in the normal secretory patterns of hormones can lead to toxicity. However, little is known concerning exposure of the endocrine system to toxins. Therefore, many of the proposed methods still require careful testing and validation. For example, some substances can interfere with the stimulation of adenylate cyclase activity by thyrotropin in *in vitro* thyroid membrane preparations; however, whether this effect occurs *in vivo* with resultant toxicity needs to be established in animals. The potential for *in vitro* metabolic tests is great since they are relatively inexpensive and require little time. Conceivably, such analyses could be used to screen potential toxins and certainly to examine their mechanisms of action (Clark and van Leeuwen, Chapter 14, this volume). The limitations of *in vitro* tests are considerable, however, since they give no information concerning the pharmacokinetics of the test substance or the likelihood of interactions via indirect actions.

3.4.2 Reproductive system

The reproductive system depends on the interplay between hormones and target organs and many of the biochemical and metabolic consequences are known. Methods for the examination of hormone receptor binding are well known and toxic substances may act at this level. Such actions of toxins may decrease the hormone-induced response or they may mimic the response. These actions of toxins must be considered with respect to the development stage at which exposure occurs. Thus, oestrogenic toxins may have little lasting effect in the adult but may be very deleterious if exposure occurs during the fetal or neonatal period. Biochemical analysis of toxic interactions in the reproductive system will point the way for understanding mechanisms of action of toxins and should, when combined with *in vivo* studies, provide a framework upon which predictions of hazard may be made (Nadolney *et al.*, Chapter 16, this volume).

3.4.3 Nervous system

The metabolic and biochemical tests which are of potential use are numerous. These include neurotransmitter binding, turnover and post-synaptic responses. Toxins could, in theory, act at any or all of these steps and thereby interfere with nervous system function. Such tests will probably require treatment *in vivo* and subsequent *in vitro* analysis since suitable, purely *in vitro*, model systems are not available. The potential for such *in vivo–in vitro* analyses is great but much more work is necessary to validate their value to toxicology (Garattini, Chapter 13, this volume).

3.4.4 Skin

Knowledge about the passage of molecules across the skin has increased greatly in recent years. Local and systemic toxicity of substances that contact the skin depend on a chemical penetrating its multiple layers. This is a complex phenomenon involving both a passive diffusion process and metabolic processes of the skin itself that can serve both to detoxify or to activate applied chemical agents.

Measurements of the absorption of xenobiotics through skin are laborious and it is difficult to obtain consistent results (Dugard, 1983). There are a number of *in vivo* and *in vitro* techniques that have been used; of these, the *in vitro* techniques are easier to perform, more amenable to the control of experimental conditions and more precise. However, Franz (1973) noted important differences between tests conducted *in vivo* and *in vitro*; in particular, shedding of the superficial cells of the stratum corneum does not occur *in vitro*, and the role of hair follicles and sweat glands may differ.

In vitro methods to investigate percutaneous absorption involve the use of diffusion cells in which skin is mounted as the membrane with the stratum corneum side exposed to the test environment. The integrity of the skin can be verified before use by determining its permeability for tritiated water (Bronaugh *et al.*, 1981). Chemical depilatory agents should be avoided because of their ability to increase skin absorption (Andersen *et al.*, 1980). Good agreement has been obtained between *in vitro* and *in vivo* techniques for several chemicals (Bronaugh and Maibach, 1983). However, the number of validation studies available is small so that *in vitro* studies are, at present, of greatest value to supplement *in vivo* absorption studies. Although human skin is preferred, its use is not always feasible. Several animal models have been used (Bronaugh and Maibach, 1983).

Methods to study *in vivo* percutaneous absorption have been reviewed by Wester and Maibach (1983). The most commonly used methods depend upon the measurement of radioactivity in excreta following topical application of a radiolabelled compound. Other approaches include determination of the rate of loss of radioactivity absorbed from applied substances, measurement of pharmacological responses induced by the test substance and whole body autoradiography and fluorescence.

In addition to its function as a permeable membrane, the skin is also a major site of metabolism. It constitutes about 10 per cent of normal body weight and must, therefore, be considered one of the major organs of the human body. The viable layers beneath the stratum corneum are involved in numerous biochemical processes. Chemicals that penetrate the stratum corneum are subjected to the action of drug-metabolizing enzymes that can result in the metabolism of absorbed substances before they reach the underlying capillary bed. This activity has been described as 'first-pass' metabolism of topically-applied chemicals. Besides *in vivo* studies, mouse skin in organ culture may provide a good *in vitro* model for studying the interrelationship of the skin as a metabolizing and target organ and as a primary entry for xenobiotics. The *in vitro* tests are potentially adaptable for the study of interspecies differences with respect to skin metabolism and penetration but their validity needs to be better established before they can be used with confidence for risk assessment for human beings.

3.4.5 Gastrointestinal tract

The gastrointestinal tract functions as an important metabolic organ and is a major site of extrahepatic xenobiotic metabolism. In addition, the intestinal flora play an important part in the metabolism of xenobiotics. The lack of suitable techniques (the majority of bacteria in the gut are anaerobic and have specialized nutritional requirements that are largely unknown) has inhibited research on the role of the intestinal flora in xenobiotic metabolism until recently (Rafter *et al.*, 1983).

A number of techniques have been described for investigation of the absorption and metabolism of xenobiotics both *in vivo* and *in vitro*. These include pharmacokinetic studies using radiolabelled materials, transport and uptake studies using gut loops (in which each end is cannulated to allow perfusions to be carried out, but in which the blood and other vessels supplying the intestinal segment are left intact), studies using isolated organ preparations (Barltrop and Brueton, Chapter 8, this volume), as well as enterocytes dissociated from the mucosa (Hartmann *et al.*, 1982) and subcellular fractions (mitochondria, microsomes, nuclear and microvilli). However, these techniques, developed for functional studies in clinical gastroenterology, have yet to be extensively used in toxicology. Their potential appears considerable but needs validation.

3.4.6 Lung

The importance of lung in the absorption and metabolism of xenobiotics is frequently overlooked. In addition to its function in the exchange of gases, the lung has an extensive capillary bed through which the entire cardiac output passes. Because of this, it is frequently the target organ not only for inhaled substances such as gases, asbestos or smoke particulates, but also for substances to which it is exposed systemically (e.g. paraquat). The lung also has the capability to metabolize many foreign compounds which may be activated to toxic intermediates or detoxified. For a more detailed account of the toxicologic implications of lung metabolism, the reader is referred to the reviews by Philpot *et al.* (1977) and Wilson (1982).

A variety of techniques and preparations have been used to study the metabolism of xenobiotics in the lung and pulmonary vascular system. These include isolated perfused lung preparations, distribution studies in whole animals, and measurements of the disappearance of substances from the pulmonary circulation, or of the inactivation of pharmacologically active substances. Alabaster (1977) noted that distribution studies, where the xenobiotic concentration in lung tissue is determined at varying times after administration, do not reflect the ability of lung to remove the substance in one pass. He also noted that studies in homogenized tissue do not necessarily reflect the metabolizing activity of the pulmonary circulation since homogenization can expose intracellular enzyme systems not normally accessible during passage through the pulmonary circulation. Wilson (1982) reported on significant advances in determining the kinetic parameters for metabolic pathways in pulmonary tissue. This opens up new possibilities for the use of pharmacokinetic models for the pulmonary clearance of endogenous agents, and the assessment of lung damage resulting from exposure to toxic substances.

Immunologic stimulation of the lungs results in the release of potent, biologically-active substances that are important in relation to anaphylaxis and asthma of extrinsic origin. Methods for the detection and assay of released substances have been reviewed by Said (1982). Methods based on superfusion techniques and identification of humoral agents by the use of inhibitors of their biosynthesis require specialized skills and equipment. The use of radioimmunoassays has the merit of relative simplicity, sensitivity and precision (Said, 1982).

3.4.7 Liver

The liver is the most important organ with respect to both intermediary and xenobiotic metabolism. Numerous tests of proven validity are available to establish the effects of xenobiotics on: carbohydrate and protein metabolism, oxidative phosphorylation, microsomal mono-oxygenase activity, conjugation reactions, etc. Most of these tests can easily be applied to *in vivo* as well as *in vitro* toxicity experiments (Bridges, Chapter 9, this volume).

3.4.8　Haematopoietic system

Cell renewal is used in testing chemical toxicity. Impairment of metabolism causes quantitative and/or qualitative impairment of cell numbers or function, resulting in feed-back actions causing other parts of the system to respond (indirect result of direct action) (Fliedner *et al.*, Chapter 12, this volume). Metabolic effects, mainly detected *in vivo* (in man as well as in animals), are disturbance of iron uptake and haeme biosynthesis and the formation of methaemoglobin. Determination of porphyrin patterns and methaemoglobin formation can be detected easily. For the study of iron metabolism, radionuclides are indicated. These tests are expensive and time consuming. For mechanistic studies the same approach can be used in *in vitro* models (Fliedner *et al.*, Chapter 12, this volume).

3.4.9　Kidney

The kidneys receive about 20 per cent of cardiac blood output. Therefore, the kidneys are considerably exposed to chemicals in the circulation. The removal of xenobiotics from the blood via filtration, combined with the resorption of water from the filtrate in the proximal tubule, with the subsequent concentration of xenobiotics, may expose tubule cells to relatively high concentrations of these chemicals. The role of metabolic activation in nephrotoxicity has recently been reviewed (Rush *et al.*, 1984).

3.5　EVALUATION OF EFFECTS ON DIFFERENTIATION

From a single cell, the conceptus differentiates into a complex organism containing pools of stem cells which account for the cellular renewal observed in almost all tissues and organs. If the balance between cell production and removal is lost, health is impaired and a disease state introduced. Cellular differentiation which underlies embryogenesis is a most complex process, as is the de-differentiation which accounts for malignant transformation. Neither process is well understood. However models of differentiation are required as short-term tests to determine toxicity and to aid our understanding of mechanisms of toxicity.

Differentiation is usually defined superficially, which is a reflection of our lack of in-depth knowledge of the genetic, molecular and cellular processes involved. It is a finely balanced programme of cellular events, including proliferation, migration association, differentiation, senescence and cell death, precisely arranged to produce tissues and organs selected from genetic information present in all cells. This complex process involves interactions which are both time and space dependent. Adjacent cell groups interact, apparently mediated through endogenous molecular growth modifiers. Processes of cell migration, pattern formation, and the penetration of one cell group by another further characterize this process. Nuclear and non-nuclear events are involved which can be affected genetically or epigenetically. Transcriptional and translational events are likely targets of toxic chemicals. Most of these processes have been modelled in culture systems but have not been applied directly to toxicity testing.

Although cytotoxicity can affect differentiation, cellular differentiation should be clearly distinguished from cellular replication. Many test systems are available which model cellular replication and are useful predictors for cytotoxicity. However, these end-points should not be confused with indicators of abnormal differentiation. Cytotoxicity is a very general type of toxicity; abnormal differentiation is the result of a much more specific insult. The differentiation of various tissue and organ systems, embryogenesis, and cellular transformation have much more in common. Models of these processes have many advantages in toxicological studies but share definite limitations. Various events of embryogenesis have been shown to be exquisitely sensitive to exogenous influences, and the biological consequences are frequently easily recorded. Moreover, many undifferentiated cells and tissues can easily be studied *in vitro* or grafted *in vivo* at various anatomical sites. In such systems the exposure to test agents can be precise in both concentration and timing of exposure. To extrapolate such systems to the *in vivo* situation it is often necessary to supplement the *in vitro* system with a means of metabolizing the test chemical (such as hepatic S9 microsomal fraction). In some laboratories, the serum of treated animals is used in the culture media to provide the test chemicals and metabolites.

The various components of differentiation for which models for toxicity testing are sought include:

- proliferation (DNA synthesis, meiosis, mitosis);
- activation of the genome (expression of new phenotypes);
- polarization of cells (morphology, secretions);
- interactive events with other cells or with the extracellular matrix;
- migration and the attachment of cells;
- cell recognition and spatial organization;
- appearance of cell- and tissue-specific functions;
- cell death; and
- regeneration.

Knowledge concerning these events and their control systems is increasing rapidly, and models of many of these processes are being employed by biologists in their laboratories. Such models can be adopted by toxicologists to identify chemicals capable of perturbing specific steps in the differentiational process. The present situation employs much less sophisticated toxicity tests. In most cases, embryonic cells and whole tissues are used in culture to identify the effects of toxic chemicals. The endpoints are crude and lack specificity, and cytotoxic chemicals are often confused with those capable of altering differentiation.

Nevertheless, the future is encouraging. These newer systems might soon unravel some of the basic mechanisms which account for the harmful effects of chemicals, and aid in the laboratory identification of such hazards. For example, cellular events such as impaired cellular migration, abnormal cellular aggregation, and membrane changes can now be detected in *in vitro* systems.

Various mature tissues and organs offer a number of attractive models which deserve much greater emphasis on their laboratory development, and efforts to evaluate their validity for toxicity testing should be given a high priority.

3.5.1   Gut mucosa

The gut mucosa provides a classic example of differentiation at a local site. Active crypt cell proliferation generates enterocytes which undergo motivation as they migrate to the villus tip, where they are lost into the gut lumen. Monitoring histo-chemical and immunochemical function during this period therefore permits the recognition of a wide variety of toxicological effects within an extremely short time scale. The notable metabolic activity of crypt cells has only been recently appreci-ated. It is probable that their advantages and relevance as a site of primary contact with xenobiotics, when compared with the use of cells from less accessible tissues, has not been fully appreciated or exploited.

3.5.2   Liver

The liver, although capable of regeneration following damage or partial hepatec-tomy, does not appear to offer any significant model of differentiation.

3.5.3   Kidney

The developing kidney, *in vitro*, has been identified as a sensitive indicator of chemical fetotoxicity and teratogenicity (Kavlock and Gray, 1983; Kavlock *et al.*, 1982). *In vitro* models to assess organ development using organ culture (Saxén, 1983), or to assess cell differentiation using embryonic kidney anlagen in culture, have been developed in a number of laboratories with routine techniques (Saxén, 1983; Saxén, Chapter 10, this volume). These test systems seem to be of potential interest to toxicologists as suggested by studies seeking to define the toxic effects of chemicals.

3.5.4 Skin

The skin is a particularly useful organ to serve as a model system for cellular differentiation. Cultured keratinocytes are especially interesting as models for toxicity testing (Suskind, Chapter 11, this volume). These cells grow well and have defined markers of differentiation.

3.5.5 Haematopoietic system

The haematopoietic cell renewal system involves the erythrocytic, granulocytic and megakaryocytic series which differentiate from a stem-cell pool capable of unlimited self-replication. Specific stimuli trigger stem cells to differentiate into specific cell lineages (Fliedner *et al.*, Chapter 12, this volume).

Recently, tests have become available to study *in vitro* cellular differentiation (using haematopoietic progenitor cells). Mononuclear cells from human bone marrow and blood can be forced by appropriate humoral stimuli to differentiate into erythropoietic, granulocytic-macrophage, and megakaryocytic cell lines or into all three lines simultaneously. These new cell culture systems should now be adapted to evaluate the effects of chemicals on cell differentiation.

3.5.6 Immune system

The immune system, like the hematopoietic system, contains a series of cells whose continued differentiation is required to provide immune homeostasis. Morphological differences as well as functional deficits can be monitored as indicators of altered differentiation using standardized tests. Several chemicals (e.g. TCDD, benzene) have been shown to alter differentiation in cells of the immune system (Vos and Dean, Chapter 15, this volume).

3.5.7 Nervous system

The nervous system is generally presented as a non-replicating system. However, prenatal neural tissue does differentiate and can be modelled *in vitro*. Also, the supporting glial elements in the nervous system do differentiate postnatally and can be maintained in appropriate culture systems. These culture systems include whole-embryo, whole organ, organ explants, reaggregation of dispersed cells, and dispersed cell cultures.

3.5.8 Reproductive system

The reproductive system, especially gametogenesis, offers especially attractive model systems for cellular differentiation. In both the testis and ovary, stem cells differentiate during the process of spermatogenesis and oogenesis. Unique meiotic processes, thought to be particularly susceptible to chemical perturbation, occur as the haploid sperm and ova are formed. Fertilization leads to both embryonic and non-embryonic tissues which differentiate actively.

A great number of systems are available which attempt to model embryogenesis. However, most are crude and few are able to provide information concerning the specific mechanisms of differentiation which are altered by the test chemical. However, the study of trophoblast function, hormone production and implantation, has been neglected in most laboratories but offer unique test systems which are relatively easily maintained and monitored *in vitro* as well as *in vivo*.

3.5.9 Future prospects for tests for effects on differentiation

In practice, most of the screening tests for altered differentiation are still implemented *in vivo*, using pregnant laboratory animals. Although longer in duration than most *in vitro* toxicity tests and tests using perfused or cultured organ systems, a 21–30 day gestation is still, by definition, a short-term test.

Nevertheless, a great many systems have been proposed for teratogenicity testing; many fewer model systems are available for gonadal and accessory sex organ function. Recent improvements of many analytical methods for detecting qualitatively and quantitatively the toxic affects of chemicals at cell and tissue levels have increased the validity of the classic test systems. In contrast, few *in vitro* model systems have been adopted as routine tests. *In vitro* tests, however, should be thoroughly studied and their obvious advantages with regard to amount of time and resources required should be exploited in the laboratory. A primary constraint to the increased use of such *in vitro* systems is that embryonic cells and tissues may vary greatly in their sensitivity toward exogenous influences depending on their state of development. This feature requires special attention when the applicability of such models in toxicology is considered. Also to be considered is the possibility that harmful effects which occur *in vivo* might be readily reversible.

3.6 EVALUATION OF EFFECTS ON FUNCTION

Numerous function tests are currently used in mammalian toxicology and clinical medicine. In the past, the major end-points observed in toxicity testing have been degeneration and cell death, which are identified by morphological and histological changes. Cell functions are rarely addressed in this context, although they appear in many cases to be more sensitive indices and may help to elucidate the underlying mechanisms of toxicity.

3.6.1 Cellular function

It is well known in cell biology that cells have both constitutive and luxury functions. Constitutive functions are involved in the maintenance of membrane integrity and transport, energy metabolism and respiration. If constitutive functions are disrupted by chemical exposure, cytotoxicity (cell degeneration and death) results. In contrast, luxury functions involve proliferation, differentiation and other functions which specify the individual characteristics of the cell (i.e. distinguish hepatocytes from lymphocytes). Some luxury functions can be inhibited by toxic agents (e.g. lymphokine elaboration, detoxifying enzyme production, hormone production) without resulting in cell death. These luxury functions are often more sensitive indicators of toxic insult and may have greater predictive value than constitutive functions for toxicity assessment. Currently, enzyme histochemistry and immunohistochemistry procedures can be used to determine enzyme or hormone production at a cellular level whereas other sensitive function assays can measure whole organ/system performance. It has become increasingly recognized that loss of some functional reserve in an organ/system of man or rodent can occur following chemical exposure without immediate adverse clinical sequelae. However, this functional deficit should still be considered as a toxic consequence for risk assessment. To reveal loss of functional reserve, it is often necessary to optimize the test system by an appropriate challenge, stress or stimulus.

3.6.2 *In vitro* systems

Since functions are often the consequence of a complex cascade of physiological and biochemical events, often involving the cooperation of various cell types within an organ/system, it becomes essential to first establish the functional deficit in the intact animal using selected tests that measure terminal responses (e.g. resistance to infectious agent challenge, reproductive performance, etc.). Additional tests, some of which can be applied *in vitro*, can be used to dissect sequential responses and identify the specific lesion (i.e. mechanistic studies). *In vitro* function tests at present are limited because of the complexity of the organ/system from which they are derived. One advantage afforded by *in vitro* function tests are that in some systems human tissue can be utilized.

3.6.3 Organs and physiological systems

The degree to which functional tests relating to particular organs and systems can at present be applied to toxicity testing varies markedly. Thus hepatic and renal function tests are more frequently used in animal models than tests involving other organs, reflecting their known propensity for damage by toxic chemicals and the accumulation of knowledge from clinical observation. Further, tests involving the endocrine, immune, haematopoietic, and central nervous systems are now highly developed and available. However, these tests are numerous and normally undertaken in specialized laboratories. Thus, selection of appropriate tests in this context will require further validation before wider application becomes possible.

Among the remaining organs and systems, cardiopulmonary and reproductive function tests have been elaborated for studies involving humans and to a lesser extent laboratory animals. Their application in toxicity testing is at present limited and requires further development and validation. Although gastrointestinal function studies have been increasingly used in clinical medicine, similar methods for laboratory animals have seldom been applied. Similarly, ear and eye function tests common in man need to be developed for animal models.

3.6.4   Future prospects for tests for effects on function

A strategy for the future would be to incorporate more function tests in toxicity testing because of their sensitivity, relevance and information provided about the nature of the toxic lesion. Special emphasis should be given to the development and validation of *in vitro* methodology using tissues of human as opposed to animal origin. This should facilitate more accurate risk assessment.

3.7   PRACTICAL USE OF TESTS FOR ORGAN/SYSTEM SPECIFIC TOXICITY

As an increasing variety of *in vitro* and *in vivo* short-term tests becomes available, it is essential that toxicologists appreciate the strengths and weaknesses of each in order to use them appropriately. The selection of the tests to be utilized should involve consideration of factors such as the chemical and physical properties of the substance under study, the analogy with chemicals for which toxicological effects are known (for instance an organophosphorus compound must be tested for possible inhibition of cholinesterase), and the intended use of the chemical (e.g. route of administration for a drug, or condition of exposure of an environmental contaminant). It would be erroneous to believe that either a single specific test or even a preordained list of tests is likely to be an effective approach to providing precise and predictive answers about the potential target organ/system toxicity of a chemical. It is also not appropriate to lay down a rigid protocol for each test. There is a danger in encouraging the legislator and the consumer to believe that the development of a few simple tests will enable toxicologists to provide complete assurance to the public on the safety of chemicals to which man is exposed. It should be appreciated that the prediction of toxicological effects for humans is one of the most difficult and complex aspects of biology. From a safety assessment standpoint, each chemical must be regarded as an individual entity when selecting appropriate tests and test conditions.

It must be appereciated that the human being and, for that matter, any mammal is a unit, the function of which is maintained by the continuous interaction of complex regulated circuits that are able to tolerate stress even of a chemical nature. It is the goal of all predictive test systems to analyse the potentials and limitations of the entire organism or its components to tolerate environmentally induced stress and to determine the threshold values for irreversible changes of function. In addition, one should remember that the possibilities and limitations of man to tolerate exposure to chemicals is also determined by genetic factors. Thus, inter-individual differences in disposition must be taken into account when extrapolations are made from the 'pure' test system to man.

3.8   CONCLUSIONS AND RECOMMENDATIONS

3.8.1   Conclusions

The test systems outlined in Tables 3.1(A) – (H), and in the contributed papers in Part B of this volume, require intelligent use. Each system has its merits for particular purposes and its limitations for general use. It is inappropriate both at the present time, and for the foreseeable future, to rely solely on *in vitro* tests to assess potential toxic hazard to man. Until very major advances in our knowledge occur, the proof of toxicity must reside with the findings from *in vivo* tests. However *in vitro* tests may make a number of very important contributions to identifying and quantitating the toxicological properties of a chemical:

(A)   *In vitro* and *ex vivo* tests potentially enable the study of a wide range of variables which may affect the toxicity of a chemical (e.g. interactions with other chemicals or cells). They may also greatly assist in identifying those chemicals which produce subtle damage in target organs which is not immediately identifiable *in vivo* due to the organs' functional reserve.

(B)   Some of the limitations described earlier for *in vitro* tests may become advantages if efforts are made to properly understand the differences between *in vitro* and *in vivo* findings. *In vitro* tests may be especially helpful in deciding whether the organ toxicity of a chemical is a direct or an indirect effect. For instance, a chemical inducing thymic atrophy might act through a direct cytotoxic effect on the thymocytes or may activate the adrenal gland to secrete excessive amounts of corticosteroids which are thymolytic agents; a chemical which induces anaemia may do so because it impairs bone marrow functions or because it inhibits the absorption of important nutrients (e.g. vitamins). *In vitro* tests are vital in resolving the underlying cause of many such *in vivo* observations.

(C)   A major advantage of *in vitro* systems is that human cells and tissues can be utilized. This allows us to evaluate the toxic effects of chemicals directly on human cells and makes possible direct comparisons on the same cell types across animals species. The merit of this approach is already evident. Considerable differences in cell sensitivity to the same concentrations of chemicals have been documented. For example, saccharin prevents, *in vitro*, the formation of lymphoblasts obtained from rats but not from man, while levels of clofibrate, which produce considerable peroxisome proliferation in cultured rat hepatocytes, produce no such induction in man.

3.8.2 Recommendations

In order to develop better test systems it is essential to:

(A) Improve our present knowledge on mechanisms of target specific toxicity. Such information is required to identify:

- the most appropriate biological model to use in assessing a particular type of toxicity;
- the relevance of the findings to the human situation;
- the relevance of the end-points used to human disease;
- individuals at risk.

(B) Develop better procedures for maintaining in a near *in vivo* state, isolated cells and tissues from animal and human organs.

(C) Establish effective means of probing the contributions of particular cell types to toxicity within the intact tissue.

(D) Develop *in vitro* methods for replicating *in vivo* pharmacokinetics, including metabolism.

(E) Utilize developments of knowledge of living systems more effectively to develop new toxicological tests.

(F) Increase the use of sensitive function tests rather than relying on detection of gross toxic change.

REFERENCES

Alabaster, V.A. (1977). Inactivation of endogenous amines in the lungs. In: Bakhle, Y.S., and Vane, J.R. (Eds), *Metabolic Functions of the Lung*, Marcel Dekker, New York, pp. 3–31.

Anderson, K.E., Maibach, H.I., and Anjo, M.D. (1980). The guinea-pig: an animal model for human skin absorption of hydrocortisone, testosterone and benzoic acid. *B. J. Dermatol.*, **102**, 447–53.

Berndt, W.O. (1976). Renal function tests: What do they mean? A review of renal anatomy, biochemistry, and physiology. *Environ. Health Perspect.*, **15**, 55–71.

Brain, J.D., Proctor, D.F., and Reid, L.M. (Eds) (1977). *Respiratory Defence Mechanisms*, Marcel Dekker, New York.

Brody, A.R., and Davis, G.S. (1982). Alveolar macrophage toxicology. In: Witischi, H., and Netteuheim, P. (Eds), *Mechanisms in Respiratory Toxicology*, Volume II, CRC Press, Boca Raton, Florida, pp. 3–28.

Bronaugh, R.L., and Mainbach, H.I. (1983). *In vitro* percutanious absorption. In: Marzulli, F.N., and Maibach, H.I. (Eds), *Dermatotoxicology*, Second Edition, Hemisphere Publishing Company, New York, pp. 117–29.

Bronaugh, R.L., Congden, E.R., and Scheuplein, R.J. (1981). The effect of cosmetic vehicles on the penetration of N-nitrosodiethanolamine through excised human skin,. *J. Invest. Dermatol.*, **76**, 94–6.

Chaube, S., Falahee, K.J., Rose, C.S., Seifried, H.E., Taylor, T.J., and Winstead, J.A. (1982). *Dermatotoxicity*, US Environmental Protection Agency, EPA-560/11-8-002, Washington, DC.

Code of Federal Regulations (1980). Title 16, part 1500.41.

Coombs, R.R.A., and Gell, P.G.H. (1975). Classification of allergic reactions responsible for clinical hypersensitivity and disease. In: Gell, P.G.H., Coombs, R.R.A., and Lachmann, P.J. (Eds), *Clinical Aspects of Immunology*, 3rd Edition, Blackwell Scientific Publications, Oxford, Chapter 25.

Dean, J.H., Luster, M.J., and Boorman, G.A. (1982). Immunotoxicity. In: Sirois, P., Rola-Pleszczynski, M. (Eds),*Immunopharmacology*, Elsevier Biomedical Press, Amsterdam, pp. 349–97.

Dean, J.H., Murray, M.J., and Ward, E.C. (1986). Toxic responses of the immune system. In: Klaassen, C.D., Amdur, M.O., and Doull, J. (Eds), *Casarett and Doull's Toxicology: The Basic Science of Poisons*, Third Edition, MacMillan Publishing Co., New York, pp. 245–85.

Dewey, D.L., Butcher, F.W., and Galpine, A.R. (1977). Hydroxyanisole induced repression of the Harding-Passey melanoma in mice. *J. Pattiol.*, **122**, 117–27.

Draize, J.H., Woodaid, G., and Calvery, H.O. (1944). Methods for the study of irritation and toxicity of substances applied topically to the skin and mucous membranes. *J. Pharmacol. Exp. Ther.*, **82**, 377–90.

Dugard, P.H. (1983). Skin permeability theory in relation to measurements of percutaneous absorption in toxicology. In: Marzulli, F.N., and Maibach, H.I. (Eds), *Dermatotoxicology*, Second Edition, Hemisphere Publishing Company, New York, pp. 91–116.

European Chemical Industry Ecology and Toxicology Centre (ECETOC) (1985). Acute toxicity tests, LD50 (LC50) determinations and alternatives, Monograph No. 6, Brussels, Belgium, 38p.

Epstein, J.H. (1983). Photocontact allergy in humans. In: Marzulli, F.N., and Maibach, H.I. (Eds), *Dermatoxicology*, Second Edition, Hemisphere Publishing Company, New York, pp. 391–404.

Evans, M.J (1982). Cell death and cell renewal in small airways and alveoli. In: Marzulli, F.N., and Maibach, H.I. (Eds), *Dermatoxicology*, Second Edition, Hemisphere Publishing Company, New York, pp. 189–218.

Franz, T.J. (1973). Percutaneous absorption: on the relevance of *in vitro* data. *J. Invest. Dermatol.*, **64**, 190–95.

French, J.G., Lowrimore, G., Nelson, W.C., Finklea, J.F., English, T., and Hertz, M. (1973). The effect of sulfur dioxide and suspended sulfates on acute respiratory disease. *Arch. Env. Health.*, **27**, 129–133.

Gaginella, T.S., Haddad, A.C., Go, V.L.M., and Phillips, S.F. (1977). Cytotoxicity of ricinoleic acid (castor oil) and other intestinal secretagogues on isolated intestinal epithelial cells. *J. Pharmacol. Exp. Therap.*, **201**, 259–66.

Gellin, G.A., and Maibach, H.I. (1983). Detection of environmental depigmenting chemicals. In: Marzulli, F.N., and Maibach, H.I. (Eds), *Dermatotoxicology*, Second Edition. Hemisphere Publishing Company, New York, pp. 443–57.

Goldstein, E., Jordan, G.W., MacKenzie, M.R., and Osebold, J.W. (1976). Methods for evaluating the toxicological effects of gaseous and particulate contaminants on pulmonary microbial defense systems. *Ann. Rev. Pharm. Tox.*, **16**, 447–63.

Goyer, R.A. (1983). Environmental factors in renal disease. In: Kolber, A.R., Wong, T.K., Grant, L.D., DeWoskin, R.S., and Hughes, T.J. (Eds), *In Vitro Toxicity Testing of Environmental Agents: Current and Future Possibilities*, Part A: Survey of Test Systems, Plenum Press, New York, pp. 511–22.

Graham, J.A., Gardner, D.E., Waters, M.D., and Coffin, D.L. (1975). Effect of trace metals on phagocytosis by alveolar macrophages. *Infect. Immun.*, **11**, 1278–83.

Greenspan, B.J., and Morrow, P.E. (1984). The effects of *in vitro* and aerosol exposures to cadmium on phagocytosis by rat pulmonary macrophages. *Fund. Appl. Toxicol.*, **4**, 48–57.

Harber, L.C. (1981). Current status of mammalian and human models for predicting drug photosensitivity. *J. Invest. Dermatol.*, **77**, 65–70.

Harber, L.C., Shalita, A.R., and Armstrong, R.B. (1983). Immunologically mediated contact photosensitivity in guinea-pigs. In: Marzulli, F.N., and Maibach, H.I. (Eds), *Dermatotoxicology*, second Edition. Hemisphere Publishing Corp., New York, pp. 357–74.

Hartmann, F., Owen, R., and Bissell, D.M. (1982). Characterization of isolated epithelial cells from rat small intestines. *Am. J. Physiol.*, **242**, G147–155.

Hayes, J.A. (1983). Systemic responses to toxic agents. In: Homburger, F., Hayes, J.A., and Pelikan, E.W. (Eds), *A Guide to General Toxicology*, Karger, New York, pp. 92–129.

Henderson, R.F., Rebar, A.H., Pickrell, J.A., Brownstein, D.G., and Muhle, H. (1979). Endo-bronchial lavage fluid as an indicator of acute lung damage-effect of species, age and method of lavage on baseline values. *Toxicol. Appl. Pharmacol.*, **48**(1), 64.

Kaidbey, K. (1983). The evaluation of photoallergic contact sensitizers in man. In: Marzulli, F.N., and Maibach, H.I. (Eds), *Dermatotoxicology*, Second Edition, Hemisphere Publishing Company, New York, pp. 405–14.

Kammuller, M.E., Penninks, A.H., and Seinin, W. (1984). Spanish toxic oil syndrome is a chemically induced GVHD-like epidemic. *Lancet*, **i**, 1174–5.

Kavlock, R.J., and Gray,, J.A. (1983). Morphometric, biochemical and physiological assessment of perinatally induced renal dysfunction. *J. Toxicol. Environ. Health*, **11**, 1–13.

Kavlock, R.J., Chernoff, N., Rogers, E., Whitehouse, D., Carver, B., Gray, J., and Robinson, K. (1982). An analysis of fetotoxicity using biochemical endpoints of organ differentiation. *Teratol.*, **26**, 183–94.

Klecak, G. (1983). Identification of contact allegens: predictive tests in animals. In: Marzulli, F.N., and Maibach, H.I. (Eds), *Dermatotoxicology*, Second Edition, Hemisphere Publishing Company, New York, pp. 193–236.

Kornhauser, A., Warmer, W., and Giles, A. (1983). Light-induced dermal toxicity: effects on the cellular and molecular level. In: Marzulli, F.N., and Maibach, H.I. (Eds), *Dermatotoxicology*, Second Edition, Hemisphere Publishing Company, New York, pp. 323–55.

Kutz, S.A., Hinsdill, R.D., and Weltman, D.J. (1980). Evaluation of chemicals for immuno-modulatory effects using an *in vitro* antibody-producing assay. *Environ. Research*, **22**, 368–76.

Lunn, J.E., Knowelden, J., and Handyside, A.J. (1967). Patterns of respiratory illness in Sheffield infant schoolchildren. *Br. J. Prev. Soc. Med.*, **21**, 7–16.

Maibach, H.I., and Marzulli, F.N. (1983). Photoxicity (photoirritation) of topical and systemic agents. In: Marzulli, F.N., and Maibach, H.I. (Eds), *Dermatoxicology*, Second Edition, Hemisphere Publishing Company, New York, pp. 375–389.

Mansur, J.D., Fukuyama, K., Gellin, G.A., and Epstein, W.L. (1978). Effects of 4-tertiary butyl catechol on tissue cultured melanocytes. *J. Invest. Dermatol.*, **70**, 275–9.

Mathias, C.G.T. (1983). Clinical and experimental aspects of cutaneous irritation. In: Marzulli, F.N., and Maibach, H.I. (Eds), *Dermatotoxicology*, Second Edition, Hemisphere Publishing Company, New York, pp. 167–83.

McCreesh A.H., and Steinberg, H. (1983). Skin irritation testing in animals. In: Marzulli, F.N., and Maibaech, H.I. (Eds), *Dermatotoxicology*, Second Edition, Hemisphere Publishing Company, New York, pp. 147–66.

Metcalfe, D. (1977) *Hemopoietic Colonies*, Springer, Berlin.

Mishell, R.I., and Dutton, R.W. (1967). Immunization of dissociated spleen cell cultures from normal mice. *J. Exp. Med.*, **126**, 423–42.

National Academy of Sciences (1977). *Principals for Evaluating the Toxicity of Household Substances*, NAS, Washington, D.C.

Organization for Economic Cooperation and Development (OECD) (1981). *Guidelines for the Testing of Chemicals*, OECD, Paris.

Paganuzzi-Stammati, A., Silan, V., and Zucco, F. (1981). Toxicology investigations with cell culture systems. *Toxicol.*, **20**, 91–153.

Philopot, R.M., Anderson, M.W., and Eling, T.E. (1977). Uptake, accumulation and metabolism of chemicals by lung. In: Bakhle, Y.S., and Vane, J.R. (Eds), *Metabolic Functions of the Lung*, Marcel Dekker, New York, pp. 123–71.

Plaa, G.L., and Hewitt, W.R. (1982). Detection and evalution of chemically induced liver injury. In: Hayes, A.W. (Ed.), *Principles and Methods of Toxicology*, Raven Press, New York, pp. 407–45.

Porter, G.A. (Ed.) (1982). *Nephrotoxic Mechanisms of Drugs and Environmental Toxins*. Plenum Medical Book Co., New York, 466 p.

Rafter, J.J., Bakke, J., Larsen, G., Gustafsson, B., and Gustafsson, J.A. (1983). Role of the intestinal microflora in the formation of sulfur-containing conjugates of xenobiotics. *Rev. Biochem. Toxicol.*, **5**, 387–408.

Rush, G.F., Smith, J.H., Newton, J.R., and Hook, J.B. (1984). Chemically induced nephrotoxicity: role of metabolic activation. *CRC Critical Reviews in Toxicology*, **13**(2), 99–160.

Said, S.I. (1982). Release of pharmacological agents and mediators from the lungs. In: Witschi, H., and Nettlesheim, P. (Eds), *Mechanisms of Respiratory Toxicology*, volume I, CRC Press, Boca Raton, Florida, pp. 63–83.

Saxén, L. (1983). *In vitro* model systems for chemical teratogenesis. In: Kolber, A.R., Wong, T.K., Grant, L.D., DeWoskin, R.S., and Hughes, T.J. (Eds), *In Vitro Toxicity Testing of Environmental Agents: Current and Future Possibilities*, Part B: Development of Risk Assessment Guidelines. Plenum Press, New York, pp. 173–90.

Steinkamp, J.A., Wilson, J.S., and Svitra, Z.V. (1979). Detection of early changes in lung cell cytology by flow-systems analysis techniques. DOE report LA-7983-PR, Los Alamos Scientific Laboratory, National Technical Information Service, Springfield, Virginia.

Till, J.E., and McCulloch, E.A. (1961). A direct measurement of the radiation sensitivity of the normal bone marrow cells. *Radiat. Res.*, **14**, 213–22.

Tucker, A.N., Sanders, V.M., Mallet, P., Kauffman, B.N., and Munson, A.E. (1982). *In vitro* immunotoxicological assays for detection of compounds requiring metabolic activation. *Environ. Health Perspect.*, **43**, 123–7.

Uyeki, E.M., Ashkar, A.E., Shoemau, D.W., and Bisle, T.V. (1977). Acute toxicity of benzene inhalation to haemopoietic precursor cells. *Toxicol. Appl. Pharmacol.*, **40**, 49–57.

van Furth, R. and van Zwet, T.L. (1973). *In vitro* determination of phagocytosis and intracellular killing by polymorphonuclear and mononuclear phagocytes. In: Weir, D.M. (Ed.), *Handbook of Experimental Immunology*, 2nd Edition, Blackwell Scientific, Oxford, Chapter 36.

Wester, R.C., and Maibach, H.I. (1983). *In vivo* percutaneous absorption. In: Marzulli, F.N., and Maibach, H.I. (Eds), *Dermatotoxicology*, Second Edition, Hemisphere Publishing Company, New York, pp. 131–46.

Wilson, A.G.E. (1982). Toxicokinetics of uptake, accumulation and metabolism of chemicals by the lung. In: Witschi, H., and Nettlesheim, P. (Eds), *Mechanisms of Respiratory Toxicology*, volume I, CRC Press, Boca Raton, Florida, pp. 161–85.

Witschi, H. (1976). Proliferation of type II alveolar cells: a review of common responses in toxic lung injury. *Toxicology*, **5**, 267–77.

Short-term Toxicity Tests for Non-genotoxic Effects
Edited by P. Bourdeau *et al.*
© 1990 SCOPE. Published by John Wiley & Sons Ltd

CHAPTER 4

Methods to Predict Toxicity

4.1 QUANTITATIVE STRUCTURE–ACTIVITY RELATIONSHIPS

Quantitative structure–activity relationships (QSAR) are quantitative models which relate the variation in measures of activity in a series of chemical compounds to the variation in chemical structure between compounds in the series. The use of QSAR in the study and identification of potentially toxic chemicals is receiving increased attention, as demonstrated by several recent reviews (for example, McKinney, 1985; Hansch, 1985; Enslein, 1984; Birge and Cassidy, 1983).

Although most extensively applied to drug design, QSAR is now being effectively exploited by other fields from anticancer research (Nasr *et al.*, 1984) to aquatic toxicology (Birge and Cassidy, 1983). The major limiting factor in the application of QSAR systems appears to be the inability to delineate biological responses quantitatively to the same degree of precision as is possible for molecular descriptors (Birge and Cassidy, 1983). This is due to the fact that many of the biological responses so far used in QSAR systems are the result of the interaction of a variety of toxic manifestations and, therefore, are not as absolute as physiochemical parameters used to define molecule descriptors.

The models used in QSAR range from simple additivity models where each parameter is independent of all others (e.g. the Free–Wilson model (Free and Wilson, 1964)), to complicated models of pattern recognition where multivariate activity data are related to different chemical structures and physiochemical parameters. These models provide both qualitative classifications (indicating the existence of an effect or its likelihood of occurring) and quantitative data (i.e. an index of the probable severity of an effect). However, qualitative classification must be done at the same time or prior to any quantitative analysis.

In qualitative predictions, each compound is assigned to a class (active *vs.* non-active, synergist *vs.* antagonist, etc.). Usually, a compound is given a value for its probability of belonging to each class. Some method of pattern recognition—discriminant analysis—is used to determine a relation between the class assignment and the molecular descriptor which indicates physiochemical values and/or structural features of the chemical.

QSAR has potential for use in priority setting, toxicity evaluation and hazard analysis, but much more development is necessary. There are inadequacies in the toxicity data bases that are available for QSAR studies and inadequacies in the methods used for encoding chemical structures and quantifying biological activities for computer analysis which must be overcome before QSAR can be fully exploited in toxicology.

4.2 PREDICTING SAFE LEVELS OF EXPOSURE TO CHEMICALS

A major goal of toxicology is the establishment of levels of chemical exposure which will not cause irreversible harm to man. Safe levels of exposure are usually determined by extrapolation of mammalian toxicological data to the human situation.

It is often advantageous to predict safe levels of chemical exposure based on short-term test results, or before a full safety evaluation has been completed. Such situations include:

- the laboratory and pilot production stage in the development or manufacture of a new chemical;
- when only very small quantities of a chemical are to be produced;
- when short-term or limited exposure is expected during the use of the chemical;
- when accidental release of or exposure to a chemical occurs before the safety evaluation is completed.

A variety of methods have been proposed for estimating safe exposure levels for chemicals (see Sanockij, Chapter 20, this volume). However, these methods are restricted to families of chemicals with well understood properties and which are not suspected of having delayed or long-term effects. The primary limitation to the routine establishment of safe exposure levels from short-term tests is the lack of sufficient validation of the correlation of short-term tests with long-term effects. It is often difficult or impossible at present to extrapolate dose–effect (response) relationships in the whole organism from short-term tests, with any degree of precision or confidence.

REFERENCES

Birge, W.J. and Cassidy, R.A. (1983). Structure–activity relationships in aquatic toxicology. *Fund. App. Toxicol.*, **3**, 359–68.

Enslein, K. (1984). Estimation of toxicological endpoints by structure–activity relationships. *Pharmacol. Rev.*, **36**(2), 131S–135S.

Free, S.M. and Wilson, J.W. (1964). A mathematical contribution to structure-activity studies. *J. Med. Chem.*, **7**, 395–9.

Hansch, C. (1985). The QSAR paradigm in the design of less toxic molecules. *Drug Metab. Rev.*, **15**(7), 1279–94.

McKinney, J.D. (Ed.) (1985). Monograph on structure–activity correlation in mechanism studies and predictive toxicology. *Environ. Health Perspect.*, **61**,

Nasr, M., Paull, K.D. and Narayanan, V.L. (1984). Computer-assisted structure–activity correlations. *Adv. Pharmacol. Chemo.*, **20**, 123–90.

Short-term Toxicity Tests for Non-genotoxic Effects
Edited by P. Bourdeau *et al.*
© 1990 SCOPE. Published by John Wiley & Sons Ltd

CHAPTER 5

*Short-term Tests in Ecotoxicology**

5.1 INTRODUCTION

Human toxicology, by definition, is concerned with the effects of chemicals on a single species—man. Research and testing are undertaken with one major objective, protection of the health and safety of the individual. In contrast, ecotoxicology not only deals with the impact of chemicals on individuals of an immense number of species, but also deals with the influence of chemicals on supra-organismal levels of biological organization. Thus, it is concerned with the potential impact of chemicals on populations, communities and ecosystems as well as on individual species and the individual organisms of those species. This introduces a great deal of complexity because of the great variety of environmental factors, and their interactions, that have to be taken into account (Levin and Kimball, 1983; Vouk and Sheehan, 1983; Sheehan *et al.*, 1984, Vouk *et al.*, 1985).

In ecotoxicology, the main objective of testing procedures is to evaluate hypotheses about the potential for chemical agents to exert adverse effects, the outcomes of which might be serious not only in respect to ecosystem structure and function, but also with respect to the health and welfare of human beings as a component of that ecosystem. Thus, in addition to investigations aimed at elucidating the potential effects of a chemical on individual species, testing methods should also provide data suitable to predict effects and impacts on higher levels of biological organization and complexity. This represents a challenge since our current understanding of the subject is limited and the acquisition of experience, gained through observation of adverse effects caused by past events, may, in reality, require many decades.

Ecotoxicologic tests are important for regulatory decisions relating to the registration of pesticides, for the generation of pre-manufacturing or pre-marketing data to support approval of new chemicals in commerce, for management decisions affecting the use of land, air and water and to protect the quality of these media by controlling pollution, and for monitoring the effectiveness of remedial measures to restore or improve a previously impacted site. Thus, there are many needs for

---

*This chapter was prepared by a Workgroup comprised of the following members: P. Bourdeau, G. C. Butler, D. Calamari, J.W. Gillett, V. Landa, D. Peakall, P. Sheehan, G. Persoone, R Truhaut and P. Wells.

ecotoxicologic tests and any improvement in the predictive power,* efficiency and interpretive capability of these tests will have direct economic and social benefits and serve to increase credibility in the scientific and technical assessments that are based upon them. In this way, the questions which ecotoxicologic tests propose to answer have important socio-economic consequences, not least of which is the influence they may have on the cost and availability of goods and services.

For the purpose of this section, short-term tests are considered as those that can be generally completed within thirty days. Clearly, this is an arbitrary time-frame that does not take into account the widely different time scales of environmental influences on different organisms, communities or functions that may be subject to testing. Nevertheless, although arbitrary, this time-frame does fit within the time scale of many decisions relating to the screening of new chemicals with a view to their further development for commercial purposes, or for environmental management decisions in the face of real or potential deteriorating situations.

5.2 SINGLE SPECIES TESTS

Short-term, single species tests have provided the basis for many important actions to protect and enhance the quality of life and the environment (Mount and Gillett, 1982). They have been adopted in screening procedures for selection of new chemicals which meet essential needs or provide useful products to improve the quality of life, and they have been adopted as part of the regulatory controls that have been implemented to prevent degradation of vital ecosystem functions.

Laboratory experiments of relatively short duration on single species have provided helpful information, especially in relation to the aquatic environment. In particular, one may observe that single species tests have been widely used in the assessment of the following (as discussed by Persoone *et al.*, Chapter 18, this volume):

- prediction of lethality and other effects (e.g. avoidance) for the tested species under field conditions, including information on the concentrations of a chemical which cause these effects;
- prediction of interactions and synergistic properties of mixtures of chemicals;
- probability of toxicity under different physiochemical conditions;
- prediction of toxicity (by extrapolation) to other species;
- determination of acute-to-chronic toxicity ratios and their use as 'application factors' for setting water quality objectives and effluent limits;
- measurements of short-term developmental responses (as compared to long-term, life-cycle responses);

---

*Predictive power covers a variety of different extrapolations that are made on the basis of the results obtained. These include extrapolations from one species to another, from one chemical to another and from one set of environmental conditions to many others.

- prediction of long-term lethality based upon the shape of dose–response–time curves; and
- determination of bioconcentration factors.

Short-term, single species tests have also been used as range-finding tests for long-term studies and to provide data for the development of quantitative structure–activity relationships (QSAR) for biological responses. Short-term assays can sometimes give useful information on the rate of degradation of toxic compounds, especially if degradation results in the formation of a more toxic substance as part of the process.

Through the conduct of short-term bioassays using appropriate, preselected test species, it is possible to predict whether a chemical is selectively toxic, to estimate thresholds for harmful effects, to estimate safe concentrations, and to set limits on the range and types of species likely to be affected by point sources of pollution. Results of these investigations can be used, for example, to control the disposal of industrial wastes or to establish pesticide application rates at levels which avoid serious environmental impacts.

By the use of batteries of appropriate tests, and the application of safety factors to the results obtained, specific protection of desirable resources (e.g. protection of fisheries and habitats of endangered species) can be achieved. However, the use of large, arbitrary safety factors may lead to unnecessarily stringent regulation of environmental quality with consequent economic costs and social disbenefits. With present limited knowledge, it is very difficult to judge whether safety factors used in any given situation are excessive; from limited studies, it is evident that extrapolation from laboratory test conditions to the field situation is fraught with difficulties and that potential outcomes may vary considerably between different sets of field conditions.

There are, however, a number of situations where data from single species testing failed to reveal serious and significant impacts of chemicals on the environment. These include:

(1)	shell thinning affecting raptors and pelagic seabirds;
(2)	avoidance by salmonoids of heavy metal plumes in rivers;
(3)	neurotoxic effects in mammals caused by the consumption of fish containing residues of methyl mercury;
(4)	long-term impact of oil spills on shallow water and inshore invertebrates;
(5)	impact of mirex and other pesticides on many estuarine species; and
(6)	effects of airborne pollutants on lichens and forests.

Despite these limitations, single species tests have been widely accepted in scientific and regulatory circles and this has resulted in their adoption as standardized procedures such as those published by the OECD (1982). Their use, in combination with physicochemical parameters such as the octanol–water partition coefficient (to estimate potential for bioaccumulation) and toxicokinetic studies (to estimate bio-concentration potential) can yield substantial insight into the anticipated outcome of chronic exposure, including bioaccumulation, biomagnification and food chain amplification.

5.3   MULTI-SPECIES TESTS

In order to bridge the gap between the artificial, simple conditions of laboratory test systems and the diverse, complex situation that exists in the real world of field conditions, numerous multi-species test systems have been developed and applied over the past decade (Gillett and Witt, 1979; Giesy, 1980; Hammonds, 1981). These multi-species test systems have been compared to the more traditional methods of predicting adverse outcomes in the environment with favourable results. They appear to be more relevant ecologically, and more realistic and more cost-effective in operation. However, these systems require 45–90 days minimum for each test, and experimental emphasis has tended to be given to the use of longer operating times to enhance realism and effectiveness.

Rather than effects on single species, these systems test effects on processes, structures and functions of ecological components as well as interactions between species under more realistic exposure conditions. Microcosm tests have shown impacts on primary production (plant photosynthesis), on growth, reproduction, and secondary productivity of higher animals, on nutrient cycling and on various inter-species interactions. They have been used extensively in the aquatic field for better estimates of fate and effects of pollutants.

Many phenomena cannot be effectively or efficiently quantified by single species tests in the laboratory or in the field. Because microcosms are relatively well controlled, the quality and quantity of data can be high, without risks attendant to field tests.

Originally it was hoped that, in addition to their value as an experimental research technique, microcosms and other model ecosystems might be the answer to the high costs of screening chemical substances (Draggan, 1976). Early failures due to over-expectations, limitations in duration and self-sustaining operation, and credibility has prevented wide acceptance of microcosm tests (Gillett and Witt, 1979). However, recent progress has established the role of microcosm experiments as an upper level test in a step-sequenced or tiered testing scheme. For example, the soil core microcosm has been used to evaluate the application of flyash to agricultural fields and compared favourably to tests in greenhouse flower-pots and small field test plots (van Voris *et al.*, 1983a,b). Considerable progress has also been made with the applicability of aquatic microcosms/mesocosms.

Multispecies tests are required for long-term environmental protection, to examine interspecies interactions, population and community dynamics, and ecosystem processes (Cairnes *et al.*, 1981). They must be combined with QSAR to develop more efficient approaches to the testing and evaluation of chemicals.

5.4   CONCLUSIONS AND RECOMMENDATIONS

5.4.1 Conclusions

1. There are no true short-term tests of ecosystem function. There are inherent and theoretical reasons that do not permit extrapolation from *in vivo* and *in vitro* tests to higher levels of biological organization and across taxa, and the lack of field-to-field and lab-to-field validation efforts further hamper predictive capabilities.
2. Deficiencies in knowledge of ecosystem structure and function is obviously limiting, but, more critical to the purposes of this report, there is an explicit absence of data and understanding linking many lower level tests (physiochemical, physiological, and single species) with higher level tests (population, community and ecosystem). This deficiency is further affected by lack of adequate knowledge of the behaviour of chemicals and organisms relative to exposure, especially in heterogeneous environments (such as soil and sediment).
3. Two major areas, however, show substantial promise for shortening the time-to-decision, lessening resource requirements, and providing more incisive information relative to outcomes hypothesized for a chemical substance in the environment:

   (a) quantitative structure–activity relationships (QSAR) (particularly for properties important to prediction of environmental behaviour) and the prediction of environmental concentrations and dosages; and
   (b) multi-species test systems (including microcosms or other model ecosystems) for studying ecological processes and chemical disposition.

4. Single species tests are the only ones widely accepted and employed at present, although they are not sufficient for purposes of ecotoxicologic assessment without the use of large and arbitrary 'safety factors'.
5. Multi-species tests have been developed for a variety of natural systems, but have not been widely employed with a great number of types and classes of chemicals and have not been recognized officially by any regulatory body. In spite of the more limited experience and greater technical requirements of these test systems, they have been found to be more incisive and cost-effective than simpler tests.

5.4.2   Recommendations

1. A concerted effort should be made to make proprietary data, in the hands of governments and private organizations and companies, more available in order to establish better QSAR for both chemical fate and biological effects.

   (a) The potential for using QSAR and 'pre-biological' estimates of effect should be pursued and elaborated upon by specific research and testing efforts at both the single-species and multiple-species levels.

(b) Research to establish understanding of the linkages of these properties and molecular structure to toxicologic effect must be pursued.

2. Improvements in testing effectiveness and efficiency will require better linkage between single species tests (both laterally between taxa and vertically between levels of biological organization) and multiple species tests. This is particularly important in establishing actions which should be taken (regulatory action, further testing, waiving of further testing, etc.) on the basis of test results.

3. Research and development must extend and expand multiple species tests (microcosms, mesocosms, and similar test vehicles), specifically to enhance the range of chemical classes considered and of geographic/ecologic zones represented. Efforts must be made to extend the time over which such systems are representative of natural environments.

4. Perhaps most importantly, in terms of enhanced efficiency of resource use and information obtained, an improved contextual basis for the use of ecotoxicologic tests must be created. This will require research into the connections between tested outcomes and those factors resulting in action to avoid or correct problems ('regulatory end-points'), and harmonization of testing and evaluation schemes.

5. Specific development of single species assays for particular types of questions will continue to be needed, so these should be pursued in research and development activities. Examples noted include plant life cycle bioassays, honeybee tests, earthworm tests and aquatic invertebrate tests. However, testing of more species or development of new types of tests need not be pursued simply to broaden the testing base. The standardization of many existing tests, and inter-laboratory calibration of these is needed. Of special interest are short-term aquatic embryo-larval systems because of their focus on sensitive developmental stages.

6. Specific attention must be given to research to develop better powers of extrapolation from one test system to another, requiring further research in biometrics, ecology, and biogeographical relationships.

REFERENCES

Cairnes, J. Jr., Alexander, M., Cummin, K.W., Edmonson, W.T., Goldman, R., Harte, J., Isensee, A.R., Levin, R., McCormick, J.F., Peterle, T.J. and Zar, J.H. (1981). *Testing for Effects of Chemicals on Ecosystems*, National Academy Press, Washington, D.C.

Draggan, S. (1976). The microcosm as a research tool for estimation of environmental transport of toxic material. *Intern. J. Environ. Studies*, **10**, 5–10.

Giesy, J. (1980). *Microcosms in Ecological Research*. DOE Symposium No. 52, U.S. National Technical Information Service, Springfield, Virginia.

Gillett, J.W. and Witt, J.M. (1979). *Terrestrial Microcosms*, NSF-RA-79 0034, National Science Foundation, Washington, D.C.

Hammonds, A. (Ed.) (1981). *Methods for Ecological Toxicology—A Critical Review of Laboratory Multi-Species Tests*, Ann Arbor Science Publishers, Woburn, MA.

Levin, S.A. and Kimball, K.D. (1983). *New Perspectives in Ecotoxicology*, Ecosystems Research Centre, Cornell University, Ithaca, NY.

Mount, D.I. and Gillett, J.W. (1982). Progress in research on ecotoxicology. In: Mason, W.T. (Ed.), *Research on Fish and Wildlife Habitat*, EPA-600/8-82-022. US Environmental Protection Agency, Washington, D.C., pp. 143–64.

Organization for Economic Cooperation and Development (OECD) (1982). *Guidelines for Ecotoxicologic Testing of Chemicals*, OECD, Paris.

Sheehan, P.J., Miller, D.R., Butler, G.C. and Bourdeau, P. (Eds) (1984). *Effects of Pollutants at the Ecosystem Level*, SCOPE 22, John Wiley & Sons, New York.

van Voris, P., Arthur, M.F. and Tolle, D.A. (1983a). *Field and Laboratory Evaluation of Terrestrial Microcosms for Assessing Ecological Effects of Utility Wastes*, Project Report 124–5, Electric Power Research Institute, Palo Alto, CA.

van Voris, P., Tolle, D.A., Arthur, M.F., Chesson, J. and Brocksen, R.W. (1983b). Terrestrial microcosms: Validation, applications and cost-benefit analysis. Presented at the 4th annual meeting of the Society of Environmental Toxicology and Chemistry, Arlington, VA.

Vouk, V.B. and Sheehan, P.J. (Eds) (1983). *Methods for Assessing the Effects of Chemicals on Reproductive Functions*, SCOPE 20, John Wiley & Sons, New York.

Vouk, V.B., Butler, G.C., Hoel, D.G. and Peakall, D.B. (Eds) (1985). *Methods for Estimating Risks of Chemical Injury: Human and Non-Human Biota and Ecosystems*, SCOPE 26, John Wiley & Sons, New York.

PART B

CONTRIBUTED PAPERS

Short-term Toxicity Tests for Non-genotoxic Effects
Edited by P. Bourdeau *et al.*
Published by John Wiley & Sons Ltd

CHAPTER 6

*Conceptual Approaches to Methodology Development**

ALAN M. GOLDBERG AND ANDREW N. ROWAN

6.1   INTRODUCTION

There is a societal need and responsibility for public authorities to attempt to ensure that individuals in society are protected from harm. Given the current state of our knowledge, this necessitates some testing in animals and extrapolation of the results, no matter how difficult, to predict likely human responses. We are still far too ignorant to predict the toxic effects of a compound from first principles. Therefore, we have to fall back on appropriate models of the human system to identify possible hazards. By necessity, this leads to the use of mammals or other species that often respond in a sufficiently similar manner to humans to provide an index of the potential hazard.

Nevertheless, the problems of extrapolation and evaluation are formidable. Thousands of new chemicals need to be evaluated every year while only a fraction of the estimated 65 000 chemicals (Maugh, 1978) in use today have been subject to testing according to available public information (National Research Council, 1984). In addition, the present animal testing techniques are generally crude, cumbersome and costly and there is growing public criticism of such use of animals.

Among toxicologists, there are some who see animal testing as an unsatisfactory answer to toxicology's problems. Thus, in 1971, Rofe, in an excellent but little-cited review of the use of tissue culture in toxicology, stated that:

In seeking to bridge the gap between the effects of foreign substances on animals and their effects on man, it seems unlikely that a substantial contribution to the problem can be made by prolonging the conventional toxicological procedures or including additional organ function tests.

*Reproduced, with permission, in abridged form from the *Annual Review of Pharmacology and Toxicology*, Volume 25, © 1985 Annual Reviews, Inc.

Others, scientific and non-scientific, have also criticized animal testing (Rofe, 1971; Melmon, 1976; Muul *et al.*, 1976; Zbinden, 1976; Heywood, 1978; Stevenson, 1979; Efron, 1984), commenting variously that toxicology has sometimes created more problems than it has solved in the last decade, that toxicology is a science without scientific underpinning, and that we should move towards the development of an appropriate battery of short-term tests, using both *in vitro* and *in vivo* approaches, to assess product safety.

The techniques most commonly highlighted as having potential for the future are (i) cell and organ culture, (ii) computer modelling, and (iii) the use of less invasive animal procedures and endpoints producing little stress or suffering. There have already been a number of reviews of the cell and organ culture in toxicology investigations beginning with a seminal paper by Pomerat and Leake in 1954, followed by a number of reviews after 1970 (Rofe, 1971; Dawson, 1972; Worden, 1974; Nardone, 1977; Berky and Sherrod, 1978; Tardiff, 1978; Deutsche Pharmakologische Gesellschaft, 1980; Stammati *et al.*, 1981; Zucco and Hooisma, 1982; Ekwall, 1983; Grisham and Smith, 1984). However, judging from the number of citations to these papers, none have had impact. According to the records of the *Science Citation Index*, Rofe's 1971 review has been cited less than twenty times in the following twelve years with a high of three citations each in 1976 and 1980. Although more and more toxicological research is being conducted *in vitro*, the potential of cell culture as applied to toxicological evaluation and hazard assessment is only now beginning to be tested and assessed. This is the result of public pressure, the availability of funds for such studies, and increased concern among scientists.

However, the use of cell cultures in toxicology testing and hazard assessment must be developed and implemented cautiously. Obviously, a single cell culture cannot accurately mimic the complex interactions of all the cell types in the body no matter how exquisite the experimental design. *In vivo* metabolism may be simulated to some extent but not completely (Fry and Bridges, 1977) and other integrating functions (e.g. hormones, immune reactions, phagocytosis) are not included. In addition, a cell culture is a relatively static system in which the dose of the test chemical reaching the target system and the duration of contact may not be the same as those that occur in the *in vivo* test. There are also physical problems regarding solubility, stability and biophysical effects of the test compound.

On the other hand, the technique of cell culture has great potential once investigators have acquired the background knowledge to ask highly focused and specific questions. The static nature of cell culture is also an advantage in that the dose and duration of contact of a test chemical can be precisely determined. Much less test chemical is required to carry out cell culture investigations than to conduct tests *in vivo*. Replicate cultures can be set up with ease and generate more data in a short time.

One of the most exciting aspects of cell culture studies in toxicology is that one can use human tissue. Such studies have been limited in the past because of the difficulty of maintaining and growing differentiated human cell types in culture but the technical problems are being steadily overcome. For example, important developments in the last years include improvements in the quality control of media and plasticware provided by manufacturers, improved quality control in the laboratory, better media formulations (Barnes and Sato, 1980) for the growth of normal cells as well as for cells exhibiting specialized functions (e.g. heart cell contractility and melanin production by melanocytes), and improvements in cell separation and cloning techniques (cf. Nardone and Bradlaw, 1983).

Nardone and Bradlaw (1983) describe four interfaces between *in vitro* methodology and animal toxicology—screening tests, mechanistic studies, personnel monitoring and considerations for risk assessment. They note that screening tests are the most developed and are likely to remain the major focus of *in vitro* toxicology. However, mechanistic studies probably will become steadily more important, both in toxicological evaluations and for risk assessment. One could also classify *in vitro* methodology according to whether the approach is empirical, model development or mechanistic (Goldberg, 1984a).

The empirical approach for the development of methodology is problematic. The questions asked are generally not focused and the intent is to develop correlations prior to fundamental understandings. Additionally, the results tend to be somewhat unpredictable. Should this be the case in the development of *in vitro* toxicological methods, we will have, unfortunately, provided supplementary testing strategies but not replacement testing strategies. This will leave us with the dilemma of attempting to use the *in vitro* methodologies without being able to rely on them.

Model development attempts to utilize systems that mimic the *in vivo* systems. Generally, the model system is neither complete nor faithful in all aspects of the system being modelled, but it tends to provide useful information if the data are not over-interpreted. In those model systems where a single aspect of an integrated response is examined and the data are interpreted, it can provide meaningful inferences for the evaluation of chemical effects.

The mechanistic approach in the development of *in vitro* methodologies should be based on a thorough knowledge of the underlying metabolism, kinetics and biology in the system or species to be examined. If the metabolic pathways are understood, or if it is known that the parent compound produces the toxicological insult, then one can develop a system to examine the mechanisms by which the chemical(s) works. That is, one can examine the adverse chemical or physical effects that lead to a significant functional loss in the tissue or system. This approach allows the *in vitro* system to be derived from the species under study. It also provides a better understanding of the chemical–biological interaction and the consequences of that interaction. Once a mechanism has been identified, it may then be possible to develop appropriate, interpretable, simple and reliable *in vitro* methodologies.

From a scientific viewpoint, the mechanistic approach is not only preferable but necessary. *In vitro* methods will be more acceptable and will develop rapidly when the knowledge base has advanced far enough to permit a focus on mechanisms.

6.2   ALTERNATIVES IN TOXICOLOGY

Toxicity testing on animals may be divided into acute, subacute and chronic tests. Acute tests are those in which the animals are dosed with one or a few doses of the test compound and kept for at most a few weeks. Such tests include protocols for determining the various LD50s as well as eye and skin irritancy tests. Up to 50 per cent of all animals used in toxicology testing are killed in acute tests (Rowan, 1984). Subchronic tests last from a few weeks to several months. Chronic tests last for more than three months and include tests for reproductive and carcinogenic effects among others. The search for new approaches in all these areas will continue to evolve. However, at the present time, our lack of knowledge about the mechanisms of possible toxic insults is such that some animal testing is going to be required.

6.2.1   Acute toxicity testing

In acute tests, the investigator is observing an immediate response in which the orgnaism's defence mechanisms are rapidly overwhelmed. Where specific end-points are being determined (e.g. eye irritancy) it may well be possible to develop an adequate *in vitro* alternative based on one or more screening systems. However, one of the functions of acute testing is the identification of unexpected toxic effects. The empiricism of this approach requires that a relatively good model for the whole human being be used. This generally means using a whole mammal because the metabolism and response of other mammals is at least sufficiently similar to human responses to provide an index of hazard. However, there are acute tests for which the prospect of either reducing the number of animals used, or for developing an adequate *in vitro* test are relatively good and these are discussed below.

6.2.1.1   *LD50 testing*

The calculation of the median lethal dose (LD50) for the measurement of toxicity was introduced in 1927 (Trevan, 1927). At that time, determination of the LD50 was used to standardize such potent biologicals as digitalis, insulin and diptheria toxin. With time, however, the LD50 came to be used as a standard measure by which the toxicity of all chemicals was assessed. In 1968, Morrison, Quinton and Reinert questioned this use of the LD50 (Morrison *et al.*, 1968), arguing that the classical test used too many animals and that the statistical figure resulting was quite mean-ingless. They contended that a figure, generated from the use of 6–10 animals, was the best that could be achieved given the inadequacies of the test system (Hunter *et al.*, 1978). There have been several recent criticisms of the LD50 (Zbinden and Flury-Roversi, 1981; Rowan, 1983; Goldberg, 1984b). As a result of scientific criticism, coupled with political pressure from the animal welfare movement, the classical LD50 test (with a few specific exceptions) appears to be on its way out as a regulatory requirement. For example, the German authorities state that they are accepting acute toxicity test data using a small number of animals (Bass *et al.*, 1982; Veberla and Schnieders, 1982) and the Food and Drug Administration has now explicitly stated that it has no requirement for LD50 tests and that acute toxicity data from alternative tests may well be acceptable (Food and Drug Administration, 1984).

The alternatives that are being considered all require the use of far fewer animals. Bruce (1985) has proposed the use of six to ten animals in the Up–Down method (Dixon and Mood, 1948) although it cannot be recommended for testing materials where delayed deaths (more than a few days) are the rule. Several simplifications of the standard method, all of which require fewer animals, have recently been proposed (Muller and Kley, 1982; Schutz and Fuchs, 1982; Tattersall, 1982; Lorke, 1983) and the last (Lorke, 1983), which recommends the use of only thirteen animals, is claimed to be suitable for industrial use where a variety of chemicals of widely differing toxicities must be assessed. Where only an estimate is required, the method proposed by Deichmann and LeBlanc offers yet another choice (Deichmann and LeBlanc, 1943).

Another approach which has also been suggested is the use of a structure–activity computer model to estimate LD50s (Enslein and Craig, 1978; Enslein *et al.*, 1983). This approach has been criticized because the chemicals used to design the models were not congeneric and because the biological end-point (death) used is not the function of a single active site in a well-defined system (Rekker, 1980). The developers of the model argue that there is no question that the use of a congeneric set of chemicals would produce tighter estimates but that this is insufficient reason not to explore a model based on heterogeneous collections of chemicals. As this field of quantitative structure–toxicity relationships (QSTR) develops, one can anticipate major strides in the use of these systems as predictors of toxicity (Golberg, 1983).

There have been several papers which have correlated the results of cytotoxicity assays with animal LD50s (Barile and Hardegree, 1970; Sako, 1977; Autian and Dillingham, 1978; Ekwall, 1980; Balls and Bridges, 1984) but the development of an adequate cell culture alternative is very unlikely. There are many different toxic effects, and a crude cytotoxicity assay is unlikely to be successful as a general screen for acute toxicity. In addition, these non-mechanistic tests may result in the identification of an excessive number of false-positives and false-negatives and efforts to correlate cytotoxicity data with questionable LD50 figures are unlikely to yield significant toxicological insights. Nevertheless, there is a clear need for good cytotoxicity data and for the development of reliable measures of cytotoxicity (cf. Autian and Dillingham, 1978; Balls and Bridges, 1984).

Therefore, the present state of development of alternative approaches to the classical LD50 test is focused on the use of fewer animals (up to a 90 per cent reduction) with more attention being paid to morbidity and symptoms than a statistical estimate of the median lethal dose. For most purposes, the use of small numbers of animals to estimate the median lethal dose appears to be a satisfactory alternative. Cell culture systems have been investigated but they cannot provide the breadth of coverage of possible toxic insults of a simple *in vivo* mammalian organism. A computer model for estimating LD50s has been developed (Enslein *et al.*, 1983). While it allows one to estimate the toxicity of a new substance quickly, the computer model suffers limitations as a possible replacement to the animal test.

6.2.1.2 *Ophthalmic irritancy testing*

The classic method for assessing the potential for ophthalmic irritancy of chemicals is the Draize eye irritancy test (Draize *et al.*, 1944; Freidenwald *et al.*, 1944). In recent years, this test has been criticized by both scientists (Weil and Scala, 1971; Griffith *et al.*, 1980) and by animal welfare groups (Rowan, 1981). In fact, in 1978, Smyth commented that the Draize eye irritancy test was one area where a search for a non-animal alternative had a real chance of success (Smyth, 1978). A recent review of eye irritation testing outlines some of the difficulties in identifying eye irritants and the specific historical background of, and problems with the Draize Eye Irritancy test (Falahee *et al.*, 1981). For example, one of the main difficulties with this test as a regulatory tool is identified as the subjective nature of scoring and evaluating the test response.

Pressure from animal welfare campaigns has, in recent years, resulted in the support of a number of projects to seek an alternative to the Draize eye irritancy test with promising results. The projects can be divided into those investigating modifications of the test which would result in less animal distress, and those investigating *in vitro* and protozoan systems as possible replacements (cf. Nardone and Bradlaw, 1983).

(*a*) Refinements to the classical Draize eye irritancy test. The test modifications which have been proposed include the use of smaller volumes (Griffith *et al.*, 1980), which would reduce the severity of the reaction as well as permitting the investigator to develop dose–response curves, the use of local anaesthetics (Falahee *et al.*, 1981), an exfoliative cytology test which is reportedly more sensitive and more easily quantified than the classic Draize eye irritancy test (Walberg, 1983), and the identification of all severe dermal irritants as eye irritants without further testing. Griffith and his colleagues have argued, with some justification, that the use of a single 100 µl aliquot for eye irritation testing is inappropriate. They suggest that a 10 µl aliquot (and higher multiples) is retained in the eye better and that dose–response curves can be developed if necessary (Griffith *et al.*, 1980). In most cases, the use of smaller quantities of material being placed in the eye will result in less irritation and, therefore, less animal distress.

In recent years, there have been several investigations of the use of local anaesthetics in the eye during ophthalmic testing as a means of reducing animal suffering. Ulsamer *et al.* (1977) have reported that butacaine sulphate provided adequate anaesthesia without notably affecting the irritancy scores. Hoheise (personal communication, 1984) indicates that a double dose of tetracaine (separated by 10 minutes) is more effective in abolishing pain and interferes less with the irritant response, although Walberg disputes this (Walberg, 1983). Johnson (1980) reports that amethocaine HCl is also effective. In a trial of 31 substances, the anaesthetic either had no effect, or produced an increase in the irritant response and did not, therefore, mask irritancy.

Walberg (1983) has developed a very promising modification to the Draize eye irritancy test which is less stressful to the animal, more sensitive and more easily quantified. The eye is exposed to the test substances and then, at standard intervals after the exposure, exfoliated cells are retrieved from the conjunctival sac via a distilled water rinse. The number of cells retrieved is a very sensitive index of irritancy and correlates well with published Draize eye irritancy test scores. The approach needs further validation but appears to be promising as a more sensitive and more objective approach to eye irritancy testing. The greater sensitivity of the exfoliative cytology test also means that smaller or more dilute doses of irritant substances could be used, thereby causing less trauma and distress.

It has also been suggested that a rapid and simple approach to the elimination of most severe irritants from eye testing, and to reduce the number of rabbits required, would be to pre-test materials for primary skin irritation or other properties. However, Williams (1984) reports that of 60 materials that were found to be severe primary skin irritants or corrosive to the skin and that had also been tested for primary eye irritancy, only 34 were also severe eye irritants. Fifteen of the 60 were only mildly irritating or non-irritants in the eye test. Williams cautions, therefore, that it may be misleading to classify a substance as an eye irritant solely on the basis of dermal irritancy. He suggests that the 24-hour occlusion method used in skin testing may well overwhelm physiological defence mechanisms. The lack of correlation between dermal and ophthalmic scores may be due to overestimation of the dermal response by current test procedures. With regard to other properties such as pH, substances with a pH of 12 or more are usually regarded as eye irritants. However, Murphy *et al.* (1982) cautions that there is no simple rule for predicting irritancy from the pH. Acetic acid (5 per cent), with a pH of 2.7, produces substantial corneal opacity while 0.3 per cent hydrochloric acid (pH of 1.3) causes no corneal opacity. At the other end of the scale, 2.5 per cent ammonium hydroxide (pH 11.8) produced corneal opacity while 0.3 per cent sodium hydroxide (pH 12.8) did not. Nevertheless, Walz (1984) reports a clear relation between irritation (oedematous reaction after intracutaneous injection) and pH in a mouse skin test of tissue compatible buffers. Buffers with a pH of below 3 and above 11.5 caused irritation. The boundary for the alkalis was very sharp.

(*b*) Replacement methods for the classical Draize eye irritancy test. A wide range of *in vitro* and protozoan systems have been proposed as possible alternatives (at least as preliminary screens) for the Draize eye irritancy test. Nardone and Bradlaw (1983) have already reviewed many of these including the use of the enucleated eyes (rabbit), human or rabbit cornea cell cultures, other types of cell culture, and the chorioallantois of chick embryos. Some of the first attempts to devise a specific alternative to the Draize eye irritancy test were undertaken in Britain using mouse (Simons, 1980) or human buccal cavity mucosa cells (Bell *et al.*, 1979). The authors of both reports indicated that the *in vitro* approach showed promise but that much more work would be needed to develop and validate an adequate test system. While there have been a spate of recent research reports (Carter *et al.*, 1973; Burton *et al.*, 1981; McCormack, 1981; North-Root *et al.*, 1982; Scaife, 1982; Chan and Haschke, 1983; Douglas and Spilman, 1983; Leighton *et al.*, 1983; Muir *et al.*, 1983; Silverman, 1983; Borenfreund and Borrero, 1984; Muir, 1984; Shopsis and Sathe, 1984) from investigators seeking an alternative to the Draize eye irritancy test, there is still no clear indication of which approach, or approaches, might be the most effective.

Cytotoxicity and cell morphology studies appear to be the favoured approach but few of the studies have gone beyond a characterization of the *in vitro* system. Douglas and Spilman chose to develop a human ocular cell culture as an *in vitro* assay since it would retain species-specific and organ-specific characteristics (Douglas and Spilman, 1983). They chose corneal tissue since corneal damage is the most heavily weighted in scoring damage in the Draize eye irritancy test. They further required that the test system should be practical for routine use and that the assay be based on cell perturbations which are relevant to *in vivo* irritation (e.g. ^{51}Cr release, LDH release, uptake of A1B (a non-metabolized amino acid), and rhodamine uptake (as an index of mitochondrial function)). Although the preliminary results from ^{51}Cr release were promising, the project was, unfortunately, not completed.

While Douglas and others have favoured the idea of using corneal cells to match, as far as it is possible, organ-specific characteristics, Borenfreund and Borrero (1984) report that cells from different organs and species appear to give very similar results, indicating that it may not be that important to match cell culture type with the target organ. The results of Borenfreund's cytotoxicity and morphology assay indicate reasonable correlation with Draize eye irritancy test scores and also with another possible alternative based on a cellular uridine-transport assay developed in the same laboratory (Shopsis and Sathe, 1984).

Another approach has involved the use of whole enucleated rabbit (Burton *et al.*, 1981) or bovine (Carter *et al.*, 1973) eyes. Burton *et al.* (1981) report that the enucleated eyes remain viable for at least four hours and that there is good correlation of the results from this system (using a measurement of corneal swelling) with *in vivo* eye irritancy. However, although these whole eye systems may be useful as predictors of human eye irritation, Douglas and Spilman (1983) argue that such systems are poorly suited to the screening of a large number of compounds or of many replicate samples.

It has been suggested that cell culture systems are not well suited to predicting how fast the eye might recover from the toxic insult. However, Chan and Haschke (1983) are working with a corneal cell culture system which might be used to predict recovery from injury and Jumblatt and Neufeldt (1983) have described a cell culture model for wound closure studies.

Two other *in vitro* models using the chick chorioallantoic membrane (Leighton *et al*, 1983) and excised guinea-pig ileum (Muir *et al.*, 1983; Muir, 1984) have also been reported recently. Leighton *et al.*, (1983) are developing the chorioallantoic membrane (CAM) from the chick embryo as a non-sentient but intact organ which could be used to evaluate irritation and inflammation. The initial reports are based on tests conducted with fairly strong acid and alkali solutions and measurement of the size of the resultant lesion. This is an end-point which requires refinement. There have also been problems from background irritation caused by shell fragments falling on the CAM when the aperture is cut. Nevertheless, the CAM system could be a very promising model for modelling inflammatory responses provided a simple but elegant end-point can be developed.

Many new model systems have been investigated in the past few years and some already show considerable promise as improvements on the Draize eye irritancy test or as the basis for rapid screening systems. However, at the present time, none of the *in vitro* systems have yet been sufficiently validated or evaluated to be considered as replacements to the classical or modified Draize eye irritancy test.

6.2.1.3   *Dermal toxicity testing*

Some of the same approaches applied to the search for alternatives to ophthalmic irritancy testing would probably be successful for dermal irritancy testing. There are difficulties in extrapolating from animal to humans, for example (Kligman 1982; Marks 1983). However, very little research into possible *in vitro* systems for identifying skin irritants has, so far, been undertaken. There have been isolated reports of the use of *in vitro* skin cultures to study toxic reactions or mechanisms (cf. Fouts, 1982; Imokawa and Okamoto, 1983; Kao *et al.*, 1983) but there has been no concerted programme to seek an *in vitro* screening test for irritancy and cutaneous toxicity. Another area of dermal toxicity is phototoxicity which is now routinely evaluated in animals. Several alternative methods have been investigated (Weinberg and Springer, 1981; Morrison *et al.*, 1982; McAuliffe *et al.*, 1983; Tenenbaum *et al.*, 1984) but are still at a relatively early stage of development. More information on dermal toxicity is presented elsewhere in this volume.

6.2.1.4   *Other organs*

One area of acute toxicity where alternative methods may be expected to contribute to our understanding of potential chemical insult concerns the acute reactions of isolated organs or cell cultures to large doses such as might occur during unintentional exposures. The setting of public emergency limits and the development of appropriate therapies for acute poisoning cases could find data derived from *in vitro* organotypic systems to be invaluable. Little attention has been paid to this area of acute organ toxicity.

6.2.2   Chronic toxicity testing

In chronic toxicity testing where the investigator is assessing the likelihood for both targeted (e.g. carcinogenicity) and non-targeted (e.g. disorder in lipid metabolism) effects, we are much more likely to be able to predict human hazards if we understand the mechanism of the toxic insult than if we continue to rely on empirical testing approaches. In the acute toxicity field discussed above, there has been a focused, funded effort to find alternatives following both empirical and mechanistic lines. In chronic toxicity testing, a similar effort is underway to develop short-term tests to identify mutagens, carcinogens and teratogens, but not to investigate organ-specific effects. We will be discussing some of the issues in developing alternatives in chronic toxicity testing, specifically for hepatotoxicity, neurotoxicity and teratogenicity but will not discuss carcinogenicity and mutagenicity. Other chapters in this volume will discuss specific organ systems.

6.3   CONCLUSION

This brief review of alternative approaches to acute toxicity tests and eye irritancy testing provides an introduction to some new conceptual approaches to toxicology testing. A simple empirical search for *in vitro* tests that correlate with various toxic endpoints will not only be insufficient, it will be detrimental. The possibility of developing superior methods for safety evaluation is much more likely to be realized if mechanistic approaches are used when investigating *in vitro* tests. For cell cultures, both animal and human, to be used to their full potential, the culture techniques must be considerably improved. Fully defined growth media must be developed which will support the growth of a wide range of defined cells. It is now possible to maintain and grow many different types of cells which express differentiated function *in vitro*. For example, changing culture conditions allowed one group of investigators to establish a thyroid cell line which expressed differentiated thyroid cell characteristics even after three years of continuous culture (Ambesi-Impiombata *et al.*, 1980). Also, beating heart cells can be maintained for a week in good condition and have been used to investigate anaesthetic (Miletich *et al.*, 1983) and isoproterenol (Ramos *et al.*, 1983) cardiotoxicity.

Computer-assisted structure–activity relationships in toxicology have not yet been developed. As toxicology data bases and our understanding of mechanisms improve, so will the potential applicability of quantitative structure–toxicity relationships (Craig, 1983; Golberg, 1983; Wold *et al.*, 1983).

With the exciting advances now taking place in the disciplines that contribute to toxicology (e.g. molecular biology, cell biology), the time is opportune for academic, industrial and regulatory toxicologists to explore new avenues for safety evaluation. This will mean discarding tests which no longer do what they are meant to and developing new ones which provide better assessments of potential human hazards.

REFERENCES

Ambesi-Impiombata, F.S., Parks, L.A.M. and Coon, H.G. (1980). Culture of hormone-dependent functional epithelial cells from rat thyroids. *Proc. Nat. Acad. Sci.*, **77**, 3455–9.

Autian, J. and Dillingham, E.O. (1978). Overview of general toxicity testing with emphasis on special tissue culture tests. In: Berky, J. and Sherrod, C. (Eds), *In Vitro Toxicity Testing 1975–1976*, Franklin Institute Press, Philadelphia, pp. 23–49.

Balls, M. and Bridges, J.W. (1984). The FRAME research program on *in vitro* cytotoxicology. In: Goldberg, A.M. (Ed.), *Acute Toxicity Testing: Alternative Approaches*, Mary Ann Liebert, New York, pp. 61–79.

Barile, M.F. and Hardegree, M. (1970). A cell culture assay to evaluate the toxicity of Arlacel. *Proc. Soc. Exp. Biol. Med.*, **133**, 222–8.

Barnes, D. and Sato, G. (1980). Serum-free culture: a unifying approach. *Cell*, **22**, 649–55.

Bass, R., Gunzel, P., Henschler, D., Konig, J., Lorke, D., Neuberg, D., Schutz, E., Schuppan, D. and Zbinden, G. (1982). LD50 versus acute toxicity: critical assessment of the methodology currently in use. *Arch. Toxicol.*, **51**, 183–6.

Bell, M., Holmes, P.M., Nisbet, T.M., Uttley, M. and Van Abbe, N.J. (1979). Evaluating the potential eye irritancy of shampoos. *Int. J. Cosmet. Sci.*, **1**, 123–31.

Berky, J. and Sherrod, C. (Eds) (1978). *In Vitro Toxicity Testing 1975–1976*, Franklin Institute Press, Philadelphia.

Borenfreund, E. and Borrero, O. (1984). *In vitro* cytotoxicity assays: Potential alternatives to the Draize occular irritancy test. *Cell Biol. Toxicol.*, **1**, 33–9.

Bruce, R.D. (1985). An up and down procedure for acute toxicity testing. *Fundam. Appl. Toxicol.*, **5**, 151–7.

Burton, A.B.G., York, M. and Lawrence, R.S. (1981). The *in vitro* assessment of severe eye irritants. *Fd. Cosmet Toxicol.*, **19**, 471–80.

Carter, L.M., Duncan, G. and Rennie, G.K. (1973). Effects of detergents on the ionic balance and permeability of isolated bovine cornea. *Exp. Eye Res.*, **17**, 409–16.

Chan, K.Y. and Haschke, R.II. (1983). Epithelial-stromal interactions: Specific stimulation of corneal epithelial cell growth *in vitro* by a factor(s) from cultured stromal fibroblasts. *Exp. Eye. Res.*, **36**, 231–46.

Craig, P.N. (1983). Mathematical models for toxicity evaluation. *Ann. Rep. Med. Chem.*, **18**, 303–6.

Dawson, M. (1972). *Cellular Pharmacology*, Charles Thomas, Springfield, Maryland.

Deichmann, W.B. and LeBlanc, T.J. (1943). Determination of the approximate lethal dose with about six animals. *J. Ind. Hyg. Toxicol.*, **25**, 415–17.

Deutsche Pharmakologische Gesellschaft, Toxicology Symposium (1980). Isolated cell systems as a tool in toxicology research. *Arch. Toxicol.*, **44**, 1–210.

Dixon, W.J. and Mood, A.M. (1948). A method of obtaining and analyzing sensitivity data. *J. Am. Stat. Assoc.*, **43**, 109–26.

Douglas, W.H.J. and Spilman, S.D. (1983). *In vitro* ocular irritancy testing. In: Goldberg, A.M. (Ed.), *Product Safety Evaluation*, Mary Ann Liebert, New York, pp. 205–30.

Draize, J.H., Woodard, G. and Clavery, H.O. (1944). Methods for the study of irritation and toxicity of substances applied topically to the skin and mucous membranes. *J. Pharmacol. Exp. Ther.*, **82**, 377–90.

Efron, E. (1984). *The Apocalyptics: Politics, Science and the Big Cancer Lie*, Simon & Schuster, New York.

Ekwall, B. (1980). Screening of toxic compounds in tissue culture. *Toxicol.*, **17**, 127–142.

Ekwall, B. (1983). Screening of toxic compounds in mammalian cell cultures. In: Williams, G.M., Dunkel, V. and Ray, V.A. (Eds), *Cellular Systems for Toxicity Testing, Ann. N.Y. Acad. Sci.*, **407**, 64–77.

Enslein, K. and Craig, P.N. (1978). A toxicity prediction system. *J. Environ. Toxicol.*, **2**, 115–21.

Enslein, K., Lander, T.R., Tomb, M.E. and Craig, P.N. (1983). A predictive model for ·estimating rat oral LD50 values. *Benchmark Papers in Toxicology*, volume 1, Princeton Scientific Publishers, Princeton.

Falahee, K.J., Rose, C., Olin, S.S. and Siefried, H.E. (1981). *Eye Irritation testing: An assessment of methods and guidelines for testing materials for eye irritancy*, Office of Pesticides and Toxic Substances, US Environment Protection Agency (EPA-560/11-82-001), Washington, D.C.

Food and Drug Administration (1984). Final Report on Acute Studies Workshop, February 23, Washington, Office of Science Co-ordination, U.S. Food and Drug Administration.

Fouts, J.R. (1982). The metabolism of xenobiotics by isolated pulmonary and skin cells. *Trends in Pharmac. Sci.*, **3**, 164–6.

Friedenwald, J.S., Hughes, W.F. and Herrmann, H. (1944). Acid-base tolerance of the cornea. *Arch. Ophthalmol.*, **31**, 279–83.

Fry, J.R. and Bridges, J.W. (1977). The metabolism of xenobiotics in cell suspension and cell culture. In: Bridges, J.W. and Chausseaud, L.F. (Eds), *Progress in Drug Metabolism*, volume 2, John Wiley & Sons, London, pp. 71–118.

Golberg, L. (Ed.) (1983). *Structure-Activity Correlation As a Predictive Tool in Toxicology: Fundamentals, Methods and Applications*, Hemisphere Publishing Corporation, Washington, D.C., 330 p.

Goldberg, A.M. (1984a). Approaches to the development of *in vitro* toxicological methods. *Pharmacol. Rev.*, **36**, 173S–5S.

Goldberg, A.M. (Ed.) (1984b). Acute Toxicity Testing: Alternative Approaches, *Alternative Methods in Toxicology*, volume 2, Mary Ann Liebert, New York.

Griffith, J.F., Nixon, G.A., Bruce, R.D., Reer, P.J. and Bannan, E.A. (1980). Dose–response studies with chemical irritants in the albino rabbit eye as a basis for selecting optimum testing conditions for predicting hazard to the human eye. *Toxicol. Appl. Pharmacol.*, **55**, 501–13.

Grisham, J.W. and Smith, G.J. (1984). Predictive and mechanistic evaluation of toxic responses in mammalian cell culture systems. *Pharmacol. Rev.*, **36**, 151S–75S.

Heywood, R. (1978). Animal studies in drug safety evaluation. *J. Roy. Soc. Med.*, **71**, 686–9.

Hunter, W.J., Lingk, W. and Rekcht, P. (1978). Intercomparison study on the determination of single administration toxicity in rats. *J. Assoc. Off. Anal. Chem.*, **62**, 864–73.

Imokawa, G. and Okamoto, K. (1983). The effect of zinc pyrithione on human skill cells *in vitro. J. Soc. Cosmet. Chem.*, **34**, 1–11.

Johnson, A.W. (1980). Use of small dosage and corneal anaesthetic for eye testing *in vivo*. In: *Proceedings of the CTFA Ocular Safety Testing Workshop: In Vivo and In Vitro Approaches*, Oct. 6 and 7, Cosmetic, Toiletry and Fragrance Foundation, Washington.

Jumblatt, M.M. and Neufeldt, A.H. (1983). Corneal epithelial wound closure: a tissue culture model. *Invest. Ophthalmol. Vision Sci.*, **24 (Suppl.)**, 44.

Kao, J., Hall, J. and Holland, J.M. (1983). Quantitation of cutaneous toxicity: an *in vitro* approach using skin organ culture. *Toxicol. Appl. Pharmacol.*, **68**, 206–17.

Kligman, A.M. (1982). Assessment of mild irritants. In: Frost, P. and S.N. Horwitz (Eds), *Principles of Cosmetics for the Dermatologist*, Mosby, St. Louis, pp. 265–73.

Leighton, J., Nassauer, J., Tchao, R. and Verdone, J. (1983). Development of a procedure using the chick egg as an alternative to the Draize rabbit test. In: Goldberg, A.M. (Ed), *Product Safety Evaluation*, Mary Ann Liebert, New York, pp. 163–77.

Lorke, D. (1983). A new approach to practical acute toxicity testing. *Arch. Toxicol.*, **54**, 275–87.

Marks, R. (1983). Testing for cutaneous toxicity. In: Balls, R.J., Riddell, A.N. and Worden (Eds), *Animals and Alternatives in Toxicity Testing*, Academic Press, London, pp. 313–27.

Maugh, T.M. (1978). Chemicals: How many are there? *Science*, **199**, 162.

McAuliffe, D.J., Morrison, W.L. and Parrish, J.A. (1983). An *in vitro* test for predicting the photosensitizing potential of various chemicals. In: Goldberg, A.M. (Ed.), *Product Safety Evaluation*, Mary Ann Liebert, New York, pp. 285–307.

McCormack, J. (1981). A procedure for the *in vitro* evaluation of the eye irritation potential of surfactants. In: *Trends in Bioassay Methodology: In Vivo, In Vitro and Mathematical Approaches*, National Institutes of Health (NIH Publ. No. 82–2382), Washington, D.C., pp. 177–86.

Melmon, K.L. (1976). The clinical pharmacologist and scientifically unsound regulations for drug development. *Clin. Pharmacol. Ther.*, **20**, 125–9.

Miletich, D.J., Khan, A., Albrecht, R.F. and Jozefiak, A. (1983). Use of heart cell cultures as a tool for the evaluation of halothane arrhythmia. *Toxicol. Appl. Pharmacol.*, **70**, 181–7.

Morrison, J.K., Quinton, R.M. and Reinert, M. (1968). The purpose and value of LD50 determination. In: Boyland, E. and Goulding, R. (Eds), *Modern Trends in Toxicology*, volume 1, John Wiley & Sons, Chichester, pp. 1–17.

Morrison, W.L., McAuliffe, D.J., Parrish, J.A. and Bloch, K.B. (1982). *In vitro* assay for phototoxic chemicals. *J. Invest. Dermatol.*, **78**, 460–463.

Muir, C.K. (1984). Further investigations on the Ileum model as a possible alternative to *in vivo* eye irritancy testing. *ATLA*, **II**, 129–34.

Muir, C.K., Flower, C. and Van Abbe, N.J. (1983). A novel approach to the search for *in vitro* alternatives to *in vivo* eye irritancy testing. *Toxicol. Lett.*, **18**, 1–5.

Muller, H. and Kley, H.P. (1982). Retrospective study of the reliability of an 'approximate LD50' determined with a small number of animals. *Arch. Toxicol.*, **51**, 189–96.

Murphy, J.C., Osterberg, R.E., Seabaugh, V.M. and Bierbower, G.W. (1982). Ocular irritancy responses to various pH's of acids and bases with and without irritation. *Toxicol.*, **23**, 281–91.

Muul, I., Hegyeli, A.F., Dacre, J.C. and Woodard, G. (1976). Toxicological testing dilemma. *Science*, **193**, 834.

Nardone, R.M. (1977). Toxicity testing *in vitro*. In: Rothblatt, R.M. and Cristofala, V.J. (Eds), *Growth, Nutrition and Metabolism of Cells in Culture*, volume 3, Academic Press, New York, pp. 471–96.

Nardone, R.M. and Bradlaw, J.A. (1983). Toxicity testing with *in vitro* systems: I. Ocular tissue culture. *J. Toxicol.-Cut. Ocular Toxicol.*, **2**, 81–98.

National Research Council (1984). *Toxicity Testing: Strategies to Determine Needs and Priorities*, Washington, D.C., National Academy of Sciences.

North-Root, H., Yackovitch, F., Demetrulias, J., Gracula, M. and Heinze, J.E. (1982). Evaluation of an *in vitro* cell toxicity test using rabbit corneal cells to predict the eye irritation potential of surfactants. *Toxicol. Letts.*, **14**, 207–12.

Pomerat, C.M. and Leake, D.C. (1954). Short-term cultures for drug assay. *Ann. N.Y. Acad. Sci.*, **53**, 1110–28.

Ramos, K., Combs, A.B. and Acosta, D. (1983). Cytotoxity of isoproterenol to cultured heart cells: Effects of antioxidants on modifying membrane damage. *Toxicol. Appl. Pharmacol.*, **70**, 317–23.

Rekker, R.F. (1980). LD50 values: Are they about to become predictable? *Trends Pharmac. Sci.*, **1**, 383–4.

Rofe, P.C. (1971). Tissue culture and toxicology, *Fd. Cosmet. Toxicol.*, **9**, 683–96.

Rowan, A.N. (1981). The Draize Test: Political and scientific issues. *Cosmetic Technol.*, **3**(7), 32–7.

Rowan, A.N. (1983). Shortcomings of LD50 values and acute toxicity testing in animals. *Acta Phamacol. Toxicol.*, **52 (Suppl. 2)**, 52–64.

Rowan, A.N. (1984). *Of Mice, Models and Men: A Critical Analysis of Animal Research*, State University of New York Press, Albany, New York.

Sako, F. (1977). Effects of food dyes on *Paramecium caudatum:* Toxicity and inhibitory effects on leucine aminopeptidase and acid phosphatase activity. *Toxicol. Appl. Pharmacol.*, **39**, 111–17.

Scaife, M.C. (1982). An investigation of detergent action on cells *in vitro* and possible correlations with *in vivo* data. *Int. J. Cosmet. Sci.*, **4**, 179–83.

Schutz, E. and Fuchs, H. (1982). A new approach to minimizing the numbers of animals used in acute toxicity testing and optimizing the information of test results. *Arch. Toxicol.*, **51**, 197–200.

Shopsis, C. and Sathe, S. (1984). Uridine uptake inhibition as a cytotoxicity test: Correlations with the Draize test. *Toxicol.*, **29**, 195–206.

Silverman, J. (1983). Preliminary findings on the use of protozoa *(Tetrahymena thermophila)* as models for ocular irritation testing in rabbits. *Lab. Animal Sci.*, **33**, 56–9.

Simons, P.J. (1980). An alternative to the Draize tests. In: Rowan, A.N. and Stratmann, C.J. (Eds), *The Use of Alternatives in Drug Research*, Macmillan, London, pp. 147–51.

Smyth, D.H. (1978). *Alternatives to Animal Experiments*, Scolar Press, London, p. 68.

Stammati, A.P., Silano, V. and Zucco, F. (1981). Toxicology investigations with cell culture systems. *Toxicol.*, **20**, 91–153.

Stevenson, D.E. (1979). Current problems in the choice of animals for toxicity testing. *J. Toxicol. Environ. Health*, **5**, 9–15.

Tardiff, R.G. (1978). *In vitro* methods of toxicity evaluation. *Ann. Rev. Pharmacol. Toxicol.*, **18**, 357–69.

Tattersall, M.L. (1982). Statistics and the LD50 study. *Arch. toxicol., Suppl.*, **5**, 267–70.

Tenenbaum, S., DiNardo, J., Morris, W.E., Wolf, B.A. and Schnetzinger, R.W. (1984). A quantitative *in vitro* assay for the evaluation of phototoxic potential of topically applied materials. *Cell. Biol. Toxicol.*, **1**, 1–9.

Trevan, J.W. (1927). The error of determination of toxicity. *Proc. Roy. Soc. Lond. B.*, **101**, 483–514.

Ulsamer, A.G., Wright, P.L. and Osterberg, R.E. (1977). A comparison of the effects of model irritants on anaesthetized and non-anaesthetized rabbit eyes. *Society of Toxicology*, 16th Annual Meeting, Abs. 143.

Veberla, K. and Schnieders, B. (1982). In reference to the paper by Bass *et al.*, *Arch. Toxicol.*, **51**, 187.

Walberg, J. (1983). Exfoliative cytology as a refinement of the Draize eye irritancy test. *Toxicol. Letts.*, **18**, 49–55.

Walz, D. (1984). Towards an animal-free assessment of topical irritancy. *Trends Pharmac. Sci.*, **5**, 221–4.

Weil, C.S. and Scala, R.A. (1971). Study of intra- and inter-laboratory variability in the results of rabbit eye and skin irritation test. *Toxicol. Appl. Pharmacol.*, **19**, 276–360.

Weinberg, E.H. and Springer, S.T. (1981). The evaluation *in vitro* of fragrance materials for phototoxic activity. *J. Soc. Cosmet. Chem.*, **32**, 303–15.

Williams, S.J. (1984). Prediction of ocular irritancy potential from dermal irritation test results. *Fd. Chem. Toxicol.*, **22**, 157–61.

Wold, S., Hellberg, S. and Dunn, W.J. (1983). Computer methods for the assessment of toxicity. *Acta Pharmacol. Toxicol.*, **52 (Suppl. 2)**, 158–89.

Worden, A.N. (1974). Tissue culture. In: Boyland, E. and Goulding, R. (Eds), *Modern Trends in Toxicology*, volume 2, Butterworths, London, pp. 216–49.

Zbinden, G. (1976). A look at the world from inside the toxicologist's cage. *Eur. J. Clin. Pharmacol.*, **9**, 33–8.

Zbinden, G. and Flury-Roversi, M. (1981). Significance of the LD50 test for the toxicological evaluation of chemical substances. *Arch. Toxicol.*, **47**, 77–99.

Zucco, F. and Hooisma, J. (Eds) (1982). Proceedings of the Second International Workshop on the Application of Tissue Culture in Toxicology. *Toxicol.*, **25**, 1–74.

Short-term Toxicity Tests for Non-genotoxic Effects
Edited by P. Bourdeau *et al.*
© 1990 SCOPE. Published by John Wiley & Sons Ltd

CHAPTER 7

Toxicity Tests with Mammalian Cell Cultures

B. Ekwall, V. Silano, A. Paganuzzi-Stammati and F. Zucco

7.1   INTRODUCTION

Cell culture can be used to screen for toxicity both by estimation of the basal functions of the cell (i.e. those processes common to all types of cells) or by tests on specialized cell functions (Ekwall, 1983b). General toxicity tests, aimed mainly at detection of the biological activity of test substances, can be carried out on many cell types (e.g. fibroblasts, HeLa and hepatoma cells). A number of parameters including vital staining, cytosolic enzyme release, cell growth and cloning efficiency are used as end-points to measure toxicity. Organ-specific toxic effects are tested using specialized cells by measuring alterations in membrane and metabolism integrity and/or in specific cell functions (e.g. glycogen metabolism in primary hepatocyte cultures, beating rate in mixed myocardial cells or myocytes, and phagocytosis in macrophages).

Major problems in the interpretation of results obtained *in vitro* to identify cell-specific effects are as follows:

(1)   Since basal cell functions always support specific cell functions, chemicals that are capable of affecting basal cell functions are also likely to affect the specialized ones;

(2)   The effects of a test substance on a cell system may be different depending on the conditions of incubation (e.g. incubation time and concentration of toxicant). Therefore, unless a set of favourable circumstances occurs and a well-planned experimental design is adhered to, it may prove difficult to distinguish between basal and organ-specific effects.

Cytotoxicity tests using specialized cells have proved most useful when the *in vivo* toxicity of a chemical is already well established and where *in vitro* investigations using specialized cell cultures have been used to clarify the mechanisms of toxic action on the target tissue. These tests have also provided useful insight into the pathogeneses of some human diseases (e.g. for liver diseases, see Klaassen and Stacey, 1982, and for coeliac disease, see Auricchio *et al.*, 1985).

75

The assessment of the significance of the results of *in vitro* tests in relation to the *in vivo* situation presents another major problem. Much can be learned from past experience with drugs which indicates that intrinsic cell sensitivity is only one factor, and not necessarily the most important, in determining specificity of toxic action of chemicals. Other factors, more directly related to chemical kinetics such as rates of absorption, biotransformation, distribution and excretion, which influence the exposure at the level of target cells *in vivo* cannot, at present, be adequately simulated *in vitro*. Furthermore, even when the appropriate cell type is used, intrinsic cell sensitivity depends on a number of cell characteristics which are likely to be preserved only in part *in vitro*; these include chemical biotransformation and binding, membrane permeability characteristics and surface determinants, intracellular synthetic pathways and adaptive and recovery mechanisms. For some toxic chemicals, it is the functional status of the cell rather than the cell type that determines the extent to which the inhibition of a given biochemical mechanism is critical to the function and survival of the cell.

For a more detailed discussion of cytological and biochemical differences responsible for selective toxicity of chemicals, the textbooks by Albert (1979) and Schwartz and Mihic (1973) can be consulted. Some anti-cancer drugs will be discussed here to illustrate the biological base for selective toxicity and some uses and limitations of *in vitro* cytotoxicity testing. Cancer cells are normally highly-specialized cells which have regressed to a much simpler, more primitive stage and which, unlike the normal parent, divide continuously, although inefficiently. Because a much higher proportion of cancer cells are undergoing active division, they are more vulnerable than most normal cells to anti-cancer drugs. However, normal tissues with high mitotic indices (e.g. bone marrow, spleen, thymus and intestinal epithelium) are also more susceptible to anti-cancer drugs. Both in normal and in neoplastic proliferating tissues, the toxicity of many of these drugs appears to be related to effects on the mitotic spindle and replicating DNA. Chemicals capable of a direct attack on the microtubules or the mitotic spindle (e.g. colchicine or the vinca alkaloids) are selective for proliferating cells, but only rarely are they more selective for tumour tissues. The selective toxicity on tumours observed for some of the chemotherapeutic agents, depends more on pharmacokinetic and metabolic factors in target cells than on the direct proximal action of the agent. The alkylating and intercalating drugs, which act directly at the level of DNA, and the mitotic poisons have been shown to produce a fairly uniform response in mammalian replicating cells, i.e. clumping and fragmentation of the chromatin (Schwartz and Mihic, 1973). Differential cell lethality in the presence of alkylating agents is probably due to differences in repair mechanisms as related to the cell's demand for functional DNA (Alexander, 1969). Thus, a slow rate of repair in rapidly dividing cells will be more critical than the same repair rate in slowly dividing or non-proliferating cells. A number of DNA antimetabolites, co-factor analogs and enzyme inhibitors, which inhibit enzymes involved in the synthesis of DNA or its precursors, cause characteristic lesions in proliferating cells with a scatter of toxicity in non-proliferating ones. In many cases, the selectivity of action of these agents depends mainly on the fact that normal proliferating tissues have distinctive physiological or biochemical characteristics that affect drug actions (Schwartz and Mihic, 1973).

For the sake of completeness, it should be mentioned that, in addition to cytotoxicity testing, cell culture systems are also useful to carry out metabolism studies including biotransformation, interaction with endogenous metabolites, binding to cells, and induction of metabolism.

This chapter is an overview of the present state of the art of *in vitro* testing of cell toxicity of chemicals. Available cell culture systems and methodologies are discussed in the light of present experimental trends. Furthermore, the significance of cell systems as alternatives to whole animal systems for predicting toxic potential of chemicals with respect to selected end-points and for selecting priority among existing chemicals are examined together with possible future developments.

7.2 CELL CULTURE SYSTEMS AND METHODS

The growing use of *in vitro* systems in biomedical research has accentuated the need for standardization and clarification of the terms more frequently used by researchers working in this field. In 1964, a Terminology Committee of the Tissue Culture Association was set up in order to recommend a generally acceptable terminology. The final report of the Committee was accepted at the annual meeting of the Tissue Culture Association in 1966 (Fedoroff, 1966). This nomenclature was subsequently revised in 1984 (Schaeffer, 1984). Primary cell cultures, cell lines and cell strains have been defined as follows:

- A primary cell culture is 'a culture started from cells, tissues or organs taken directly from organisms. A primary culture may be regarded as such until it is successfully subcultured for the first time. It then becomes a cell line'.
- A cell line 'arises from a primary culture at the time of the first successful subculture. The term, cell line, implies that cultures from it consist of numerous lineages of cells originally present in the primary culture. The terms, finite, or continuous, are used as prefixes if the status of the culture is known. If not, the term line will suffice'.
- A cell strain 'derives either from a primary culture or a cell line by the selection or cloning of cells having specific properties or markers. The properties or markers must persist during subsequent cultivation'.

Cell lines may be finite or continuous. A finite cell line is generally diploid and, in this case, no less than 75 per cent of all the cells must be of the same standard karyotype as the parent species; its lifespan is approximately 40–50 divisions (Fedoroff, 1966; Hayflick and Moorhead, 1961). A continuous cell line derives from primary cultures or diploid cell lines by transformation processes which are either spontaneous, or induced by viruses, chemical or physical agents (Fedoroff, 1977).

When a cell line derives from a single cell, it is called a clonal cell line. Clonal cell lines can be obtained by several techniques, starting from primary cultures, diploid cell lines or established cell lines. They are not necessarily homogeneous populations and only frequent cloning can keep culture heterogeneity to a minimum.

Available cell lines are collected by the American Type Culture Collection which provides a catalogue listing of every cell type with its history and information concerning viability, growth medium, growth characteristics, plating efficiency, age of culture since origin, morphology, karyology, sterility tests and virus susceptibility.

Primary cell cultures have morphological and biochemical characteristics that are more similar to those of the original tissue; however, problems with obtaining reproducible results may negate these advantages. Nevertheless, primary cultures offer the only possibility for comparative studies of some specialized tissues taken from different animal species where cell lines and strains from the same tissues are not available. Primary cultures are generally more sensitive to the effects of toxic chemicals than are cell lines because, while exposed, they have also to adapt to culture conditions. The main limitations of primary cultures are low homogeneity and a tendency to rapid loss of specialization under culture conditions. Cell lines offer the advantage of being more homogeneous and standardized than primary cultures. They are well characterized, easy to cultivate and reproducible results are easier to obtain. On the other hand, they may be quite different from the original tissue due to the fact that established cell lines have undergone a number of transformations.

Cell strains have the advantage of being more homogeneous populations from the point of view of selected characteristics, but they present the same disadvantages as cell lines from which they derive.

Compared with cells from normal adult tissues, embryo and tumour cells are more easily cultured because they have a higher growth capability and adapt more readily to variations in external factors. The setting up of primary cell cultures and, to a larger extent, of continuous cell lines imply some loss of differentiation, but there are many cell types that display highly specialized biological activities *in vitro* that are characteristic of their original tissues or organs (Sato and Yasumura, 1966). Some examples were reported in the review of Paganuzzi-Stammati *et al.* (1981). A growing number of cell types have been shown more recently to retain some specialized functions in culture. Some examples include:

(1) Endothelial cells *in vitro* display several specialized functions including a non-thrombogenic surface to platelets, Factor VIII antigen, the surface angiotensin-converting enzyme, and synthesis of fibronectin and collagen (Striker *et al.*, 1980).

(2) Adult cardiac myocytes from different animal species retain several biochemical, morphological and physiological characteristics (Lieberman *et al.*, 1980).

(3) Human epidermal keratinocytes are capable of terminal differentiation in

culture; in particular, they produce keratin and the cells of the upper layer of the colonies lose their ability to divide and develop a cornified cell envelope.

(4) Mouse secondary cultures of Schwann cells are still able to synthesize enzymes typical of myelin-forming cells (White *et al.*, 1983).

Some tumour cell lines can, under some culture conditions, retain a degree of differentiation *in vitro*. Engvall *et al.* (1984) obtained sublines from mouse teratocarcinoma-derived endodermal cell line PF Mr-9, that possess a number of protein markers of the parent cells, for example, the two intermediate filament proteins Endo A and B. They also produce a large amount of laminin and a small amount of fibronectin as well as Type IV collagen and heparan-sulphate proteoglycans.

New and sophisticated *in vitro* techniques are very useful to maintain the specialized functions of cells. Among these is the use of serum-free media consisting of a nutrient basal medium supplemented with hormones and growth factors necessary to the various cell types.

These selective media facilitate adaptation of cells to the culture and allow a better standardization of experimental conditions. Serum is a very complex and poorly characterized mixture, the composition of which may vary according to the commercial batch; some components essential for cell growth may be absent. Serum may contain naturally-occurring substances (Barnes and Sato, 1980b) or microbiological contaminants (e.g. mycoplasma, viruses, endotoxins) that are toxic for certain types of cultures (Higuchi, 1976).

Serum-free media facilitates the isolation of the desired cell type and, in setting up primary cell cultures, they almost completely eliminate the overgrowth of fibroblasts that, usually, grow rapidly in serum-supplemented media. Moreover, these selective media are useful to study interactions of cells with hormones or drugs and to perform cell nutrition studies (Barnes and Sato, 1980a). Examples of the advantages of serum-free (or low serum) media include the establishment of differentiated rat thyroid cells in hormone-supplemented medium containing only very small amounts of serum (Ambesi-Impiombato *et al.*, 1980). Other cell types can also be grown more efficiently and in a more differentiated way in serum-free media. For example, the MC84 5 line forms villus-like secretory structures (Murakami and Masui, 1980), the HLE 222 human lung epidermoid carcinoma cells produce extensive keratinization (Barnes *et al.*, 1980), rat granulosa cells synthetize large amounts of progestins and oestrogens after stimulations by follicle-stimulating hormone (FSH) (Orly *et al.*, 1980); additional examples are reported by Barnes and Sato (1980a).

Much attention has been given to the identification of factors such as hormones, growth factors, binding proteins, attachment and spreading factors, which are essential for the replacement of the various functions carried out by serum. Some (e.g. insulin, transferrin) are common to most cell types whereas others are specific for particular cultures (Barnes and Sato, 1980b). Often the various factors effective for a given cell line have also been shown to be useful for the primary culture from the same tissue (Barnes and Sato, 1980b). Many investigations have been devoted to the development of selective media for primary cultures (Sato *et al.*, 1982).

Cell lines are more widely used for general toxicity studies than primary cell cultures because they are well characterized and more easily cultured. The more commonly used cell lines include diploid human fibroblast lines (e.g. WI-38) and tumour cell lines (e.g. HeLa). When the mechanism of toxicity of a chemical is under investigation and it becomes necessary to take into account specific characteristics of specialized cell types, primary cell cultures of the target organ or tissue are often used in conjunction with cell lines from the same origin.

7.3   *IN VITRO* TESTING OF CELL TOXICITY OF CHEMICALS: METHODOLOGICAL ASPECTS

The first and most readily observed effect following exposure of cells to toxicants is morphological alteration in the cell layer and/or cell shape in monolayer culture. Therefore, it is not surprising that morphological alterations are used as an index of toxicity. A systematic appraisal of cell injury has been attempted to allow a greater standardization of the observations. A checklist suitable for computer-based programmes has been proposed (Walton and Buckley, 1975; Walton, 1975). Different types of toxic effects may require investigative tools of different levels of sensitivity. Gross modifications such as blebbing or vacuolization can be observed using light microscopy (Ekwall, 1983b) whereas fine ultrastructural modifications require analysis by transmission or scanning electron microscopy.

Another indicator of toxicity is altered cell growth. The effect of chemicals on the capability of cells to replicate is used as an index of toxicity; the concentration of the substances at which 50 per cent of the cells do not multiply is called the median inhibitory dose (ID_{50}). A more specific measure of replication is plating efficiency—the ability of cells (100–200 per dish, 60 mm diameter) to form colonies after 10–15 days of culture in the presence of a toxic agent gives more complete information, indicating both cell survival and ability to reproduce (Nardone, 1977). Cell reproduction can be measured by several parameters including cell count, DNA content, protein content, or enzyme activity (e.g. ornithine-decarboxylase; Costa, 1979). Each of these parameters can be measured by more or less sophisticated means. Examples are the assay of DNA content by biochemical methods and incorporation of radiolabelled precursors.

Another crude index of toxicity is cell viability measured by using vital dyes such as trypan blue which enters dead cells only or neutral red that is actively taken up by living cells; the latter is commonly used in biomaterial testing by the agar overlay method (Guess *et al.*, 1965). A count of dead and vital cells in comparison with the control provides an index of lethality of the test compound. The release of ^{51}Cr is another index of lethality measuring membrane functions (Holden *et al.*, 1973).

Other indices of toxicity to basal cell functions involve measurement of biochemical or metabolic cell alterations. The pathways of energy transmission and their alterations, O_2 consumption or ATP levels are usually measured by the Clark electrode (Harmon and Sanborn, 1982; Yoshida *et al.*, 1979) and by the luciferin–luciferase assay respectively (Waters *et al.*, 1975). High pressure liquid chromatography has been used to measure the pool of DNA and RNA precursors whose imbalance is considered an important toxicity indicator (Bianchi *et al.*, 1982; Bianchi, 1982). Acid phosphatase activity has been used as an index of cell damage (Bitensky, 1963). Lactate dehydrogenase activity in the culture medium, usually measured as the NADH–NAD conversion needed to convert pyruvate into lactate (Elferink, 1979; Acosta *et al.*, 1978), has been used as an index of membrane damage.

Cells derived from different organs or tissues, that retain some specialized functions *in vitro* or that maintain specialized structures, have also been widely used in toxicology. For these cells, effects on more specialized functions and/or structures have usually been taken into account in addition to effects on basic ones; specific end-products, metabolic pathways, membrane functions or structures have been tested. A tentative grouping of possible specific end-points used for some cell types is shown in Table 7.1.

Table 7.1   End-points more commonly used as markers of toxic effects in specialized cells*

Synthesis or release of specific molecules
Collagen mat, heme, haemoglobin, albumin, urea, lipoprotein, α-aminolevulinic acid, bile salts, metallothionein, glycosaminoglycans, proline and hydroxyproline, energy-dependent choline accumulation, histamine release and c-AMP.

Synthesis, activity or release of specific enzymes
β-glucuronidase, lactate-dehydrogenase, oubain-insensitive ATPase, G-6-P dehydrogenase, ASAL, glycogen phosphorylase, glutamic-oxalacetic transaminase, glutamic-pyruvic transaminase, acetylcholinesterase, and renin.

Interactions of compound with cells
Phagocytosis, cytoplasmic inclusions, intracellular accumulation, siderosome formation, uptake and/or binding of compound to cytosol and lipoproteins, mitogenic response.

Alterations of metabolic pathways
Methaemoglobin reduction, glucose-transport, 5-methyltetrahydropholate accumulation, hormone-stimulated gluconeogenesis, lipid peroxidation, fat accumulation and glucosamine and galactose incorporation.

Cell surface activities
Adhesiveness, Con-A agglutination, antibody-mediated rosette formation, complement deposition on treated cell membrane, chemotactic migration, antagonism with Histidine-H1 receptor, GABA-mediated postsynaptic inhibition, spike frequency, membrane polarization, fibre retraction or outgrowth, and electrophysiological alteration.

---

* For references see Paganuzzi-Stammati *et al.* (1981).

Because some cell systems do not possess an efficient metabolism (see also Section 7.4), *in vitro* testing may require some form of metabolic activation. This is usually done in one of three ways:

(1)   By the addition of S-9 fraction from rat liver; usually the mixed function oxidases are pre-induced by treating the animals with phenobarbital, β-naphthaflavone or Aroclor (Dolfini *et al.*, 1973);

(2)   By pre-incubation of the test substance with a primary hepatocyte culture and addition of the pre-incubated medium to the test culture (Moldeus *et al.*, 1978).

(3)   By co-culture of the target cell with hepatocytes in the presence of the test substance (Grisham, 1979).

The physicochemical properties of test compounds determine exposure conditions and the concentration of toxic agents in the culture medium. The medium is usually an aqueous saline solution with the addition of serum at concentrations ranging from 2 to 15 per cent. Only hydrophilic test compounds can be completely solubilized. For gaseous toxic agents, special incubation equipment is available to ensure a constant exposure with time provided the partition coefficients and solubilities are known. Similar problems apply to hydrophobic test compounds or mineral particulates. Lipophilic substances can be solubilized in ethanol, methanol or dimethylsulphoxide before addition to the medium; a control using the carrier solvent alone must be used.

In order to increase comparability of results and optimize testing procedures, standardization and harmonization of the experimental approaches and procedures is desirable. The use of well characterized cell lines, possibly of a human origin, is necessary and basic and specific toxicity end-points, as well as the most suitable assay methods, should be agreed upon. Cell cultures should be examined periodically for possible contamination with micro-organisms or for cross-contamination with other mammalian cell types. Periodic checks of the karotype would be appropriate. Reports should provide details of exposure conditions including information on the purity of the test compound. Moreover, the measurement of the concentration of the compound at the beginning and at the end of the experiment (and the reporting of concentrations as 'molarity', whenever possible), would simplify the comparison of results from one laboratory to another.

7.4   PRESENT TRENDS OF TOXICOLOGY INVESTIGATIONS WITH CELL CULTURE SYSTEMS

A literature survey on present trends in toxicology investigations using cell cultures has been published (Paganuzzi-Stammati *et al.*, 1981). These authors identified three major research areas where cell culture systems have proved to be extremely useful: (1) clarification of action mechanisms of toxic substances with specialized cell systems; (2) clarification of the effects on basic cell functions mainly with fibroblasts and epithelioid cells; and (3) in metabolism investigations.

7.4.1 Investigations with specialized cell systems

Several specialized cell types have been used in toxicology investigations. Among the more widely used are cells derived from liver, lung, heart, muscle and nervous and reticuloendothelial systems (Table 7.2). Primary cultures or isolated cells are widely used because the cells retain their specialized functions better.

An examintion of publications since 1981 did not reveal major new trends although some interesting new approaches were noted.

Interaction of xenobiotics with nerve-growth-factor induced fibre outgrowth in nervous cells have been investigated (Nakada *et al.*, 1981). Some studies on the synthesis of prostaglandins (Burstein *et al.*, 1983) and alterations in oxidative response have been recently reported in macrophages (Castranova *et al.*, 1980; Hoidal *et al.*, 1981; Williams and Cole, 1981; Garrett *et al.*, 1981) and more attention has been recently paid to peroxidation and effects on phospholipase in hepatocytes (Stacey and Klaassen, 1981a, 1981b; Stacey *et al.*, 1982; Lamb and Schwartz, 1982). Substances that have been most frequently studied are generally already well known for their systemic effects on specific organs or tissues (e.g. pesticides on nervous systems and liver cells, dusts on macrophages, metals on liver and kidney cells).

7.4.2 Investigations with non-specialized cells

These investigations have been based on fibroblast, epithelioid and other cell lines.

Table 7.2   Specialized cells commonly used in toxicology

Organ of origin	Primary cultures or isolated cells	Cell lines
Nervous system	Chick embryo ganglia; chick embryo brain cells; mouse and rat cerebellum cells	C 1300 (mouse); C 6 (rat)
Lung	Human, rabbit and rat alveoloar macrophages	P 388D1 (mouse); A 549 (human)
Reticuloendothelial system	Human, mouse lymphocytes and erythrocytes; rat and mouse peritoneal macrophages	—
Liver	Rat and chick embryo hepatocytes	Chang (human); CC1144 (rat); ARL (rat); RLC-GA (rat)

The aim has been to study the effects of test substances on structures and functions common to most types of cells, i.e., basal cytotoxicity (Ekwall, 1983b). Substances under investigation mainly have been chemicals subject to registration procedures in many countries such as drugs and pesticides. Effects have been studied by monitoring rather simple parameters such as cell growth or viability on cell lines such as HeLa, CHO, 3T3, WI-38, human skin fibroblasts and BHK. Some of these investigations have been undertaken to validate the use of the cell systems as screening procedures. Such studies will be described in more detail in Section 7.5.

7.4.3   Metabolism investigations

Metabolism has been investigated *in vitro* with systems of different complexity by using, for instance, liver slices, hepatocytes or purified microsomes. Liver slices or hepatocytes have been extensively used in the investigation of metabolic pathways, and in the identification of intermediates or secondary products. A number of investigations have been devoted to the preparation of isolated hepatocytes preserving their metabolic activities. Recently, the very rapid decay of Phase I enzymes in culture systems has been prevented by using special media; monoxygenase levels were kept near to the values *in vivo* for quite a long time (Grisham, 1979). Microsome preparations, first introduced for mutagenicity assays, have also been used as activating systems in cytotoxicity investigations; however, they may themselves contribute some cytotoxic activity (Balls and Bridges, 1983). Although the importance of metabolism in liver cells is well known, cell types derived from other organs or tissues such as lung (Baird *et al.*, 1980; Tell and Douglas, 1980), aorta (Baird *et al.*, 1980) intestine (Schiller and Lucier, 1978), and ovary (Drake *et al.*, 1982) also display metabolic activities which may have a major significance in determining toxicity. Phase I and II metabolic reactions have been studied *in vitro* by co-cultivating human adult hepatocytes and rat liver epithelial cells for several weeks (Begue *et al.*, 1983).

It is well known that metabolism may differ significantly among various animal species (Miller and Miller, 1971; Weisburger *et al.*, 1964; Quinn *et al.*, 1958; Hucker, 1970). For this reason, it is highly desirable to use human cells for metabolism investigations. However, because of difficulties associated with the availability of material and standardization of techniques, only a few papers have been published in this area (Guillouzo *et al.*, 1982; Guguen-Guillouzo *et al.*, 1988).

7.5   CELL SYSTEMS AS ALTERNATIVES TO WHOLE ANIMAL SYSTEMS FOR PREDICTING TOXIC POTENTIALS OF CHEMICALS WITH RESPECT TO SELECTED END-POINTS

The objectives of toxicity tests, whether conducted in the whole animal or in cell systems, must be to predict the adverse effects of the tested compound in human beings both in a qualitative and quantitative way. To this end, both animal and cellular tests try to simulate aspects of the human body. The animal is a more complete model of the human body, which includes basic and specific cell functions as well as almost all human organizational functions (Ekwall, 1983b), including pharmacokinetic determinants. The cell culture is a model of a target tissue in the human body and mimics the response of human cells to exposure to chemicals. Provided that time and degree of exposure (dosage for animals and concentration/ exposure time in cell tests) in the experiments correspond to human exposure, both models can potentially predict any type of chemical interference with corresponding aspects of the human body.

There are interesting differences between whole animal and cellular systems with respect to the different types of toxic action measured. In principle, the whole animal model measures the critical toxicity of a chemical, i.e. the one or two toxic effects that appear first when a dose to an animal is gradually increased. These critical effects often overshadow many other potential toxic effects, which are thus not recorded by the whole animal experiment. Relatively subtle species differences in receptor affinity or metabolic pathways may influence which of the many kinds of potential effects are observed so that whereas animal experiments have the advantage of predicting, in many cases, the critical effects in the human body, they could fail to do so because of species differences. Cell cultures, on the other hand, will only measure potential toxic effects. The critical toxicity for the human body must then be judged by a comparison of tissue culture results with actual human exposure to the chemicals. In the case of local toxicity, this may be relatively simple but in the case of systemic toxicity, concentrations of the toxicants in human tissues or the dose and the pharmacokinetics of the compounds must be known. However, for screening purposes, it will suffice to compare the cell toxicity with possible exposures to chemicals *in vivo*.

Tissue culture tests will not reveal toxicity due to disturbance of extracellular, organizational functions in the human body. Therefore, they must remain complementary to whole animal tests. The extent to which they can be relied upon as alternatives to animal screening tests depends on how frequently chemicals affect organizational aspects of the body. As with animal tests, most tissue culture tests of acute toxicity are optimal in the sense that they involve concentrations and exposure times directly transferable to the human condition in contrast to the case for the short-term mutagenicity and carcinogenicity screening tests (Bartsch and Tomatis, 1983).

There are two types of cellular models, i.e. undifferentiated and differentiated cells, used in acute toxicity testing (Ekwall, 1983b). Of these two types, the simple systems measuring basal cytotoxicity are probably the more useful in the sense that a central toxic effect is measured. This type of test is multi-purpose, and can be used to test both essential traits of local toxicity as well as various forms of systemic toxicity, including teratogenicity. The use of specialized cells for screening purposes will probably be determined by the cost and benefit of each model. Further research on differential cytotoxicity (comparison of results from parallel testing of substances in different cell systems, e.g., a cell line and hepatocytes as described by

Ekwall and Acosta, 1982) will show how often local irritancy to corneal, gingival or dermal cells actually is caused by selective cytotoxicity, not measured by basal cytotoxicity tests. Likewise, the frequency of organ-specific cytotoxicity to the liver, nervous system (Nardone, 1983), kidney, and so forth, will be determined. Until the frequency of selective cytotoxicity to different organs is fairly well known, the use of organ-specific tests for screening purposes is difficult to define (Ekwall and Ekwall, 1988).

The potential for cytotoxicity tests to supplement or provide an alternative to the use of laboratory animals in toxicity investigations has been discussed recently (Lindgren *et al.*, 1983; Williams *et al.*, 1983; Goldberg and Liebert, 1983; Balls *et al.*, 1983). Their use in range-finding and screening tests is tending to increase for scientific, ethic and economic reasons. Some current trends are described in the following paragraphs.

7.5.1   Implants

The most traditional use of tissue cultures in toxicology is the testing of implants, including dental materials for local irritancy (Ekwall, 1980; Browne and Tyas, 1979; Kasten *et al.*, 1982). Two studies (Hensten-Pettersen and Helgeland, 1977, 1981) compared different systems and cell types (including cell lines and secondary cultures of human gingival fibroblasts) in the prediction of local irritancy. Differences in methods (rather than in cell types used) caused differences in the results obtained; predictability was generally low; the reason may be the attempt to extrapolate from short-term incubation *in vitro* to long-term effects *in vivo* and the fact that true concentrations were not tested and that circulation may rapidly remove some substances from the local site *in vivo*. Because of the unreliability of various methods to produce comparable results, the US Commission on Dental Materials, Instruments and Therapeutics (COMIET) recommended the use of three standard tissue culture tests in 1978 (Stanford, 1980). These methods are a ^{51}Cr-release method (Spangberg, 1973), a millipore filter test (Wennberg *et al.*, 1979), and the widely-used agar-overlay test (Autian, 1977). These recommendations are now followed by all professional workers involved in testing dental materials. This must ultimately lead to long series of compounds tested by each method, a prerequisite for large-scale evaluation of results.

7.5.2   Eye and skin irritants

The Draize test to assess the local irritancy of chemicals in the rabbit eye has been criticized for cruelty and the subjectiveness of scoring, the latter probably contributing to the large inter-laboratory variability of results (Williams *et al.*, 1982; Wahlberg, 1983; Swanston, 1983). Alternative tests with enucleated rabbit eyes (Burton *et al.*, 1981; York *et al.*, 1982) or with rabbit ileum (Muir, 1983; Muir, 1984) have been proposed. Trials using culture tests for eye irritancy testing have given equivocal (Krejci, 1976; Scaife, 1983) or clearly positive results (North-Root *et al.*, 1982; Kemp *et al.*, 1983a; Kemp *et al.*, 1983b; Shopsis and Sathe, 1984; Borenfreund and Borrero, 1984; Selling and Ekwall, 1985). Borenfreund tested 34 toxicants in an assay using a number of cell types, including epithelial rabbit corneal cells, and found the same degree of toxicity in all cell systems tested. It seems that permanent cell lines are as good indicators of eye irritancy as more organ-specific cells (Kemp *et al.*, 1983b; Shopsis and Sathe, 1984; Borenfreund and Borrero, 1984; Selling and Ekwall, 1985); this implies that the basal cytotoxic action of most toxicants is the critical feature in irritancy. It is probable that a battery of simple cell cultures could be substituted in place of the Draize test but a large-scale evaluation involving more classes of chemicals is required to establish this. Success in using culture methods as a replacement for the *in vivo* method must be attributed to comparable incubation times *in vitro* and *in vivo* and also to the direct application of the toxicant on the target tissue *in vivo*, thereby avoiding distortion of *in vitro* results due to deficient absorption or local pharmacokinetics. Corresponding research to evaluate dermal irritation by use of tissue cultures is not so advanced (Kao *et al.*, 1983), neither can eye irritancy be predicted by skin irritancy of chemicals (Williams, 1984).

7.5.3 Inhalable pollutants

Screening techniques to detect local toxicity have been used to investigate the effects of various substances on the lung. These include tobacco smoke (Chamson *et al.*, 1982; Curvall *et al.*, 1984), diesel exhausts (Zamora *et al.*, 1983; Lundborg *et al.*, 1983), and various dusts and fibres (Garrett *et al.*, 1981). One study (Brown and Poole, 1983) compared 21 mineral dusts in four different cell systems from various laboratories, and a similarity between toxicity to different cells, such as macrophages, V79-4 Chinese hamster fibroblasts, and erythrocytes was demonstrated. Comparison of the *in vitro* toxicity with the *in vivo* pathogenicity was hampered by sparsity of *in vivo* data. In another study (Curvall *et al.*, 1984), the toxicity of more than 300 tobacco chemicals was tested in four different cell systems; good agreement was obtained between systems and it was noted that biological activity could be related to chemical structure for many of the chemicals tested. It is unfortunate that these authors did not attempt to compare their results with the *in vivo* activity of the same compounds; by the use of test substances with a known and varied human lung toxicity, the same efforts would have resulted in more valuable information about the reliability of the methods.

7.5.4 Systemic toxicity

Several workers have attempted to predict acute systemic toxicity in man using various cellular systems (Allred *et al.*, 1982; Rodgers *et al.*, 1983; Johnson and Knowles, 1983; Wenzel and Cosma, 1983; Walum and Peterson, 1984; Reinhardt *et al.*, 1982). In many instances, relatively few substances have been tested by the new methods and the experimental protocols did not provide for evaluation of the method by examination of the correlation between *in vitro* and *in vivo* toxicity. However, Walum and Peterson (1984) tested 35 common chemicals for their toxicity to neuroblastoma C1300 cells using a cell detachment method. For 30 of these substances, a positive correlation was found between cytotoxicity and the oral LD50 in rats; a very poor correlation was noted for five substances and this was attributed, in part, to the limited metabolic capacity of neuroblastoma cells. The authors concluded that batteries of cell tests are necessary to compensate for inaccurate predictions that might occur based on the results of a single test. Reinhardt *et al.* (1982) tested seven substances for toxicity in baby hamster kidney cells, as measured by cell detachment and cloning efficiency; both assays ranked all compounds tested according to their systemic *in vivo* toxicity. The relatively close relation between *in vitro* cytotoxicity and high (lethal) systemic toxicity found in these two studies confirms earlier studies (Lindgren *et al.*, 1983; Ekwall, 1983a,b) and is probably due to a very high frequency with which common chemicals exert a basal cytotoxic action at lethal doses for animals and man (Ekwall, 1983b). Thus, it would appear that screening procedures based on measurement of cytotoxicity in simple cell cultures can be used to detect chemicals that have acute systemic toxicity in man. Only a few substances exhibiting organizational toxicity, or which need metabolic activation for expression of their toxicity, or which otherwise have an organ-selective cytotoxicity will not be detected. This is different from the overall picture with short-term carcinogenicity tests, in which the group of chemicals requiring metabolic activation to express their carcinogenicity is fairly large. However, groups of chemicals, selected for specific biological activities, such as drugs and pesticides, are likely to include a higher percentage of members with an organizational toxicity than other groups so that the methods are likely to be less reliable in these cases.

A recent development is the use of rat hepatocytes for screening purposes (Cantilena *et al.*, 1983; Gray *et al.*, 1983; Story *et al.*, 1983; Tyson *et al.*, 1983). Story *et al.* (1983) tested 34 chemicals for cytotoxicity in rat hepatocytes, as measured by transaminase leakage after two and five hours of incubation. Good correlation between hepatotoxicity in an *in vitro* system and hepatotoxic responses *in vivo* was found. In a study of five haloalkanes, Tyson *et al.* (1983) showed that isolated hepatocyte systems have value for ranking structurally-related chemicals as to their cytotoxicity, even though their mechanisms of action may differ. For most compounds, the hepatocyte system probably measures basal cytotoxicity. Only studies of the apparent differences in toxicity between hepatocytes and undifferentiated cells *in vitro* (Ekwall and Acosta, 1982) or, more specifically, *in vitro/in vivo* comparisons can demonstrate the frequency of occurrence of organ-selective hepatotoxicity. One difficulty in interpreting the results of studies using hepatocytes is the time necessary for specific metabolite-mediated hepatotoxicity to be expressed clinically, compared with the relatively short incubation time used in the above discussed studies.

Testicular cell cultures (mixed cultures of Sertoli and germ cells) have recently been prepared and their response to some model testicular toxins studied (Gray and Beamand, 1984). Although this culture system has proved useful for limited series of congeners suspected to cause the testicular injury, its more general applicability remains unknown. In screening compounds with unknown toxicity, the use of such specific systems will not be cost-efficient since very few positives will result; at the same time, they are also laborious to carry out.

The most effective strategy for using tissue cultures for toxicity screening is to develop batteries of simple cell tests that measure basal cytotoxicity. It is probable that this can already be done with confidence for screening for eye irritant properties of chemicals. The battery should include hepatocytes, to estimate aspects of metabolically-induced toxicity, and possibly other systems of important organ-specific cells, too, if it is to be used to predict acute systemic toxicity. In addition to their use as screening tests basal cytotoxic and organ-selective cell tests can be used as analytical tools in conjunction with conventional animal toxicity tests to provide additional information on potential cytotoxicity and on mechanisms of toxic action.

7.6 *IN VITRO* CYTOTOXICITY AS A CRITERION FOR SELECTING 'PRIORITY CHEMICALS'

Chemical inventories, available in several countries including the US, Japan and EEC countries, indicate that a very large number of chemicals is being produced and marketed in many countries. For instance, about 55 000 commercial substances are listed in the US EPA TSCA inventory. Although about 9.5 per cent of the total number of substances reported (i.e. about 5000 chemicals) account for 99.9 per cent of the total production (Blair and Bowman, 1983) it is evident that exposure to relative low volume chemicals could be a major health problem for specific population groups under certain circumstances.

Toxicological data are currently either inadequate or non-existent for most existing chemicals (Grossblatt *et al.*, 1984; Silano *et al.*, 1986). In the absence of data concerning the health-related parameters, *in vitro* cytotoxicity data, which can be produced in a relatively short time and at a low relative cost, could be very useful for ranking chemicals with a similar exposure potential according to their potential toxicity and, possibly, to confirm other predictions based on consideration of their chemical structures. *In vitro* cytotoxicity data could also indicate the need for specific kinds of additional toxicity tests that would be required. Since industrial chemicals are not primarily of interest because of their specific biological activities, *in vitro* cytotoxicity data may provide a more useful criterion for priority ranking these chemicals than for other groups of chemicals such as drugs or pesticides. The use of a battery of tests with different cell types would be more appropriate than a single test in carrying out these screening tests. An established cell line, human diploid fibroblasts and rat hepatocytes could be used to provide tests with little variation, normal basic functions and metabolic capacity, respectively (see also Section 7.5).

Another possible approach is that used in the FRAME Research Programme on *in vitro* cytotoxicology (Balls and Bridges, 1983). FRAME has established a multi-centre research programme in partnership with a number of industrial companies, to determine whether cell cultures can be used reliably in place of live animal methods currently used in routine acute toxicity tests. Two parallel thrusts are involved: (1) a co-ordinated attempt to devise a simple, rapid and inexpensive method for evaluating the gross toxic effects of chemicals on the fundamental properties of cultured cells; and (2) an attempt to increase the range of methods available to study the effects of chemicals on differentiated tissue-type specific properties of cells from common target organs. A human embryo lung fibroblast-like cell strain (BCL-D1) was used to detect the 'gross' toxic effects of chemicals on the 'fundamental' properties of cells, whereas eight additional cell types were selected for the study of the effects of chemicals on the specific properties of 'differentiated' cells. A xenobiotic metabolizing system was included in the *in vitro* cytotoxicity test protocol (Balls and Bridges, 1983).

7.7 FUTURE DEVELOPMENTS

There have been a number of important meetings in recent years that have discussed the use of tissue cultures in toxicology (Lindgren *et al.*, 1983; Williams *et al.*, 1983; Goldberg and Liebert, 1983; Balls *et al.*, 1983). These include 4 biannual European conferences on the use of tissue cultures in toxicology from 1980 to 1988 (published in *Toxicology and Xenobiotica*), and the annual conferences on methods and strategies for general toxicity testing with cell systems, arranged by the Scandinavian Society for Cell Toxicology, from 1983 to 1989 (published in *ATLA*). As time goes by, the research field thus begins to be structured by consensus among researchers. As mentioned in Section 7.4, three areas of research are now fairly well separated; toxicity testing, studies of toxic effects and mechanisms, and lastly, studies of metabolism of compounds.

A common problem to all areas and types of cell systems is the lack of standardization of procedures. Now, almost all laboratories produce results that are difficult to compare because of variations in methodology. Such results do not contribute to the common pool of knowledge of cytotoxicity, nor can they be collectively used in large-scale validation studies (Ekwall, 1980; Paganuzzi-Stammati *et al.*, 1981).

Another problem is the lack of good evaluation studies, designed to prove the value of tissue cultures in testing procedures. Such studies must be planned to account for basal cytotoxicity and selective cytotoxicity versus organizational toxicity, and also be performed on a rather large scale with many classes of chemicals. All forms of toxicity to human beings, acute and chronic, direct and indirect, various types of local and systemic toxicity, must be separately validated by systematic *in vitro*/*in vivo* comparisons since the success of tissue culture methods in predicting one type of toxicity in humans does not imply a similar success in predicting another type.

A third obstacle to the greater use of cytotoxicity testing today is confusion about the best use of different cell types and end-points of cellular toxicity (Ekwall and Ekwall, 1988). Basal toxicity is often measured in elaborate, organ-specific culture systems, while undifferentiated cells are used to measure organ-selective or even organizational toxicity in man. Inappropriate specific end-points are sometimes used to measure the gross inflammatory capacity of chemicals, while growth parameters are used to measure injury.

Future development within the area of toxicity testing will progress on several lines:

(1)   Greater standardization of the methodology; standards for cells, media, and end-points must be established. Once this is done, more researchers will use established and documented methods in their work.

(2)   Extensive validation of methods. The programme of the English organization FRAME has already made some progress in this respect and another collaborative validation study has recently been launched within the teratogenicity field—a long list of well-known teratogens with good animal data has been developed to be used in validation of tissue culture teratogenicity tests (Smith *et al.*, 1983). The Scandinavian Society of Cell Toxicology is now organizing a multilaboratory study by which a large number of toxicants with well-defined human acute toxicity can be tested *in vitro* (the multi-center evaluation of *in vitro* cytotoxicity, MEIC) (Bernson *et al.*, 1987, Bondesson *et al.*, 1989; Ekwall *et al.*, 1989). Studies of this kind could lead to a more definite opinion on the utility of cell culture tests in toxicological investigations. The outcome of these validation studies could also elucidate the current confusion about which cells and culture methods to use for various kinds toxicity testing, and assist in the development of test batteries for screening purposes.

REFERENCES

Acosta, D., Anuforo, D., and Smith, R.V. (1978). The use of primary liver cell culture to study hepatotoxic agents. *Toxicol. Appl. Pharmacol.*, **45**, 262–3.

Albert, A. (1979). *Selective Toxicity. The Physico-chemical Basis of Therapy*, Chapman & Hall, London.

Alexander, P. (1969). Comparison of the mode of action by which some alkylating agents and ionizing radiations kill mammalian cells. *Ann. N.Y. Acad. Sci.*, **163**, 652–75.

Allred, L.E., Oldham, J.W., Milo, G.E., Kindig, O., and Capen, C.C. (1982). Multiparametric evaluation of the toxic responses of normal human cells treated *in vitro* with different classes of environmental toxicants. *J. Toxicol. Environ. Health*, **10**, 143–56.

Ambesi-Impiombato, F.S., Parks, L.A.M., and Coon, H.G. (1980). Culture of hormone-dependent functional epithelial cells from rat thyroids. *Proc. Nat. Acad. Sci.*, *USA*, **77**, 3455–9.

Auricchio, S., De Ritis, G., De Vincenzi, M., and Silano, V. (1985). Toxicity mechanisms of wheat and other cereals in celiac disease and related enteropathies. *J. Pediatr. Gastroenterol Nutr.*, **4**, 923–30.

Autian, J. (1977). Toxicological evaluation of biomaterials: Primary acute toxicity screening programme. *Artific. Organs*, **1**, 53–60.

Baird, W.M., Chemerys, R., Grinspan, J.B., Mueller, S.N., and Levine, E.M. (1980). Benzo(a)pyrene metabolism in bovine aortic endothelial and bovine lung fibroblast-like cell culture. *Cancer Res.*, **40**, 1781–6.

Balls M. and Bridges, J.W. (1983). The FRAME Research Programme on *in vitro* cytotoxicology. In: Goldberg, A.M., and Liebert, M.A. (Eds), *Alternative Methods in Toxicology*, volume 2, New York.

Balls, M., Ridell, R.J., and Worden, A. (Eds) (1983). *Animals and Alternatives in Toxicity Testing*, Academic Press, London.

Barnes, D., and Sato, G. (1980a). Methods for growth of cultured cells in serum-free medium. *Anal. Biochem.*, **102**, 255–70.

Barnes, D., and Sato, G. (1980b). Serum-free cell culture: a unifying approach. *Cell*, **22**, 649–55.

Barnes, D., Van der Bosch, J., Masui, H., Miyazaki, K., and Sato, G. (1980). The culture of human tumor cells in serum-free medium. In: Perstka, S. (Ed.), *Interferons, Methods in Enzymology*, volume 79. Academic Press, New York.

Bartsch, H., and Tomatis, L. (1983). Comparison between carcinogenicity and mutagenicity based on chemicals evaluated in the IARC monographs. *Environ. Health Perspect.*, **47**, 305–17.

Begue, J.M., Le Bigot, J.F., Guguen-Guillouzo, C., Kiechel, J.R., and Guillouzo, A. (1983). Cultured human adult hepatocytes: A new model for drug metabolism studies. *Biochem. Pharmacol.*, **32**, 1643–6.

Bernson, V., Bondesson, I., Ekwall, B., Stenberg, K., and Walum, E. (1987). A multicentre evaluation study of in vitro cytotoxicity *ATLA*, **14**, 144–6.

Bianchi, V. (1982). Nucleotide pool unbalance induced in cultured cells by treatments with different chemicals. *Toxicol.*, **25**, 13–18.

Bianchi, V., Debetto, P., Zantedeschi, A., and Levis, A.G. (1982). Effects of hexavalent chromium on the adenylate pool of hamster fibroblasts.*Toxicol.*, **25**, 19–30.

Bitensky, L. (1963). The reversible activation of lysosomes in normal cells and the effects of pathological conditions. In: de Renk, A.U.S., and Cameron, M.F. (Eds), *Lysosomes*, Churchill, London, pp. 362–75.

Blair, E.H., and Bowman, C.M. (1983). Control of existing chemicals. *ACS Symposium*, 67–79.

Bondesson, I., Ekwall, B., Hellberg, S., Romert, L., Stenberg, K., and Walum, E. (1989). MEIC—A new international multicenter project to evaluate the relevance to human toxicity of in vitro cytotoxicity tests. *Cell Biol. Toxicol.*, **5**, 331–47.

Borenfreund, E., and Borrero, O. (1984). *In vitro* cytotoxicity assays: Potential alternatives to the Draize ocular irritancy test. *Cell Biol. Toxicol.*, **1**, 33–9.

Brown, R.C., and Poole, A. (1983). The *in vitro* effects of mineral dusts. *ATLA*, **11**, 79–86.

Browne, R.M., and Tyas, M.J. (1979). Biological testing of dental restorative materials *in vitro*—A review. *J. Oral Rehabil.*, **6**, 365–74.

Burstein, S., Hunter, S.A., and Olzman, H. (1983). Prostaglandins and Cannabis. XII. The effects of cannabinoid structures on the synthesis of prostaglandins by human lung fibroblast. *Mol. Pharmacol.*, **23**, 121–6.

Burton, A.B.G., York, M., and Lawrence, R.S. (1981). The *in vitro* assessment of severe eye irritants. *Fd. Cosmet. Toxicol.*, **19**, 471–80.

Cantilena, L.R. Jr., Stacey, N.H., and Klassen, C.D. (1983). Isolated rat hepatocytes as a model system for screening chelators for use in cadmium intoxication. *Toxicol. Appl. Pharmacol.*, **67**, 257–63.

Castranova, V., Bowman, L., Reasor, M.J., and Miles, P.R. (1980). Effects of heavy metal ions on selected oxidative metabolic processes in rat alveolar macrophages. *Toxicol. Appl. Pharmacol.*, **53**, 14–23.

Chamson, A., Frey, J., and Hivert, M. (1982). Effects of tobacco smoke extracts on collagen biosynthesis by fibroblast cell cultures. *J. Toxicol. Environ. Health*, **9**, 921–32.

Costa, M. (1979). Levels of ornithine decarboxylase activation used as a simple marker of metal induced growth arrest in tissue culture. *Life Sci.*, **24**, 705–14.

Curvall, M., Enzell, C.R., and Pettersson, B. (1984). An evaluation of the utility of four *in vitro* short-term tests for predicting the cytotoxicity of individual compounds derived from tobacco smoke. *Cell Biol. Toxicol.*, **1**, 173–93.

Dolfini, E., Martini, A., Donelli, M.G., Morasca, L., and Garattini, S. (1973). Method for tissue culture evaluation of the cytotoxic activity of drugs active through the formation of metabolites. *Eur. J. Cancer*, **9**, 375–8.

Drake, S., Burns, R.L., and Nelson, J.A. (1982). Metabolism and mechanisms of action of 9-(tetrahydro-2-furyl)-6-mercaptopurine in chinese hamster cells. *Chem. Biol. Interact.*, **41**, 105–16.

Ekwall, B. (1980). Screening of toxic compounds in tissue culture. *Toxicol.*, **17**, 127–42.

Ekwall, B. (1983a). Correlation between cytoxocity *in vitro* and LD50 values. In: Lindgren, P., Thelestam, M., and Lindquist, N.G. (Eds), *First CFN Symposium on LD50 and Possible Alternatives. Acta Pharmacol. Toxicol.*, **52**, Suppl. 2, 80–99.

Ekwall, B. (1983b). Screening of toxic compounds in mammalian cell cultures. *Ann. N.Y. Acad. Sci.*, **407**, 64–77.

Ekwall, B., and Acosta, D. (1982). *In vitro* comparative toxicity of selected drugs and chemicals in HeLa cells, Chang liver cells and rat hepatocytes. *Drug Chem. Toxicol.*, **5**, 219–31.

Ekwall, B., Bondesson, I., Castell, J.V., Gómez-Lechón, M.J., Hellberg, S., Högberg, J., Jover, R., Ponsoda, X., Romert, L., Stenberg, K., and Walum, E. (1989). Cytotoxicity evaluation for the first ten MEIC chemicals: Acute lethal toxicity in man predicted by cytotoxicity in five cellular assays and by oral LD50 in rodents. *ATLA*, **17**, 83–100.

Ekwall, B., and Ekwall, K. (1988). Comments on the use of diverse cell systems in toxicity testing. *ATLA*, **15**, 193–200.

Elferink, J.G.R. (1979). Chlorpromazine inhibits phagocytosis and exocytosis in rabbit polymorphonuclear leukocytes. *Biochem. Pharmacol.*, **28**, 965–8.

Engvall, E., Oshima, R.G., Brennan, M.J. and Ruoslahti, E. (1984). Clonal tumorigenic endodermal cell lines producing basement membrane components. *Exp. Cell Res.*, **150**, 258–67.

Fedoroff, S. (1966). Proposed usage of animal tissue culture terms. *In vitro*, **2**, 155–9.

Fedoroff, S. (1977). Primary cultures, cell lines and cell strains: Terminology and characteristics. In: Fedoroff, S., and Hertz, L. (Eds), *Cell, Tissue and Organ Cultures in Neurobiology*, Academic Press, New York, San Francisco and London, pp. 265–86.

Garrett, N.E., Campbell, J.A., Stack, H.F., Waters, M.D., and Lewtas, J. (1981). The utilization of the rabbit alveolar macrophage and chinese hamster ovary cell for evaluation of the toxicity of particulate materials. I. Model compounds and metal-coated fly ash. *Environ. Res.*, **24**, 345–65.

Goldberg, A.M., and Liebert, M. (1983). Alternative methods in toxicology. In: *Product Safety Evaluation*, New York.

Gray, T.J.B., and Beamand, J.A. (1984). Effect of some phthalate esters and other testicular toxins on primary cultures of testicular cells. *Fd. Chem. Toxicol.*, **22**, 123–31.

Gray, T.J.B., Lake, B.G., Beamand, J.A., Foster, J.R., and Gangolli, S.D. (1983). Peroxisome proliferation in primary cultures of rat hepatocytes. *Toxicol. Appl. Pharmacol.*, **67**, 15–25.

Grisham, J.W. (1979). Use of hepatic cell cultures to detect and evaluate the mechanisms of action of toxic chemicals. *Int. Rev. Exp. Pathol.*, **20**, 123–210.

Grossblatt, N., Whittenberger, J.L., Bailar, J.C., Doull, J., Pfitzer, E.A., and Upton, A.C. (1984). Toxicity testing—Strategies to determine needs and priorities. National Academy Press, Washington, D.C.

Guess, W.L., Rosenbluth, S.A., Schmidt, B., and Autian, J. (1965). Agar diffusion method for toxicity screening of plastics on cultured cell monolayers. *J. Pharm. Sci.*, **54**, 1545–7.

Guguen-Guillouzo, C., Gripon, P., Vandenberghe, Y., Lamballe, F., Ratanasavanh, D., and Guillouzo A. (1988). Hepatotoxicity and molecular aspects of hepatocyte function in primary culture. *Xenobiot.*, **18**, 773–83.

Guillouzo, A., Le Bigot, J.F., Guguen-Guillouzo, C., and Kiechel, J.R. (1982). Presence of Phase I and Phase II drug metabolizing enzymes in cultured human foetal hepatocytes. *Biochem. Pharmacol.*, **31**, 2427–9.

Harmon, H.J., and Sanborn, M.R. (1982). Effect of naphthalene on respiration in heart mitochondria and intact cultured cells. *Environ. Res.*, **29**, 160–73.

Hayflick, L., and Moorhead, P.S. (1961). The serial cultivation of human diploid cell strains. *Exp. Cell. Res.*, **25**, 585–621.

Hensten-Pettersen, A., and Helgeland, K. (1977). Evaluation of biologic effects of dental materials using four different cell culture techniques. *Scand. J. Dent. Res.*, **85**, 291–6.

Hensten-Pettersen, A., and Helgeland, K. (1981). Sensitivity of different human cell lines in the biologic evaluation of dental resin-based restorative materials. *Scand. J. Dent. Res.*, **89**, 102–7.

Higuchi, K. (1976). Cultivation of mammalian cell lines in serum free chemically defined medium. *Methods Cell Biol.*, **14**, 131–43.

Hoidal, J.R., Fox, R.B., Le Marbe, P.A., Perri, R., and Repine, J.E. (1981). Altered oxidative metabolic response *in vitro* of alveolar macrophages from asymptomatic cigarette smokers. *Am. Rev. Resp. Dis.*, **123**, 85–9.

Holden, H.T., Lichter, W., and Siegel, M.M. (1973). Quantitative methods for measuring cell growth and death. In: Kruse, P. Jr., and Patterson, M.K. Jr. (Eds), *Tissue Culture: Methods and Applications*, Academic Press, New York, pp. 408–11.

Hucker, H.B. (1970). Species differences in drug metabolism. *Ann. Rev. Pharm.*, **10**, 99–118.

Johnson, T.L., and Knowles, C.O. (1983). Effects of organotins on red platelets. *Toxicol.*, **29**, 39–48.

Kao, J., Hall, J., and Holland, J.M. (1983). Quantitation of cutaneous toxicity: An *in vitro* approach using skin organ culture. *Toxicol. Appl. Pharmacol.*, **68**, 206–17.

Kasten, F.H., Felder, S.M., Gettleman, L., and Alchediak, T. (1982). A model culture system with human gingival fibroblasts for evaluating the cytotoxicity of dental materials. *In Vitro*, **18**, 650–60.

Kemp, R.B., Meredith, R.W.J., Gamble, S., and Frost, M. (1983a). A rapid cell culture technique for assessing the toxicity of detergent-based products *in vitro* as a possible screen for eye irritancy *in vivo*. *Cytobios*, **36**, 153–9.

Kemp, R.B., Meredith, R.W.J., Gamble, S., and Frost, M. (1983b). Toxicity of detergent-based commercial products on cells of a mouse line in suspension culture as a possible screen for the Draize rabbit eye irritation test. *ATLA*, **11**, 15–21.

Klaassen, C.D., and Stacey, N.H. (1982). Use of isolated hepatocytes in toxicity assessment. In: Plaa, G., and Hewitt, W.R. (Eds), *Toxicology of the Liver*, Raven Press, New York, pp. 147–79.

Krejci, L. (1976). Effect of eye drugs on corneal epithelium. Comparative test on tissue cultures. *Cesk. Oftalmol.*, **32**, 163–8.

Lamb, R.G., and Schwartz, D.W. (1982). The effects of bromobenzene and carbon tetrachloride exposure *in vitro* on phospholipase C activity in rat liver cells. *Toxicol. Appl. Pharmacol.*, **63**, 216–29.

Lieberman, M., Adam, W.J., and Bullock, P.N. (1980). The cultured heart cell: problems and prospects. In: Harris, C.C., Trumpand, B.F., and Stoner, G.D. (Eds), *Methods in Cell Biol.*, Academic Press, New York, p. 187.

Lindgren, P., Thelestam, M., and Lindquist, N.G. (Eds) (1983). First CFN Symposium on LD50 and possible alternatives. *Acta Pharmacol. Toxicol.,* **52**, Suppl. II.

Lundborg, P., Cederberg, I., Wiklund, L., and Petterson, B. (1983). Effects of waste incineration combustion emissions measured by some toxicity test systems. *Toxicol. Lett.,* **19**, 97–107.

Miller, J.A., and Miller, E.C. (1971). Chemical carcinogenesis: Mechanisms and approaches to its control. *J. Nat. Cancer Inst.,* **47**, V–XIV.

Moldeus, T., Jones, D.P., Ormstad, K., and Orrenius, S. (1978). Formation and metabolism of a gluthatione-S-conjugate in isolated rat liver and kidney cells. *Biochem. Biophys. Res. Commun.,* **83**, 195–200.

Muir, C.K. (1983). The toxic effects of some industrial chemicals on rabbit ileum *in vitro* compared with eye irritancy *in vivo. Toxicol. Lett.,* **19**, 309–12.

Muir, C.K. (1984). Further investigations on the ileum model as a possible alternative to *in vivo* eye irritancy testing. *ATLA,* **1**, 129–34.

Murakami, H., and Masui, H. (1980). Hormonal control of human colon carcinoma cell growth in serum-free medium. *Proc. Nat. Acad. Sci. ISA,* **77**, 3464–8.

Nakada, S., Saito, H., and Imura, N. (1981). Effects of methylmercury and inorganic mercury on the nerve growth factor-induced neurite outgrowth in chick embryonic sensory ganglia. *Toxicol. Lett.,* **6**. 23–28.

Nardone, R.M. (1977). Toxicity testing *in vitro.* In: Rothblat, G.H., and Cristofalo, J. (Eds), *Growth, Nutrition and Metabolism of Cell in Culture,* volume III, Academic Press, New York, San Francisco, London, pp. 471–95.

Nardone, R.M. (1983). Neurotoxicity testing: An *in vitro* strategy. *Ann. N.Y. Acad. Sci.,* **407**, 458–9.

North-Root, H., Yackovich, F., Demetrulias, J., Gacula, M. Jr., and Heinze, J.E. (1982). Evaluation of an *in vitro* cell toxicity test using rabbit corneal cells to predict the eye irritation potential of surfactants. *Toxicol. Lett.,* **14**, 207–12.

Orly, J., Sato, G., and Erickson, G. (1980). Serum suppresses the expression of hormonally-induced functions in cultured granulosa cells. *Cell,* **20**, 817–27.

Paganuzzi-Stammati, A., Silano, V., and Zucco, F. (1981). Toxicology investigations with cell culture systems. *Toxicol.,* **20**, 91–153.

Quinn, G.P., Axelrod, J., and Brodie, B.B. (1958). Species, strain and sex differences in metabolism of hexobarbitone, amidopyrine, antipyrine and aniline. *Biochem. Pharmacol.,* **1**, 152–9.

Reinhardt, C.A., Schawalder, H., and Zbinden, G. (1982). Cell detachment and cloning efficiency as parameters for cytotoxicity. *Toxicol.,* **25**, 47–52.

Rodgers, C.G., Héroux-Metcalf, C., and Iverson, F. (1983). *In vitro* cytotoxicity of polychlorinated biphenyls (Aochlors 1016, 1242, 1254 and 1260) and their effect on phospholipid and neutral lipid composition of Chinese hamster ovary (CHO-K1) cells. *Toxicol.,* **26**, 113–24.

Sato, H.G., and Yasamura, Y. (1966). Retention of differentiated function in dispersed cell culture. *Trans. N.Y. Acad. Sci.,* **28**, 1063–79.

Sato, G.H., Pardee, A.B., and Sirbasku, D.A. (Eds) (1982). Growth of cells in hormonally defined medium. Cold Spring Harbor Conference on cell proliferation, Vol. 9, Book A and B, Cold Spring Harbor Laboratory.

Scaife, M.C. (1983). *In vitro* studies on ocular irritancy. In Balls, M., Ridell, R.G., and Worden, A. (Eds), *Animals and Alternatives in Toxicity Testing,* Academic Press, London, pp. 367–71.

Schaeffer, W.I. (1984). Usage of vertebrate, invertebrate and plant cell, tissue and organ culture terminology. *In Vitro,* **20**(1): 19–24.

Schiller, C.M., and Lucier, G.W. (1978). The differential response of isolated intestinal crypt and tip cells to the inductive action of 2,3,7,8-tetrachlorodibenzo-*p*-dioxin. *Chem. Biol. Interact.,* **22**, 199–209.

Schwartz, H.S., and Mihic, E. (1973). Species and tissue differences in drug selectivity. In: Mihic, E. (Ed.), *Drug Resistance and Selectivity. Biochemical and Cellular Basis*, Academic Press, News York, pp. 413–49.

Selling, J., and Ekwall, B. (1985). Screening for eye irritancy using cultured HeLa cells. *Xenobiot.*, **15**, 713–17.

Shopsis, C., and Sathe, S. (1984). Uridine uptake inhibition as a cytotoxicity test: correlations with the Draize test. *Toxicol.*, **29**, 195–206.

Silano, V., Stammati-Paganuzzi, A., and Vittozzi, L. (1986). Possibilities for in vitro methods. In: *Chemicals Testing and Animal Welfare, Proceedings*, Swedish National Chemicals Inspectorate, Stockholm. pp. 152–182.

Smith, M.K., Kimmel, G.L., Kochhar, D.M., Shepard, T.H., Spielberg, S.P. and Wilson, J.G. (Eds) (1983). A selection of candidate compounds for *in vitro* teratogenesis test validation. *Teratog. Carcinog. Mutagen.*, **3**, 461–80.

Spangberg, L. (1973). Kinetic quantitative evaluation of material cytotoxicity *in vitro*. *Oral Surg.*, **35**, 389.

Stacey, N.H., and Klaassen, C.D. (1981a). Comparison of the effects of metals on cellular injury and lipid peroxidation in isolated rat hepatocytes. *J. Toxicol. Environ. Health*, **7**, 139–47.

Stacey, N.H., and Klaassen, C.D. (1981b). Inhibition of lipid peroxidation without prevention of cellular injury in isolated hepatocytes. *Toxicol. Appl. Pharmacol.*, **58**, 8–18.

Stacey, N.H., Ottenwalder, H., and Kappas, H. (1982). CCl_4-induced lipid peroxidation in isolated rat hepatocytes with different oxygen concentration. *Toxicol. Appl. Phrmacol.*, **62**, 421–7.

Stanford, J.W. (Ed.) (1980). Recommended standard practices for biological evaluation of dental materials. *Int. Dent., J.*, **30**, 140–88.

Story, D.L., Gee, S.J., Tyson, C.A., and Gould, D.H. (1983). Response of isolated hepatocytes to organic and inorganic cytotoxins. *J. Toxicol. Environ. Health*, **11**, 483–501.

Striker, G.E., Harlan, J.M., and Schwartz, S.M. (1980). Human endothelial cells *in vitro*. In: Harris, C.C., Trump, B.F., and Stoner, G.C. (Eds), *Methods in Cell Biology*, Academic Press, New York, London, Toronto, Sydney, San Francisco, p. 135.

Swanston, D.W. (1983). Eye irritancy testing. In: Balls, M., Ridell, R.J., and Worden, A. (Eds), *Animals and Alternatives in Toxicity Testing*, Academic Press, London, pp. 337–65.

Tell, R.W., and Douglas, W.H.J. (1980). Aryl hydrocarbon hydroxylase activity in Type II alveolar lung cells. *Experimentia*, **36**, 107.

Tyson, C.A., Hawk Prather, K., Story, D.L., and Gould, D.H. (1983). Correlations of *in vitro* and *in vivo* hepatotoxicity for five haloalkanes. *Toxicol. Appl. Pharmacol.*, **70**, 289–302.

Wahlberg, J.A. (1983). Exfoliative cytology as a refinement of the Draize eye irritancy test. *Toxicol. Lett.*, **18**, 49–55.

Walton, J.R. (1975). The systemic appraisal of cellular injury. *Agents and Actions*, **5**, 394–400.

Walton, J.R., and Buckley, I.K. (1975). Cell models in the study of mechanisms of toxicity. *Agents and Actions*, **5**, 69–88.

Walum, E., and Peterson, A. (1984). Acute toxic action of chemicals in cultures of mouse neuroblastoma C 1300 cells. *J. Toxicol. Environ. Health*, **13**, 511–20.

Waters, M.D., Vaughan, T.O., Abernethy, D.J., Garland, H.R., Cox, C.C., and Coffin, D.L. (1975). Toxicity of platinum (IV) salts for cells of pulmonary origin. *Environ. Health Perspect.*, **12**, 45–56.

Weisburger, H.H., Grantham, P.H., and Weisburger, E.R. (1964). Metabolism of N-2-fluorenylacetamide in the hamster. *Toxicol. Appl. Pharmacol.*, **6**, 427–33.

Wennberg, A., Hasselgren, G., and Tronstad, L. (1979). A method for toxicity screening of biomaterials using cells cultured on millipore filters. *J. Biomed. Mater. Res.*, **13**, 109–20.

Wenzel, D.G., and Cosma, G.N. (1983). A quantitative metabolic inhibition test for screening toxic compounds with cultured cells. *Toxicol.,* **29**, 173–82.

White, F.V., Ceccarini, C., Georgieff, I., Matthieu, J.-M., and Costantino-Ceccarini, E. (1983). Growth properties and biochemical characterization of mouse Schwann cells cultured *in vitro. Exp. Cell Res.,* **148**, 183–94.

Williams, A.J., and Cole, P.J. (1981). *In vitro* stimulation of alveolar macrophage metabolic activity by polystyrene in the absence of phagocytosis. *Br. J. Exp. Pathol.,* **62**, 1–7.

Williams, G.M., Dunkel, V.C., and Ray, V.A. (Eds) (1983). Cellular systems for toxicity testing. *Ann. N.Y. Acad. Sci.,* p. 407.

Williams, S.J. (1984). Prediction of ocular irritancy potential from dermal irritation test results. *Fd. Chem. Toxicol.,* **22**, 157–61.

Williams, S.J., Graepel, G.J., and Kennedy, G.L. (1982). Evaluation of ocular irritancy potential: interlaboratory variability and effect of dosage volume. *Toxicol. Lett.,* **12**, 235–41.

York, M., Lawrence, R.S., and Gibson, G.B. (1982). An *in vitro* test for the assessment of eye irritancy in consumer products—Preliminary findings. *Int. J. Cosmet. Sci.,* 223–34.

Yoshida, M., Onaka, M., Fujita, T., and Nakajima, M. (1979). Inhibitory effects of pesticides on growth and respiration of cultured cells. *Pesticide Biochem. Physiol.,* **10**, 313–21.

Zamora, P.O., Benson, J.M., Marshall, T.C., Mokler, B.V., Li, A.P., Dahl, A.R., Brooks, A.L., and McClellan, R.O. (1983). Cytotoxicity and mutagenicity of vapor-phase pollutants in rat lung epithelial cells and chinese hamster ovary cells grown on collagen gels. *J. Toxicol. Environ. Health,* **12**, 27–38.

Short-term Toxicity Tests for Non-genotoxic Effects
Edited by P. Bourdeau *et al.*
© 1990 SCOPE. Published by John Wiley & Sons Ltd

CHAPTER 8

The Gastrointestinal Tract and Short-term Toxicity Tests

DONALD BARLTROP AND MARTIN J. BRUETON

8.1 INTRODUCTION

The primary role of the gastrointestinal tract is the digestion and absorption of nutrients. This is critical for normal body homeostasis. The gastrointestinal tract also forms a barrier against unwanted materials, and is a major site of biotransformation and excretion. Its immunological function is defence against infection and the prevention of hypersensitivity reactions are dependent upon effective microenvironmental immunoregulation at the mucosal level. The implications of the symbiotic relationships of the gastrointestinal microflora are still being elucidated, while the complexities of the overall control of gut motility, secretion and growth are now recognized to depend on interactions between the autonomic nervous system and the neuroendocrine connections of the peptidergic nerves.

The importance of the gut with respect to toxicology arises from its central role in the absorption of ingested materials. It is the major portal of entry for a wide variety of compounds including those which have no nutritional or other functional value (xenobiotics). Most of our knowledge about absorption, transport and metabolism of xenobiotics relates to the normal adult gut, however, the expected effects following ingestion of a particular compound depend on the integrity of the intestinal mucosa. In infancy, many aspects of gut function are immature and, at any age, there are many situations in which mucosal function is compromised; infections, hypersensitivity reactions and malnutrition can all alter permeability of the gut due to epithelial cell damage, with varying effects on absorption of the compound in question.

8.2 THE NORMAL GASTROINTESTINAL TRACT

8.2.1 Structure

The inner surface area of the gastrointestinal tract is vastly increased by the convolutions of the valvulae conniventes, villi and microvilli. The villi are covered by columnar epithelial cells (enterocytes) which are renewed every 24–48 hours. They originate in the crypts, proliferate and migrate up the villi, differentiating as they progress to the villus tip. These enterocytes are covered by microvilli whose surface membranes are phospholipid bilayers within which there are electronegative pores. These pores or discontinuities in the membrane are wider (7.5–8.0 Ångström units) in the upper small bowel than in the ileum or colon. Extending from the microvillus membrane is the glycocalyx which is characterized by hydrophilic molecules with lipophilic bases resting within the lipid membrane. An unstirred water layer external to the glycocalyx prevents immediate contact with the cell surface.

The enterocytes themselves are of similar origin to hepatocytes and contain comparable subcellular structures rich in enzyme activity relating to synthesis, metabolism and secretion. Between the epithelial cells lie goblet cells; they secrete mucins which contribute to local protection.

The muscularis mucosae is a thin layer of smooth muscle which separates the epithelium from the lamina propria. This extends into the core of each villus and contains capillaries, lacteals and numerous mononuclear cells including macrophages, polymorphs, mast cells and lymphocytes. The lymphocytes are also distributed throughout the epithelium itself and occur as aggregates in the Peyer's patches, appendix and tonxils. They, in effect, form a lymphoid organ. Thus gut associated lymphoid tissue (GALT) determines the recognition of antigen and controls a subtle balance of responses such as the generation of mucosal and/or systemic immunity, tolerance or hypersensitivity reactions of various types. The outer muscle layer of the gut contains both longitudinal and circular fibres which are richly innervated.

8.2.2. Uptake, transfer and metabolism

Digestion in the lumen is dependent upon secretions from the stomach, liver and pancreas. The enterocytes with their microvilli also produce numerous digestive enzymes. Access to the enterocytes will depend initially on the physicochemical characteristics of the substance concerned. Transport into cells may be by passive diffusion down a concentration gradient, by active carrier-mediated transport, by pinocytosis or, in the case of very lipophilic compounds, by micelle solubilization in bile acid mediated diffusion. Para-cellular entry may also be gained by diffusion through the tight junctions between cells.

Although our knowledge of normal digestive function is now extensive, the handling of foreign compounds which do not have nutritional value or functional importance is less well understood. Materials which are antigenic to the immune system have been particularly studied. They are preferentially taken up by specialized 'M' epithelial cells which overlie the Peyer's patches.

Discerning the actual fate of individual foreign compounds is further complicated by numerous other factors which may affect absorption and metabolism. These include binding to nutritional constituents, the generation of toxic metabolites, gastric emptying and small bowel transit times, the dilutional and pH effects of the lumenal contents, blood flow, interaction with the gut microflora, gastrointestinal disease states, and the nutritional and maturational status of the mucosa.

Once within the enterocytes, the fate of xenobiotics is dependent on the enzymatic processes of the subcellular membranes. Biotransformation into water-soluble products may result in transport into the portal circulation and hence to the liver. Lipophilic compounds may travel within chylomicrons into the lymphatics. Some compounds such as benzo(a)pyrene are metabolized in the cell and the products are secreted back into the lumen of the gut (Hietanen, 1980).

The enterocytes are rich in enzyme activity. Synthetic enzymes catalysing acetylation, *O*-methylation and glutathione transfer are present, as well as non-synthetic enzymes concerned with hydrolysis and reduction. The smooth endoplasmic reticulum contains cytochrome P-450 acting as an oxygen activator and NADPH cytochrome P-450 reductase supplying electrons for mono-oxygenation. The microsomes have the highest specific activity of metabolizing enzymes within the enterocytes. Several types of mono-oxygenases occur. They can act on lipophilic xenobiotics to produce polar hydroxyl groups which can be acted upon by the conjugation enzymes leading to hydrophilic products (Hoensch, 1982). Conjugation can lead to reduced bioavailability of compounds in the systemic circulation, for example, glucuronic acid conjugation of morphine and terbutaline, and sulphate conjugation of ethyl oestradiol (Back *et al.*, 1981). Conversely, deconjugation by intestinal bacteria may reduce water solubility and promote absorption (Hoensch and Hartmann, 1981).

8.2.3 Immunological considerations

Nutrients and xenobiotics may generate immunological reactions. It is currently suspected that immunologically mediated allergic mechanisms underlie many unexpected reactions to oral antigen. The responses of the GALT to antigen are complex. Humoral IgA immunity was initially studied, secretory IgA not only protects against infection by preventing bacterial adhesion and neutralizing viruses and toxins, but it can complex with specific antigens and prevent their absorption. Cellular immune mechanisms continue to be elucidated and it is clear that T cell control can result in immunity or tolerance that is a specific unresponsiveness to an antigen. This tolerance is particularly generated in certain circumstances by oral exposure to the antigen while the lack of tolerance may result in the production of clinically-apparent hypersensitivity reactions. This might occur when the mucosa is damaged, or possibly in the presence of adjuvants in the gut lumen.

In the first year of life, there is an increased incidence of hypersensitivity reactions. The aetiology of these may relate to such factors as a transient deficiency of secretory IgA, an increase in receptor sites for antigen on immature enterocytes, increased macromolecular access, and decreased intralumenal degradation of antigenic material.

8.2.4 Maturational considerations

In infancy, many aspects of gut function are immature. Digestion of fats, proteins and carbohydrates are largely dependent on the development of exocrine pancreatic function. Even in full-term newborns, pancreatic function is relatively poorly developed. Lipase is low and amylase is absent, although proteases are developed fairly early and are present at birth. The neonatal pancreas is more often unresponsive to pancreozymin and shows a reduced sensitivity to secretin (Lebenthal *et al.*, 1981). Maturation of function is promoted by dietary exposure to nutrients. Brush border sucrase, maltase and alkaline phosphatase activities are high at birth; however, lactase activity is low (Moog, 1981). Different patterns of intestinal motility are also seen in infants and children, more rhythmic peristaltic waves being evident (Siegel and Lebenthal, 1981). One example of the effect of gut maturity on function may be seen in a study of lead uptake in rats in which there was a markedly reduced rate of uptake during the first 3–4 weeks of life (Barltrop, 1982).

Macromolecular transport across the intestine has been studied far more extensively in young animals than in man. In animals which receive partial passive immunity (e.g. rat) or more complete passive immunity (e.g. sheep, pig) postnatally, perinatal transport of immunoglobulin across the mucosa occurs (Morris and Morris, 1976). In animals receiving intrauterine passive immunity (e.g. rabbits, man), there is some evidence that intact proteins can penetrate the mucosal barrier of the gut of the immature animal (Udall and Walker, 1982).

8.2.5 Nutritional considerations

Malnutrition in children causes dramatic reductions in pancreatic enzyme production (Barbezat and Hansen, 1968). Animal studies have confirmed this, as well as the fact that recovery readily occurs following improvement in the diet (Schrader and Zeman, 1970). Malnutrition also comprises mucosal immunity. Thus, children suffering malnutrition encounter an increase in the number and duration of gastrointestinal infections; this further damages the mucosa and affects its capacity for absorption and metabolism.

Interaction between nutritional factors in the diet may be of importance in other respects. Lead absorption in rats has been increased by diets containing high fat, low mineral, low protein or high protein concentrations (Barltrop and Khoo, 1975; Bell and Spickett, 1983).

8.3   THE RECOGNITION OF TOXIC EFFECTS TO THE GUT

8.3.1   Introduction

Gastrointestinal symptoms are common and notoriously non-specific since their occurrence does not always imply a primary disturbance of gut function. Nausea, abdominal pain or diarrhoea frequently accompany stress in many adults, or urinary and respiratory infections in children. Similarly, substances encountered by inhalation or skin contact can be absorbed and cause secondary alimentary tract symptoms. In practice, toxic effects of many ingested compounds may not be completely evaluated since initial exposure clearly causes gastrointestinal disturbances, or macroscopic changes in the gut such as ulceration. Although the major emphasis in the literature has been placed on carcinogenesis and genotoxic mechanisms, xenobiotics have been studied in many other respects.

8.3.2   Histological studies

In man, mucosal biopsies from the oesophagus, stomach, jejunum, sigmoid colon and rectum have been studied over many years. Initially, general morphological changes were described. More exact quantification can now be applied by measuring villus height and crypt depth, by computing surface areas using light pens, and by recording cellular infiltration in terms of cell counts (related to enterocyte numbers, standard grids or calculated volumes). Individual cell types, such as mast cells, can be better identified using modern stains. Mitotic indices amongst crypt cells can be measured and monoclonal antibodies can be applied to identify lymphocyte subsets and their distribution through the mucosa. The advent of fibre-optic endoscopy has enabled macroscopic examination to complement histological appearances, and has allowed access to the rest of the colon and the terminal ileum.

Peptic ulceration is an important area of study; acrylonitrile is one substance which has a duodenal ulcerogenic action. This compound is also an interesting example since it points out the relevance of evaluating interactions with other factors. In this case, it was noted that polychlorinated phenols potentiate duodenal ulceration in rats given acrylonitrile (Szabo *et al.*, 1983). Polychlorinated phenols alone produce histological changes, gastric mucosal hyperplasia being observed in sub-human primates (Becker *et al.*, 1979).

Light microscopy may be supplemented with electron microscopy and polarizing light microscopy. The latter has been useful in demonstrating the penetration of the mucosa by particulate matter such as asbestos (Meek and Grasso, 1983). Electron microscopy of tissue residues and body fluids in man has shown that an oral intake of asbestos may results in its widespread distribution in the body (Carter and Taylor, 1980).

Two environmental toxins have been particularly implicated in causing histological damage to the mucosa and subsequent malabsorption: T-2 toxin and 2,3,7,8-tetrachlorodibenzo-*p*-dioxin (TCDD). The trichothecene T-2 toxin (derived from the fungus *Fusarium sporotrichioides*), which may occur in stored grains, causes alimentary toxic aleukia. An enteropathy is succeeded by systemic and neurological disturbances and leukopenia (Lutsky *et al.*, 1978). The mechanisms of toxicity are not known, although T-2 toxin is recognized as an inhibitor of protein synthesis and mitochondrial respiration (Schiller and Yagen, 1981). 2,3,7,8-TCDD alters fat absorption so that the mucosal cells become filled with large lipid droplets (McConnell and Shoaf, 1981).

8.3.3 Organ weights

Determination of organ weights is another long-established practice in toxicological studies. Usually, no changes have been reported in the gut except for the caecum. Many compounds, including food flavourings such as 4-methyl-1-phenylpentan-2-ol, have been shown to increase the weight of the caecum in rats (Ford *et al.*, 1983). The cause of this is disputed but physiological mechanisms involving changes in the microflora and the osmotic activity of caecal contents have been postulated (Leegwater *et al.*, 1974).

8.3.4 Gut microflora

The normal gastrointestinal tract is colonized by bacteria. Many of these are anaerobic Gram-negative organisms; their metabolism is largely reductive and hydrolytic and they may interact with a wide variety of chemicals. Enzymes present in the anaerobic flora of the caecum include nitrite reductase, azoreductase, imidazole reductase and glucosidase. In some situations, toxic compounds may be broken down; in other situations, they may be generated as in the action of bacterial glucosidase in the conversion of glycosides to toxic aglycones (Rowland, 1981; Williams, 1972). Bacterial flora can change readily for instance, in response to oral antibiotics or the ingestion of a high fibre diet, the gut microflora in rats has been shown to increase bacterial enzyme activities (Rowland *et al.*, 1983).

8.4 INTESTINAL ABSORPTION STUDIES

8.4.1 Whole body techniques

A basic approach to the clinical assessment of ingested compounds is to study absorption kinetics. This was significantly advanced when isotope labelling techniques were introduced. In man, after an oral dose of the test substance, analysis of faeces, urine, blood, saliva and expired air can be readily carried out (Walson *et al.*, 1981). Collection may be necessary for several days to ensure that delayed excretion is recognized. However, whole body analysis fails to detect localized concentrations of compounds of their metabolites in specific organs of the body.

In animals, pharmacokinetic evaluation may be extended to include tissue distribution and metabolism studies by measuring the radioactivity levels in various tissues and body fluids over time (Abou-Donia *et al.*, 1983)

8.4.2 *In vivo* techniques in animals

Transport and uptake studies may be undertaken in animals by using gut loops. A classic approach has been to construct isolated segments of small intestine. Thiry-Vella loops consist of a length of ileum, *in situ*, retaining its blood supply but externally cannulated at each end to allow perfusions to be carried out (Keren *et al.*, 1975). These preparations require a considerable amount of maintenance. For this reason, various other perfusion techniques have been developed. Triple lumen tubes may be inserted orally or, in animals, by means of a chronic jejunal fistula. After constant infusion to achieve a steady state, proximal and distal collections may be carried out to determine transport kinetics (Barbezat, 1980). Various animal models have been devised to allow *in vivo* perfusions of various lengths of gut within the abdominal cavity (Sandhu *et al.*, 1981) or in exteriorized loops for short periods; additional variants such as the effects of blood supply may also be studied (Granger *et al.*, 1976).

8.4.3 *In vitro* techniques

A basic approach has been to simply excise gut segments, tie their ends and place them in suitable media. Perfusion may be carried out by cannulating the ends of short lengths of excised gut, and perfusing them while immersed in an oxygenated medium. Various assays may be devised involving translocation of labelled compounds from the diffusing fluid to the serosal bath. Using this technique, Lyons *et al.* (1983) found that cadaverine, a substance present in spoiled fish, was able to inhibit the intestinal detoxification of histamine.

Ion transport may be studied by taking sheets of mucosa stripped of their serosal and muscle layers and mounting them in Ussing or Lucite chambers. The mucosa separates two reservoirs of oxygenated Ringer's solution, one bathing the serosal and the other the mucosal surfaces (Binder *et al.*, 1973). The potential difference across the mucosa may be monitored, and ion fluxes measured using, for instance, isotopes ^{22}Na and ^{36}Cl. Numerous compounds affect sodium, chloride and bicarbonate secretion and absorption. This can be demonstrated by adding them to the mucosal or serosal reservoirs and measuring changes in short-circuit current that reflect ion transport. Alpha-adrenergic stimulants have both anti-motility and anti-diarrhoeal activity; their effects in promoting sodium and chloride absorptions have been shown using this system (Durbin *et al.*, 1982).

Subcellular fractionation allows more detailed studies of intracellular enzyme function and dysfunction to be undertaken. The gut mucosa may be scraped off and homogenized, and subcellular fractions isolated by differential centrifugation. Studies using mitochondria, microsomes, nuclear and microvillus preparations have become practicable. Microsomes are vesicular structures visible under the electron microscope which represent the smooth endoplasmic reticulum within the cell. They are of particular importance in the current context since they carry a very high specific activity of metabolizing enzymes. Biotransformation of xenobiotics may be evaluated by incubating different substrates with microsomes (Stohs *et al.*, 1976). Amongst the various types of monooxygenase activity which have been shown to occur in intestinal tissues are: aromatic ring-hydroxylation; O-dealkylation; N-demethylation; sulphoxidation; and N-amine hydroxylation (Hoensch, 1982). Microsomal action may be influenced by many factors, for example, they are located primarily in the epithelial cells of the upper villus and may be dependent on additional factors such as dietary iron (Hoensch *et al.*, 1976). The biological effects of drugs and xenobiotics may be significantly affected by changes in intestinal metabolism, for example, phenacetin has been extensively studied and it has been found that its oxidative metabolism is increased in rats exposed to cigarette smoke (Welch *et al.*, 1972) and brassica vegetables (Pantuck *et al.*, 1976).

Enterocytes may be dissociated from the mucosa by chemical or mechanical means, and maintained in various culture systems (Hartmann *et al.*, 1982). The toxic effects of various xenobiotics on cell or organ cultures may be evaluated directly by measuring protein synthesis, enzyme activities and morphological changes using electron microscopy (L'Hirondel *et al.*, 1976). Over the last decade, enterocytes obtained from coeliac patients have been used to identify toxic fragments of ∝-gliadin; however, the difficulties encountered in obtaining sufficient cells from biopsy specimens and in standardizing the culture techniques have rendered many of these studies difficult to interpret (Falchuk *et al.*, 1974; Howdle *et al.*, 1981; Wood *et al.*, 1983).

8.5   FUNCTIONAL STUDIES IN MAN

Indirect evidence of mucosal damage may be gained from the use of conventional absorption tests and other parameters of gut function.

8.5.1   Absorption

Fat absorption is still most consistently evaluated by accurate but time-consuming measurements of intake and excretion in the stool over 3–5 days. Over the years, numerous tests to detect an increased faecal fat content have been described. More recently, specific monitoring of absorption has been undertaken using ^{14}C or stable ^{13}C labelled lipids and measuring the excreted labelled carbon dioxide in breath tests.

Changes in carbohydrate absorption can be a useful way of demonstrating enterocyte brush border damage. Lactase is a particularly vulnerable enzyme; more extensive injury will reduce sucrase and isomaltase activity, and eventually the absorption of the monosaccharides glucose and fructose can be affected. Lactose intolerance can be demonstrated on clinical challenge by the generation of watery stools of acid pH containing glucose, and confirmed by breath H_2 analysis. Disaccharidase activity may be measured directly in mucosal biopsy homogenates.

Protein absorption can be investigated laboriously using balance studies measuring N_2 excretion. A more elegant approach is to use a stable ^{15}N isotope and measuring urinary excretion after a labelled oral load. However, these methods would only indicate fairly gross evidence of mucosal damage.

8.5.2 Mucosal integrity

Various tests aim to evaluate mucosal integrity. The xylose absorption test is time honoured, but subject to various theoretical criticisms. Recently the differential absorption of two non-metabolized carbohydrate probe molecules of different molecular weight has been advocated. Lactulose, rhamnose, cellobiose or mannitol may be given orally and the urinary excretion ratio calculated. If the mucosa is damaged, more of the higher molecular weight carbohydrate is present in the urine. Polyethylene glycols of various molecular weights have also been used as probe materials. Another indirect indicator of enterocyte damage is protein loss in the stools; $\propto_1$ antitrypsin is a non-specific marker protein which can be measured.

8.5.3 Specific function

If more specific functional information is required, gastric acidity, pancreatic secretion and vitamin B_{12} absorption can all be investigated. Pancreatic function may be quantified by measuring duodenal juice lipase, trypsin, amylase and bicarbonate after intravenous injection of pancreozymin (CCK) and secretin, or after a test meal. Pancreatic function may also be measured indirectly by the *p*-aminobenzoic acid screening test. Similarly, bile acid secretions and pool size may be studied using direct analysis and isotope breath tests.

Gut motility is an area of increasing interest. Transit time measurements using carmine dye or polystyrene shapes of different sizes have been superseded by pressure manometry, electrical monitoring and the use of telemetry capsules. The normal pattern of electrical activity and motility of both the small and large bowel is now being better defined; however, disturbances associated with disease states have still not been well characterized.

8.6 CONCLUSION

It is evident from this review that a wide range of potential and practical approaches exist for the detection and evaluation of the toxicity of compounds to the gastrointestinal tract itself, and for the evaluation of factors which influence the absorption of ingested xenobiotics. At the cellular and subcellular levels, mucosal cells with intense metabolic activity and rapid turnover may be particularly appropriate for developing assay techniques. Although the intra-cellular enzyme systems of enterocytes are shared by cells in many other tissues, application to short-term *in vivo* and *in vitro* toxicity studies has yet to be adequately exploited. The demonstrable preservation of mucosal function would, nevertheless, seem to be a logical prerequisite for the evaluation of the safety of substances which may enter the body by the oral route or otherwise affect the gastrointestinal tract.

The gut is particularly vulnerable to dysfunction as a result of perturbations in both its internal and external milieu, thus enhancing its potential value for the evaluation of toxicity. Many of the organ's components and functions have similar but less accessible equivalents elsewhere in the body so that a continuous and economical alternative may be available for some test systems.

The development of new approaches to toxicity testing and safety evaluation involving the gut should, however, take account of its highly dynamic nature and overall lack of structural and functional homogeneity. Moreover, human subpopulations with developmental immaturity, particular nutritional status and with coexisting inflammatory or other enteropathic changes in the mucosa may experience modified toxicity of ingested substances. Toxicity may be modified in the gut itself, or in other organs when absorption from the gut is altered. Many of the problems identified here are at the limits of current knowledge; their elucidation will have scientific, clinical and toxicological implications.

REFERENCES

Abou-Donia, M.B., Reichert, B.L., and Ashry, M.A. (1983). The absorption, distribution, excretion and metabolism of a single oral dose of *O*-4-nitrophenyl phenylphosphonothioate in hens. *Toxicol. Appl. Pharmacol.*, **70**, 18–28.

Back, D.J., Bates, M., Breckenridge, A.M., Ellis, J.M., Hall, M., Maliver, M., Orme, L'E., and Rowe, O.H. (1981). The *in vitro* metabolism of ethinyl oestradiol, mestranol and levonorgestrel by human jejunal mucosa. *Br. J. Clin. Pharmacol.*, **11**, 275–8.

Barbezat, G.O. (1980). Triple-lumen perfusion of the canine jejunum. *Gastroenterology*, **79**, 1243–5.

Barbezat, G.O., and Hansen, J.D. (1968). The exocrine pancreas and protein-calorie malnutrition. *Pediatrics*, **42**, 77–92.

Barltrop, D. (1982). Nutritional and maturational factors modifying the absorption of inorganic lead from the gastrointestinal tract. In: Hunt, V.R., Smith, M.K., and Worth, D. (Eds), *Banbury Report II, Environmental Factors in Human Growth and Development*, Cold Spring Harbour Labortory, pp. 35–41.

Barltrop, D., and Khoo, H.E. (1975). The influence of nutritional factors on lead absorption. *Postgrad. Med. J.*, **51**, 795–800.

Becker, G.M., McNulty, W.P., and Bell, M. (1979). Polychlorinated biphenyl-induced morphologic changes in the gastric mucosa of the Rhesus monkey. *Lab. Invest.*, **40**, 373–83.

Bell, R.R., and Spickett, J.T. (1983). The influence of dietary fat on the toxicity of orally ingested lead in rats. *Food Cosmet. Toxicol.*, **21**, 469–72.

Binder, H.J., Powell, D.W., and Tai, Y.H. (1973). Electrolyte transport in rabbit ileum. *Am. J. Physiol.*, **225**, 776–80.

Carter, R.E., and Taylor, W.F. (1980). Identification of a particular amphibole asbestos fibre in tissues of persons exposed to a high oral intake of the mineral. *Environ. Res.*, **21**, 85–93.

Durbin, T., Rosenthal, L., McArthur, K., Anderson, D., and Dharmsathaphorn, K. (1982). Clonidine and lidamidine (WHR-1142) stimulate sodium and chloride absorption in the rabbit intestine. *Gastroenterology*, **82**, 1352–6.

Falchuk, Z.M., Gebhard, R.C., Sessoms, C., and Strober, W. (1974). An *in vitro* model of gluten-sensitive enteropathy. Effects of gliadin on intestinal epithelial cells of patients with gluten-sensitive enteropathy in organ culture. *J. Clin. Invest.*, **53**, 487–500.

Ford, G.P., Gopal, T., and Gaunt, I.F. (1983). Short-term toxicity of 4-methyl-1-phenylpentan-2-OL in rats. *Food Cosmet. Toxicol.*, **21**, 441–7.

Granger, D.N., Cook, B.H., and Taylor, A.E. (1976). Structural locus of transmucosal albumin efflux in canine ileum. A fluorescent study. *Gastroenterology*, **71**, 1023–7.

Hartmann, F., Owen, R., and Bissell, D.M. (1982). Characterization of isolated epithelial cells from rat small intestine. *Am. J. Physiol.*, **242**, G147–55.

Hietanen, E. (1980). Oxidation and subsequent glucuronidation of 3,4-benzopyrene in everted intestinal sacs in control and 3-methylchlanthrene-pretreated rats. *Pharmacology*, **21**, 233–43.

Hoensch, H., Woo, C.H., Raffin, S.B., and Schmid, R. (1976). Oxidative metabolism of foreign compounds in rate small intestine: Cellular localization and dependence on dietary iron. *Gastroenterology*, **70**, 1063–70.

Hoensch, H.P. (1982). Absorption and metabolism of xenobiotics in the intestine. In: Hunt, V.R., Smith, M.K., and Worth, D. (Eds), *Banbury Report II, Environmental Factors in Human Growth and Development*, Cold Spring Harbor Laboratory, pp. 89–103.

Hoensch, H.P., and Hartmann, F. (1981). The intestinal enzymatic biotransformation system: Potential role in protection from colon cancer. *Hepatogastroenterol.*, **28**, 221–8.

Howdle, P.D., Corazza, G.R., Bullen, A.W., and Losowsky, M.S. (1981). *In vitro* diagnosis of coeliac disease: an assessment. *Gut*, **22**, 939–47.

Keren, D.F., Elliott, H.L., Brown, G.D., and Yardley, J.H. (1975). Atrophy of villi with hypertrophy and hyperplasia of Paneth cells in isolated (Thiry-Vella) ileal loops in rabbits. *Gastroenterology*, **68**, 83–93.

Lebenthal, E., Lev, R., and Lee, P.C. (1981). Perinatal development of the exocrine pancreas. In: Lebenthal, E. (Ed.), *Textbook of Gastroenterology and Nutrition in Infancy*, Raven Press, New York, pp. 149–65.

Leegwater, D.C., Degroot, A.P., and Van Kalmthout-Kuyper, M. (1974). The aetiology of caecal enlargement in the rat. *Food Cosmet. Toxicol.*, **12**, 687–97.

L'Hirondel, C., Doe, W.F., and Peters, T.J. (1976). Biochemical and morphological studies on human jejunal mucosa maintained in culture. *Clin. Sci. Mol. Med.*, **50**, 425–9.

Lutsky, I., Mor, N., Yagen, B., and Joffe, A.Z. (1978). The role of T-2 toxin in experimental alimentary toxic aleukia: a toxic study in cats. *Toxicol. Appl. Pharmacol.*, **43**, 111–24.

Lyons, D.E., Beery, J.T., Lyons, S.A., and Taylor, S.C. (1983). Cadaverine and aminoguanidine potentiate: The uptake of histamine *in vitro* in perfused intestinal segments of rats. *Toxicol. Appl. Pharmacol.*, **70**, 445–58.

McConnell, E.E., and Shoaf, C.R. (1981). Studies on the mechanism of 2,3,7,8-tetrachlorodibenzo-*p*-dioxin (TCDD) toxicity lipid assimilation. 1. Morphology. *Pharmacologist*, **23**, 176.

Meek, M.E., and Grasso, P. (1983). An investigation of the penetration of ingested asbestos into the normal and abnormal intestinal mucosa of the rat. *Food Cosmet. Toxicol.*, **21**, 193–200.

Moog, F. (1981). Perinatal development of the enzymes of the brush border membrane. In: Lebenthal, E. (Ed.), *Textbook of Gastroenterology and Nutrition in Infancy*, Raven Press, New York, pp. 139–47.

Morris, B., and Morris, R. (1976). Quantitative assessment of the transmission of labelled protein by the proximal and distal regions of the small intestine of young rats. *J. Physiol. (London)*, **255**, 619–34.

Pantuck, E.J., Hsiao, K.C., Loub, W.D., Wattenberg, L.W., Kuntzman, R., and Conney, A.H. (1976). Stimulatory effect of vegetables on intestinal drug metabolism in the rat. *J. Pharmacol. Exp. Ther.*, **198**, 278–83.

Rowland, I. (1981). The influence of the gut microflora on food toxicity. *Proc. Nutr. Soc.*, **40**, 67–74.

Rowland, I.R., Wise, A., and Mallett, A.K. (1983). Metabolic profile of caecal micro-organisms from rats fed indigestible plant cell-wall components. *Food Cosmet. Toxicol.*, **21**, 25–9.

Sandhu, B.K., Tripp, J.H., Candy, D.C.A., and Harries, J.T. (1981). Loperamide: studies on its mechanism of action. *Gut*, **22**, 658–62.

Schiller, C.M., and Yagen, B. (1981). Inhibition of mitochondrial respiration by trichlothecene toxins from Fusarium sporotrichroides. *Fed. Proc.*, **40**(6), 1579.

Schrader, R.E., and Zeman, F.J. (1970). Effect of maternal protein deprivation on morphological and enzymatic development of neonatal rat tissue. *J. Nutr.*, **99**, 401–12.

Siegel, M., and Lebenthal, E. (1981). Development of gastrointestinal motility and gastric emptying during the fetal and newborn periods. In: Lebenthal, E. (Ed.), *Textbook of Gastroenterology and Nutrition*, Raven Press, New York, pp. 121–38.

Stohs, S.J., Grafström, R.C., Burke, M.D., and Orrenius, S. (1976). Xenobiotic metabolism and enzyme induction in isolated rat intestinal microsomes. *Drug Metab. Disp.*, **4**, 517–21.

Szabo, S., Silver, E.H., Gallacher, G.T., and Maull, E.A. (1983). Potentiation of duodenal ulcerogenic action of acrylonitrile by PCB or phenobarbital in the rat. *Toxicol. Appl. Pharmacol.*, **71**, 451–4.

Udall, J.N., and Walker, W.A. (1982). Macromolecular transport across the developing intestine. In: Hunt, V.R., Smith, M.K., and Worth, D. (Eds), *Banbury Report II, Environmental Factors in Human Growth and Development*, Cold Spring Harbor Laboratory, pp. 187–98.

Walson, P.D., Carter, D.E., Ryerson, B.A., Clark, D., and Parkinson, T.M. (1981). Intestinal absorption of two polymeric food dyes in man. *Food Cosmet. Toxicol.*, **19**, 687–90.

Welsh, R.M., Cavallito, J., and Loh, A. (1972). Effect of exposure to cigarette smoke on the metabolism of benzo(a)pyrene and acetophenetidin by lung and intestine of rats. *Toxicol. Appl. Pharmacol.*, **23**, 749–58.

Williams, R.T. (1972). Toxicological implications of biotransformation by intestinal microflora. *Toxicol. Appl. Pharmacol.*, **23**, 769–81.

Wood, G.M., Howdle, P.D., and Losowsky, M.S. (1983). *In vitro* toxicity of gluten fraction III on cultured coeliac biopsies shown by an effect on enzyme activities in isolated brush borders. *Gut*, **24**, A, 994.

CHAPTER 9

Specific Organ/System Toxicity: the Liver

JAMES W. BRIDGES

9.1 INTRODUCTION

Mammalian liver consists of at least fourteen different types of cells. Hepatocytes, the most common site of toxic action, account for between 60 per cent (rat) and 85 per cent (man) of the total number of cells in the liver, or 90–95 per cent of the total weight of the liver. The reticuloendothelial cells (also called Kupffer, littoral or sinusoidal cells) only constitute 5–10 per cent of liver by weight but they can comprise up to 35 per cent of the total cell population. Other cells include fat storing and pit cells.

Despite their morphological similarity, hepatocytes are not a homogeneous population. For example, those from the centrilobular region contain significantly higher levels of cytochrome P-450 (and are much more responsive to induction by phenobarbitone) than those derived from the mid-zonal or periportal regions. Cells of the periportal area tend to be more metabolically active than those of mid-zonal and centrilobular regions, probably because they are more richly endowed with blood and consequently with nutrients and oxygen.

The liver has a wide range of important physiological functions and is the site of a wide range of intermediary metabolite reactions. These functions include:

(1) synthesis of many serum proteins (such as albumin, fibronogen and clotting factors);

(2) formation and secretion of bile;

(3) storage of various substances (such as metals and vitamins);

(4) detoxification of endogenous and exogenous waste products (including drugs, environmental chemicals, active oxygen species and haem breakdown products).

The liver, despite its remarkable regenerative ability, is vulnerable to injury from many causes which may result in profound metabolic effects. These may be reversible or irreversible. Chemically-mediated liver toxicity in man may take various forms including hepatocyte necrosis, hepatitis, jaundice, vascular injury, porphyria, cirrhosis or neoplasia (see Table 9.1). Drug-induced liver damage is one of the commonest forms of iatrogenic disease. Jaundice, for example, occurs with many chemically-induced hepatic disease in man.

Pathological effects of disturbed hepatic function fall into three primary classes:

(1)   Hepatocellular failure or impaired hepatocellular function. This results from direct injury to hepatocytes leading to selective or total loss of function. It may also arise through chronic impairment of blood flow. Alterations in nitrogen metabolism, failure to remove bilirubin from blood and/or conjugate it, build up of porphyrins, reduced synthesis of plasma proteins, cyanosis and hormonal disturbances are possible consequences of hepatocellular failure.

(2)   Biliary obstruction. This may arise from blockage of the hepatic or common bile ducts or impaired flow. Consequences may include leakage of conjugated bilirubin and other bile constituents into the blood and reduced absorption of fats and fat soluble vitamins from the intestine. Prolonged cholestasis is likely to lead to hepatic necrosis.

(3)   Portal hypertension. This may develop due to obstruction of liver blood flow. As a result, blood may be shunted from the portal blood supply directly into

Table 9.1   Examples of chemically mediated hepatic injury in man

Chemical agent	Predominant effect
Acute toxicity	
Paracetamol	Necrosis
Tetracycline	Fatty change
Yellow phosphorus	Necrosis
Halothane	Necrosis
Phenylbutazone	Necrosis
Erythromycin estolate	Cholestasis
Chronic toxicity	
Methotraxate	Cirrhosis
Thorotrast	Hepatocellular/bile duct carcinoma
Vinyl chloride	Haemangiosarcoma
Chlorpromazine	Jaundice
Pyrrollizidine alkaloid	Veno occlusive disease
Alcohol	Cirrhosis
α-methyldopa	Cirrhosis
Oxy-phenisatin	Cirrhosis
Penicillin	Jaundice
Methyltestosterone	Jaundice
Triacetyloeandomycin	Jaundice
Iprindol	Jaundice
Isoniazid	Necrosis
Sulphonamides	Necrosis
p-aminosalicylic acid	Necrosis

the systemic circulation, thus by-passing the liver. These anastomoses may rupture. Toxic materials absorbed from the gut may build up in the blood due to failure of the liver to detoxify them.

9.1.1 Vulnerability of the liver

There are a number of reasons why the liver is a primary target for the toxic effects of chemical agents:

(1) Ingestion is a common route of exposure to chemicals. Chemicals absorbed in the stomach, small intestine or large intestine pass almost exclusively into the hepatic portal vein, and are transported to the liver in appreciable concentrations and amounts.

(2) The liver has a high capacity to non-specifically bind chemicals by virtue of its relatively large size and high cellular concentration of binding sites (including proteins such as ligandin, and extensive amounts of lipid-rich endoplasmic reticulum).

(3) The liver contains higher concentrations of the drug-metabolizing enzymes than any other tissue. Since these enzymes frequently cause the formation of toxic metabolites as well as bringing about detoxification, the liver is especially vulnerable to metabolite-mediated toxicity.

(4) The liver is the most biochemically diverse of all the organs, playing key roles in the utilization of absorbed nutrients, detoxification and excretion on endogenous and exogenous compounds and the synthesis of plasma proteins. This great range of activities renders the liver more vulnerable to toxins than many other organs.

9.1.2 Routes of chemical exposure of the liver

Since most of the blood supply to the gastrointestinal tract feeds into the portal circulation (it accounts for 80 per cent of the liver's blood supply), chemicals which are absorbed from the gastrointestinal tract will, in theory, expose the liver to higher concentrations of the agent than most other routes of administration.

Metabolism of some chemicals under the influence of gut microfloral metabolism will result in exposure of the liver tissue to a range of metabolites and breakdown products. Interestingly, some substances (e.g. dimethline) exhibit greater hepatoxicity by gavage than when given in the diet while the converse is true in other cases (e.g. griseofulvin).

After intraperitoneal administration, a large part of the dosage of a chemical will drain to the liver. The rate of this process will depend on the solubility of the chemical in the peritoneal fluid. The liver is also susceptible to the effects of chemicals present in the systemic circulation since it receives approximately 30 per cent of total cardiac output.

9.2 *IN VIVO* MODELS FOR LIVER TOXICITY

In vivo investigations, although usually physiologically more relevant, have a number of practical as well as ethical drawbacks:

(1) Only gross control can be exerted over the concentration of xenobiotics reaching a particular tissue site, and the time of exposure of that site to the xenobiotics.

(2) Monitoring of plasma or urine for toxic metabolites generally only picks up stable metabolites which tend to accumulate in these fluids. Metabolites which are reactive and may contribute significantly to the toxicological properties of the xenobiotic will frequently not be detected.

(3) Obfuscating factors *in vivo*, such as stress and other environmental variables, may interfere with the correct interpretation of data.

(4) Information about toxicity in man is usually the goal of toxicity studies. Many investigations cannot be made *in vivo* in man for ethical reasons.

9.2.1 Effectiveness of *in vivo* animal models for predicting hepatic toxicity in man

In some cases, *in vivo* tests using animals may fail to detect hepatic effects which do occur in man (false negative response). Such is often the case with chemically-induced hepatic disease which has an immunological basis. Drugs which induce jaundice in man (e.g. chlorpromazine, halothane, erythromycin, estolate) are very frequently not identified as having potential to cause jaundice using current methods with whole animals. Often, such effects are identified only in later clinical trials. Cirrhosis, caused by chronic alcohol poisoning, is another hepatic disease in man for which it is doubtful that a valid animal model yet exists.

There are also instances when animal tests produce hepatic disease which does not seem to occur in man (false positive responses). It would appear that a number of chemicals (e.g. clofibrate, phenobarbitone, DDT) which produce hepatocarcinoma in rodents (but are non-genotoxic in classical *in vivo* and *in vitro* tests) probably fall into this category. However, failure to identify a lesion in man may also be due to poor detection methods.

9.2.2 Methods to assess liver toxicity following *in vivo* tests

9.2.2.1 *Clinical observations*

In general, observations of animal behaviour are not helpful in distinguishing liver damage from other forms of malaise. The development of whole body proton nuclear magnetic resonance scanners suitable for small conscious animals seems likely to provide a powerful means for identifying changes in the liver and in other soft tissues. Already, such instruments are able to measure 4-mm 'slices' through the liver and measurement of 1-mm 'slices' should be possible in the near future.

9.2.2.2 *Morphology*

A number of useful morphological indices of liver damage are given in Table 9.2. Haematoxylin (H) and eosin (E) stained sections are inadequate as the sole basis for morphological assessment. For example, many of the hypolipidaemic agents, even at high doses, produce only minimal change as revealed by examination of H- and E-stained sections. In this case, however, histochemistry reveals changes in both glycogen and lipid, and electron microscopy demonstrates a very marked increase in the content of peroxisomes in the hepatocytes. Peroxisomal change is important to note since it appears to be directly related to the development of hepatic tumours.

More intelligent use of histochemical methods and development of suitable quantitative cytochemical methods are needed for toxicological studies. The increasing availability of selective antibodies and lectins also offers great potential both for selective diagnosis and for investigating mechanisms of toxicity.

9.2.2.3 *Serum biochemistry*

Serum biochemistry provides a useful indication of many types of liver damage (see Table 9.3). Important considerations in the selection of an appropriate parameter to

Table 9.2   Some important morphological indices of hepatic damage in the rat

---

Histology/histochemistry
Hypertropy
Hyperplasia
Lipofuscin
Green pigment
Eosinophilia
Necrosis
Nuclear changes (condensation, swollen and pale, fragmentation)
Balloon cell formation
Zone dependent glycogen loss
Centrilobular accumulation of fat

Electron microscopy
Peroxisome proliferation
Mitochondria proliferation
Smooth endoplasmic reticulum proliferation
Cannulicula debris
Increase in secondary lysosomes
Endoplasmic reticulum vacuolization
Lipid droplets
Disorganization of organelle relationships

Table 9.3   Serum and bile indices of hepatic damage in the rat

Index	Diagnostic value
Serum	
Alanine aminotransferase, Isocitrate dehydrogenase and sorbitol dehydrogenase	Release of cytoplasmic contents due to hepatocyte membrane damage
Glutamate dehydrogenase	Release of mitochondrial contents due to mitochondrial and plasma membrane damage
IgA, secretory component, 'bile type' 5NT and GT, alkaline phosphatase, LP-X	Cholestasis
Bile acids	Bile flow restriction/hepatic function
Albumin, γ-macroglobulin, α-fetoprotein, α-glycoprotein and heptoglobin	Acute injury anywhere
Bile	
Bile salts or bilirubin glucuronide	Hepatic damage
Serum protein, γ-glutamyl transferase	Bile duct lining cell damage
5′ nucleotidase	Hepatocyte damage

measure include:

(1) The ability of the particular index to detect liver damage (or injury to a particular type of cell) uniquely. A major problem is that a parameter which is suitable for study in one species may be unsuitable in another. For example, alanine aminotransferase found in high concentrations in the livers of rats, dogs, cats and primates is largely absent from the livers of pigs, sheep, horses and cattle.

(2) The half-life of the substance being measured. If the half-life is long, it may be difficult to relate effect to cause; with a very short half-life, the timing of the observation may be critical.

(3) Relationship of secondary consequences to the primary damage. For example, ligation of the bile duct for 24 hours causes a three-fold increase in alkaline phosphatase and a five-fold increase in bilirubin; there is also a ten-fold increase in both aspartate and alanine aminotransferases. These levels do not appear to be associated with morphological signs of injury at this time point. It has been suggested that extended cholestasis produces hepatocellular damage by causing an accumulation of dihydroxy bile acids, which cause micellar solubilization of cellular moieties. This, in turn, may result in a shift of

enzymes from organelles to cytoplasm and, hence, increased leakage from hepatocytes to the extracellular fluid.

(4) The relationship between the duration of damage and the release of a particular component into the serum. In many instances, the severity of damage may not be reflected in the levels of cellular components in the serum over prolonged periods of time. Studies of enzyme release after acute toxic liver injury in the rat have shown that there is frequently a distinct pattern of release of intra-cellular enzymes into the circulation. Cytoplasmic enzyme levels increase in serum within a few hours, followed by cytoplasmic and mitochondrial enzymes other than those of purely mitochondrial membrane origin. Subsequently, the depletion of constituents in necrotic cells leads to a decrease in the release of constituents into the serum. Hence, the direct relationship between morphological damage and serum composition no longer holds.

(5) Its stability during sample storage and sample work-up.

(6) Its ease of assay, including complexity of any sample work-up, possible presence in serum of interfering agents, etc. The sensitivity, precision and specificity of the assay needs to be defined and checked regularly.

Insufficient attention has been given to non-enzymatic proteins as an index of hepatic damage. The promise of this approach is indicated by the fact that hypolipidaemic agents induce dose-related changes in six proteins in rats detected by crossed immunoelectrophoresis. Two of these proteins appear to be specific for hypolipidaemic agents.

9.2.2.4 Tissue biochemistry

A list of useful tissue biochemistry indices of hepatic damage is given in Table 9.4. However, suitable indices of damage to non-hepatic cells are not available, nor are sensitive indices of damage to particular organelles in hepatocytes. A good specific marker for one type of organelle will not necessarily provide a suitable index of damage to that organelle. For example, succinate dehydrogenase is an excellent marker for mitochondria, but its activity is not necessarily altered following subtle mitochondrial damage.

9.2.2.5 Liver function

A number of tests of hepatic function are available although they are not generally applied in toxicology (see Table 9.5). Many of these tests are somewhat insensitive because the liver has a large functional reserve. Most commonly, an endogenous or exogenous chemical probe is employed which assesses the ability of the liver to metabolize and/or excrete (e.g. bilirubin, bromosulphthalein, radio-contrast media, bromocresol green), or assesses the rate of incorporation of precursors into macromolecules (e.g. ^{3}H-thymidine, ^{14}C or ^{35}S amino acids, etc.). It is hoped that

Table 9.4   Tissue biochemical indices of liver damage in the rat

Index	Diagnostic value
Glucose-6-phosphatase	Endoplasmic reticulum damage
Glutathione level	Production of electrophiles/free radicals
P-450 isoenzymes	Induction (certain unique forms may indicate potential chronic damaging agents)
5′ nucleotidase and ATPase	Plasma membrane damage
γ-glutamyl transferase (rats only), alkaline β-glycerophosphatase	Cell division, cholestasis
Uroporphyrin, protoporphyrin	Porphyria
β-galactosidase	Lysosome enlargement

Table 9.5   Examples of tests of liver function which may be used in the rat

Test	Diagnostic value
Bromosulphthalein, benzoic acid, indocyanin green, bilirubin	Transport and/or metabolism of added agent
Tritiated thymidine	DNA synthesis

improved understanding of membrane and cytoplasmic transport of endogenous and exogenous materials, coupled with improved microsurgical techniques, will lead to the development of more subtle and sensitive tests of liver function.

9.2.3   Chemically/surgically manipulated *in vivo* models

9.2.3.1   *Surgical preparations*

Three surgical preparations are commonly used to study effects of chemicals on the liver: biliary cannulation, cannulation of the hepatic portal vein, and partial hepatectomy. Biliary cannulation is mainly employed to determine the biliary excretion of drug metabolites. Although these models are suitable for some purposes, they have not generally mimicked fully the normal animal since specimens had to be anaesthetized or restrained. However, a number of techniques are now available which allow the animals to be unrestrained and conscious.

Cannulation of the hepatic portal vein is used to assess metabolism and/or uptake of xenobiotics by the gut or as a method by which to administer xenobiotics directly to the liver.

A favoured model for reducing the functional reserve of the liver is partial hepatectomy. This increases the liver's sensitivity to xenobiotics. Partial hepatectomy has also been used to study the effects of chemicals on cell division.

9.2.3.2 Chemically manipulated models

A wide range of chemicals have been employed to produce selective modifications in hepatic function for investigating the effects of a toxic chemical on that function. For example, modification of drug metabolizing activity can be achieved using selective enzyme inducers (such as phenobarbitone, 3-methylcholanthrene, iso-safrole, clofibrate and pregenolone carbonitrile) or inhibitors (such as cobalt chloride, piperonyl butoxide and SKF525A). Diethylmaleate is only moderately hepatotoxic and may be used to deplete glutathione thereby enabling the toxic effects of electrophiles to be more fully expressed. Chemicals such as carbon tetrachloride and paracetamol have been employed to produce selective damage in order to reduce the functional reserve of the liver. However, the effects of these chemicals tend to be rather poorly reproducible.

9.3 *IN VITRO* MODELS

There is no single ideal *in vitro* hepatic preparation for toxicological investigations, nor is there likely to be. Since no *in vitro* system can mimic all of the intricate and complex interactions which occur within an organism, only a limited assessment can be made of the adverse effects of xenobiotic *in vitro*. Therefore, the preparation must be selected in the light of the particular purpose of the intended experiment. These data can then be compared with those obtained *in vivo* and a prediction made of the compound's likely effect in a human being.

Some of the obvious limitations of the exclusively *in vitro* approach can be overcome by deriving the appropriate culture preparation from animals which have been pretreated in various ways (see 9.2.3.2 above). This approach is particularly useful where pharmokinetic considerations are critical to the expression of toxicity or where the useful lifetime of the *in vitro* preparation is rather short.

9.3.1 Perfused liver

Isolated perfused organs are particularly useful for evaluating the complex interrelationships between heterogeneous cell types or between different metabolic pathways. Variations in pharmacokinetics with time and dose are probably best studied in the perfused organ as opposed to other *in vitro* preparations. As yet, other than tissue slices, liver perfusion offers the only potential model for studying chemically-induced portal hypertension or biliary obstruction.

9.3.1.1   Perfused organ viability

Bile flow is useful as a viability index. Bile flow tends to drop with the time of perfusion since the endogenous bile acid pool is depleted during bile collection. Another easily recognizable viability criterion is perfusion flow rate. Once a stable flow is attained, the flow rate through the liver can be used as a readily available criterion for evaluating the organ's viability.

Another easily detectable criterion is visual appearance of the liver. Inadequately perfused liver gives a reddish appearance, (indicating anoxia) as well as a blotchy appearance on the surface of the liver. Oxygen consumption by the liver can also be used as a criterion for viability. Oxygen consumption can be measured by following the oxygen tension (PO_2) in the perfusate after it effuses from the liver.

A number of biochemical indices can also be used for ascertaining viability of the perfused liver including concentrations of glycolytic intermediates, respiratory quotient, and adenine nucleotide levels. A variety of other biochemical parameters may also be used, such as surface luminescence changes (which indicate cofactor status or lipid peroxidation), incorporation of ^{14}C-lysine into proteins, and activity of microsomal mixed function oxidase (MFO) and cytochrome P-450 levels. Satisfactory preservation of the hepatic MFO system is usually maintained after a 4-hour perfusion when a perfusate containing erythrocytes is used.

Biliary excretion of sulphobromophthalein (BSP) and indocyanine green have also been useful as a measure of the functional status of the isolated perfused liver. The disadvantage of using such markers for functional status is that, after establishing that they are indeed viable, the same perfused livers cannot be used for many toxicological purposes.

Although routine histological examination of perfused livers is not conducted, the technique may be useful in setting up a perfused preparation. Several authors reporting results of histological examinations of perfused livers have indicated the general usefulness of morphological examination in ascertaining the viability of perfused liver systems. However, one should be aware that morphological examinations may be of limited usefulness, since cells that appear abnormal morphologically may retain normal cellular function and, conversely, normal appearing cells may exhibit abnormal cellular functions.

9.3.1.2   Considerations and limitations of perfused liver systems

Although perfusion is a very time-consuming and relatively expensive method compared with other procedures, it is clearly of great value for studying particular aspects of toxicity, such as biliary clearance and blood-flow effects. Unfortunately, problems of technique do exist which are serious drawbacks when considering the more general applicability of the perfused liver systems. These drawbacks include: the possible interference from hormones and vasoactive factors if blood is used as the perfusate (particularly if the blood is heterologous); the problem of adequate gas exchange; the short time (less than 6 hours) during which each preparation is viable; the problem of choosing appropriate parameters of organ viability during perfusion; the difficulty in setting up more than one perfusion at a time; poor reproducibility in the hands of many workers; and the problem of adequate controls.

The predominant use of liver perfusion in toxicology to date has been to study metabolism of xenobiotics. Chemicals investigated include benzo(a)pyrene, chlorpromazine, imipramine, phenylbutazone, antipyrine, nortriptyline, *p*-nitrophenol, barbiturates and vinyl chloride.

Liver perfusion has also been used to examine the effects of: carbon tetrachloride on hepatocellular architecture and vascular resistance; sporidesmin and icterogenin on the mechanisms of bile secretion; hypoxia on lysosomal enzymes; mirex on the biliary excretion of metabolites of monochlorobiphenyl.

Particular problems exist with perfused liver systems which must be addressed. There is a need to prolong viability in order to study more than just immediate acute toxicity. Improved reproducibility between preparations is required. Development of better synthetic perfusion media offer the best prospects of achieving this latter goal. Also, better methods for handling single lobes and parts of lobes need to be developed so that perfusion studies can be applied readily to larger species, including man.

9.3.2 Cell and tissue culture

Freshly isolated tissue slices and snips have been used for a number of toxicological studies. Recently, these have been used to study the metabolism of xenobiotics and their effects on cellular respiration. Such preparations are composed of a variety of liver cell types and tend to retain the integrity of receptors. However, when cultured, these preparations tend to become necrotic at their centre and their permeability to added xenobiotics may be poor. Consequently, their useful lifetime is rather short. Improvement of systems for extending culture viability is an essential prerequisite for the more extensive adoption of tissue slices for toxicological purposes.

Isolated cells provide an excellent experimental model to study microsomal activation/deactivation of chemicals and the subsequent reactivity of metabolites with cellular macromolecules such as DNA, RNA and protein. They are especially valuable for studying mechanisms of action.

The advantages of isolated or cultured cells for investigating hepatotoxicity include:

(1)   Freedom from major variables such as hormones or nutrients. This enables problems such as hormone effects on toxicity to be investigated.
(2)   Prolonged viability of cell cultures, compared with organ perfusions.
(3)   Ready and equal access to the chemical by each cell. There is much more rigid control of dosing, concentration and time of exposure to the xenobiotic with these systems.

(4) The possibility of making direct studies of changes going on within the cells (e.g. binding of substrates to cytochrome P-450, cytochemical assessment of enzyme activity in the cells). Accumulation of metabolites or other products may be measured in the cells as well as in the medium.

(5) Direct investigation of the relationship between kinetics, metabolism and toxicity. For example, changes within the cells (such as DNA damage, DNA-repair activity, enzyme leakage, or cell-growth characteristics) can be correlated with metabolite production or metabolic inhibition. As an example of the use of metabolic inhibition, incubating cells under an atmosphere of carbon monoxide permits the identification of cell effects which are mediated by the P-450 oxidase system.

(6) Reduction of the time scale for the detection of a toxic effect.

For routine toxicological studies, it would obviously be most convenient to use a preparation of cells which readily reproduces itself *in vitro*. Dividing 'hepatocyte-like' populations may be derived from the livers of partially hepatectomized animals, from very young animals or from liver tumours.

Although culturing allows the hepatocytes to recover from the trauma of the isolation procedure (which is manifested, for example, by the initial loss of some glutathione in freshly isolated cells), the more prolonged the culture period, the greater the likelihood of some loss of normal *in vivo* characteristics. This dedifferentiation is particularly likely with dividing cell populations.

Other questions to be considered in the preparation of cell cultures include: Does the isolation procedure impair the functional capabilities of the cell? What is the viability of the cells (i.e. to what extent are the plasma membranes intact after isolation)? Of what origin are the isolated cells (are they fibroblasts, parenchymal cells or cells of the reticuloendothelial system)?

9.3.2.1 *Methods of preparation*

Tissue dispersion involves both the dissolution of the extracellular matrix and the breaking of cell-to-cell contacts without severe damage to the plasma membrane. A range of chemical, mechanical and enzymic methods have been used to separate hepatocytes. The best method involves the enzyme collagenase and starved animals. The enzyme may either be perfused through the portal vein and vena cava or added slices of liver. Perfusion produces better yields but treatment of slices is technically less demanding, cheaper and is especially suited for small biopsy samples.

Hepatocytes can be separated from other cells by differential centrifugation using gradients such as metrizamide. To check the purity of separated cells, isoenzymes of cytoplasmic pyruvate kinase have been recommended to identify hepatocytes from non-hepatocytes.

To prepare non-hepatocyte preparations, the favoured method is to incubate with pronase, which results in suspensions almost free of hepatocytes. Kupffer cells can be isolated from such preparations, since other non-hepatocytes tend not to attach to the walls of plastic culture vessels. This property of Kupffer cells can also be advantageous for removing them from cell preparations. Unfortunately, Kupffer cells tend to phagocytose during the separation and purification process resulting in accumulation of cell debris which may interfere with the assessment of the effects of exogenous chemicals. Alternatively, iron-sorbitol or triton WR 1339 can be used to load Kupffer cells to increase their density prior to centrifugation. Endothelial cells of 90 per cent purity can be produced by this approach. A centrifugal elutriator can also be employed for cell separation. Effective methods have yet to be developed for isolating bile duct lining cells.

9.3.2.2 Culture viability

It is often appropriate to check the general viability of cells both before and during a study of the effects of xenobiotics. There are no ideal viability parameters. They should be selected to suit the species of origin and the organelle or biochemical system under scrutiny (see Table 9.6). For example, for investigations of drug uptake which require information on the normality of the plasma membrane, determination of the uptake of polar dyes (e.g. trypan blue), observation of the effects of addition of endogenous chemicals on cellular performance (e.g. NADPH on ethoxycoumarin dethylase) or determination of leakage of cytoplasmic constituents into the medium (e.g. transaminases, dehydrogenases, ATP or potassium) may prove suitable. For study of the properties of the rough endoplasmic reticulum function, tests such as amino acid incorporation into proteins might be more appropriate.

For maintenance cultures, readily identifiable morphological changes can be used to monitor viability (e.g. vacuolization, granulation, blebbing, including contamination of the preparation by fibroblasts, yeasts, etc.), but more subtle dedifferentiation changes may take place. With rat hepatocytes, loss of phenobarbitone-type P-450, followed by loss of the mechanism for synthesizing particular isoforms of P-450,

Table 9.6 Parameters of hepatocyte viability

Assessment	Test substance
Vital dye uptake	Trypan blue, erythrocin B
Changes in oxygen consumption	Succinate
Enzyme leakage	Transaminases
Leakage of other constituents	Potassium
Changes in enzyme activity	NADPH, NADH or glucose-6-phosphate
Cell membrane morphology	N/A

appears to be one of the earliest changes to take place and might, therefore, be employed as a viability parameter. The relative contribution of fetal type cells can be monitored by biochemical indicators such as $\propto$-fetoprotein, alkaline phosphatase, and $\propto$-glutamyl transpeptidase. No single viability parameter is likely to be adequate.

Antibiotics such as penicillin and streptomycin are usually added to cell cultures for prolonged investigations. However, in particular studies where antibiotics may interfere (investigation of the transport of anti-cancer drugs or mixed-cell studies with mutant bacteria, for example) it is possible to work without antibiotics, provided that rigorous sterile techniques are employed.

Most maintenance-culture preparations use a solid surface onto which the cells adhere and flatten. The material used may depend on the species from which the cells were removed. For rat hepatocytes, polystyrene or collagen-coated glass or floats are generally used. Polycarbonate appears to be more effective for rabbit hepatocytes.

The requirements for maintaining dividing hepatocyte-derived lines tend to be rather similar to those for maintenance cultures, although it is important to remember that dividing cells do utilize nutrients much more rapidly than non-dividing cells.

9.3.2.3   *Current and potential* in vitro *techniques using liver cells*

Hepatocyte cell preparations have several uses in toxicology. They can be used to examine 'liver-specific' effects of chemicals. For this purpose, the hepatocytes must represent as closely as possible their state *in vivo*. They can also serve as a general model of the toxic effects in many other cell types.

Hepatocytes are a particular relevant model for chemicals which mediate their effects wholly or partly through the formation of active metabolites. Hepatocytes can be used to provide a source of toxic metabolites, the biological effects of which are monitored in a second cell type, or in the hepatocytes themselves.

Primary-maintenance cultures of adult rat hepatocytes frequently become progressively overgrown with fibroblasts. A cytotoxicity test has been devised which uses inhibition of fibroblast growth as an endpoint. Hepatocytes have also been used successfully as the metabolizing system in a number of mutagenicity tests.

A variety of methods may be used to characterize toxic effects. These methods include:

(1)   membrane change (permeability, active transport or surface-chemistry changes);
(2)   alterations in the synthesis, degradation, conformation or availability of macromolecules or growth-related factors;
(3)   modifications in intermediary metabolism;
(4)   changes in activity, growth, morphological (including organelle changes) or behavioural characteristics.

Freshly isolated hepatocytes can often be used to identify and characterize rapidly developing endpoints such as initial inhibition of protein and RNA synthesis or enzyme leakage. Primary-maintenance cultures, on the other hand, are employed to study more slowly developing lesions such as mitotic rate changes and identification of sustained alterations in organelles.

It is often possible to measure several endpoints produced by a chemical using a single preparation of hepatocytes. Positive controls can be used to ascertain the relevance of any observed changes in a preparation.

The plasma membrane is the first part of the cell to be exposed to toxins and it is, therefore, not surprising that it is a common site of toxic damage. Determinants of toxicity to the membrane include the uptake of polar dyes (such as trypan blue), co-factors (e.g. NADPH), or polar substrates (e.g. succinate). These are normally excluded from the cell by the plasma membrane. Leakage of cytoplasmic enzymes into the surrounding media has also been used by many workers as an indicator of cytotoxicity. One great advantage of studying enzyme leakage in hepatocytes is that it is a parameter which is frequently studied *in vivo*. Morphological changes in the membrane (e.g. blebbing, or rounding up of cells) may also be used as cytotoxicity criteria.

Isolated hepatocytes provide a useful model for assessing the toxicological significance of lipid peroxidation reactions. Both the drug-metabolizing enzymes and the various defense systems (e.g. catalase, superoxide dismutase, glutathione peroxidase and cellular antioxidants) bear the same quantitative relationship to one another as *in vivo*. However, few studies of lipid peroxidation have been made in isolated hepatocytes.

Many chemicals cause a significant inhibition of protein and RNA synthesis under conditions in which little or no cytotoxicity is observed. Studies on protein synthesis inhibition in hepatocytes have so far been largely restricted to measuring reduced rates of ^{14}C-leucine incorporation into acid-precipitable material.

Determination of the increased synthesis of macromolecules is liable to be a more specific indicator of selective toxicity than measurement of synthesis inhibition. Many carcinogens are known to damage DNA and therefore trigger increased unscheduled DNA repair. Hepatocytes provide a particularly relevant model in which to study such effects. DNA synthesis is minimal in hepatocytes in the absence of DNA-damaging agents (these cells have a very slow rate of cell division). This test is now widely used, with others, to identify genotoxic agents either *in vitro* or ex-*in vivo*.

Cells which have flattened out on a solid transparent surface such as collagen-coated glass or polystyrene are particularly amenable to the quantitative histochemical determination of the activity of cellular enzymes. Application of quantitative histochemical techniques to the study of toxic effects of chemicals on enzyme activity in cultured hepatocytes is still in its infancy, but early results are promising. For example, primary adult rat hepatocytes have been employed to investigate cytochrome P-450 induction by various barbiturates and benzanthracene. Primary maintenance cultures of rat hepatocytes have also been employed to test for peroxysome proliferating agents. Since this class of chemical is known to cause hepatocarcinoma, but is not detected by present genotoxicity tests, the use of hepatocytes for this purpose is important.

The identification of significant covalent binding often provides a valuable pointer to the role of active metabolites in toxicity. For example, the extent of covalent binding of ^{14}C-labelled isosafrole metabolites to hepatocyte proteins is comparable to that observed *in vivo* whereas covalent binding in liver microsomes is much higher. However, it is difficult to interpret the toxicological significance of covalent binding results unless indicators of cellular functional integrity are determined in a parallel study.

Changes in cofactor levels often result from chemical insults. ATP may be especially vulnerable. The formation of reactive metabolites may result in significant depletion of glutathione. For example, reactive metabolites of paracetamol and bromobenzene reduce glutathione levels in isolated adult rat hepatocytes, which allows increased covalent binding to cellular proteins, thereby producing cytotoxicity. BCNU also rapidly diminishes cellular glutathione. Isosafrole and safrole may exert their toxic effects, at least in part, by a similar mechanism.

Rather little attention has been paid to the use of morphological end-points as indicators of toxicity in spite of the fact that histopathology is the predominant technique in conventional toxicology for identifying toxic changes. Hepatocytes in primary culture display a very slow division rate. However, certain carcinogens can enhance the mitotic index.

A number of areas require further attention in order to improve *in vitro* techniques for toxicity studies. These areas include: the development of improved procedures for preparing and storing human hepatocytes; the extension of the useful lifetime of primary maintenance cultures in order to study the mechanisms of slow onset hepatotoxicity; the development of effective, synthetic culture media for hepatocytes; the identification of a means of preserving the constitutive P-450 isoenzymes and other drug metabolizing enzymes at the levels and activities found *in vivo* (this is particularly important for studies of metabolite mediated toxicity); development of suitable cell purification methods for the minor hepatic cell types, in particular, bile duct lining cells (this may be especially relevant to the understanding of some forms of drug-induced jaundice); improved methods for following the movement of xenobiotics and xenobiotic-endogenous macromolecular complexes (e.g. drug-receptor complexes) within cells. Modern molecular biology techniques also allow the transference of hepatic drug metabolizing enzymes to other rapidly dividing cell types.

9.3.3   Cell homogenates and fractions

The primary hepatotoxic effects of a chemical are in many cases rather specific to a particular macromolecule or organelle. Moreover, the ultimate toxin which manifests this primary effect is often created by particular isoenzymes of the drug metabolizing enzymes. Details of the processes involved are often best investigated using cell homogenates or cell fractions. This approach can be applied to the investigation of toxicity in both *in vivo* and *in vitro* systems and has been used extensively to examine the nature of the enzymes involved in the biotransformation of xenobiotics.

Methodological constraints involved in the use of cell homogenates and fractions are:

(1)　Homogenization of a tissue which contains several cell types may obfuscate understanding of the contribution of minority cell types to the process under investigation. It may also lead to the unjustified assumption that all the cells of the majority cell type are homogeneous in function.

(2)　Tissue homogenization can lead to artefactual changes in the homogenate due to hydrolytic destruction of membrane components and co-factors through the liberation of lysosomal enzymes. The homogenization procedure may also lead to activation or inhibition of various enzymes by other means. For example, the nature of the homogenizing medium used can greatly affect the functional state of mitochondria and the mitochondrial inhibition of microsomal biphenyl 2- and 4-hydroxylase activity when assayed in homogenates. Furthermore, compartmentalized endogenous inhibitors may be liberated by homogenization.

(3)　The levels of co-factors used in the incubations are generally optimal only for the enzyme(s) under study and in all probability do not correspond with levels existing within the cell. Therefore, they may give an undue emphasis to the formation of certain metabolites which are of minor significance *in vivo*. A good example here is the extremely high co-factor levels used in nitroreductase assays. Also, formation of a toxic metabolite may be of little consequence to the cell in which it is formed if it is immediately bound to a non-essential protein or is rapidly conjugated and excreted.

(4)　The use of isolated subcellular fractions will not necessarily reflect the total cellular effects of a chemical if its effects involve interactions between a number of different organelles.

(5)　Many toxic reactions depend on the entry of the xenobiotic into the cell and cannot be assessed in isolated cell fractions. Hepatocytes are readily permeable to most lipophilic xenobiotics and, therefore, it is probably uncommon for uptake to be rate limiting for toxicity. However, for metals and certain drugs, this is an important consideration. For methotrexate, for example, active transport processes govern cellular uptake.

(6)　Due consideration must be given to the importance, for the purpose of the experiment, of freedom from contamination and viability of the preparation being used.

(7)　Where *in vivo* pretreatment with a chemical precedes the liver homogenization and fractionation, attention must be given to the possibility that the treatment may modify the homogenization and separation conditions. For example, organelle membranes may become more fragile and, therefore, destroyed by the homogenization process.

Although techniques exist to separate and purify cellular components and enzymes, a number of difficulties must be overcome to improve their use in toxicology. These problems include:

(1) Improved purity and storage of organelle preparations, particularly plasma membranes, Golgi apparatus and CURL;
(2) Identification of sensitive indices of damage for each organelle;
(3) Development of techniques for transferring chemically pretreated organelles between cells in order to identify the relationship between primary and secondary lesions;
(4) Improved techniques for investigating organelle interactions;
(5) Improved techniques for enzyme and receptor extraction and purification.

9.3.3.1 *Mitochondria*

Enzymes involved in energy production, carbohydrate metabolism, haem biosynthesis, and the urea cycle are found in the mitochondria. There are a variety of biochemical parameters that can be used to assess mitochondrial function. In part, the effectiveness of these depends on the procedures used to isolate the mitochondria. Assessment of ion transport or coupling of oxidative phosphorylation with respiration are favoured methods of assessing viability.

Many of the enzymes involved in intermediary metabolism, including dehydrogenases for pyruvate, malate and glutamate, are localized in the mitochondrial matrix. Toxicant damage here has been demonstrated for agents such as arsenic, carbon tetrachloride, and methyl mercury. Trace metals such as arsenic, lead, mercury and cadmium inhibit mitochondrial respiration. For lead and arsenic, this inhibition is relatively specific for NAD-linked substrates such as pyruvate/malate.

Three of the key enzymes in the haem biosynthetic pathway are associated with the inner mitochondrial membrane. Ferrochelatase and δ-aminolevulinic acid synthetase are highly sensitive to the action of toxic trace metals (resultant increases in the urinary excretion of porphyrin precursors have proved to be useful *in vivo* biological indicators of this toxicity).

Mitochondrial swelling and contraction is caused by agents such as arsenic, carbon tetrachloride, and phosphate. These effects can be detected by measurement of light scattering in a spectrophotometer. This method is based on the increased optical density of mitochondria in a contracted state and decreased density in a swollen or orthodox configuration due to cation influx.

Movement of H^+, Na^+, K^+ or Ca^{2+} between isolated mitochondria and the surrounding medium may be monitored by specific ion electrodes. Changes in the transport of these cations have resulted from exposure to mercurials and lead. Energy-dependent mitochondrial uptake of arsenic has also been demonstrated.

Biochemical changes resulting from *in vivo* exposure to arsenate, cortisone and methyl mercury, as well as vitamin E deficiency, have been related to mitochondrial morphometry.

9.3.3.2   Lysosomes

Lysosomes are primarily involved in hydrolysis of endogenous materials. Active lysosomes (secondary lysosomes) may be cytochemically distinguished from inactive (teleolysosomes) or autophagic vacuoles by the presence of acid phosphatase activity. Lability may be determined by assessing the leakage of hydrolases from the lysosomes. The various acid hydrolase activities in lysosomes are an important means of assessing lysosome functionality. These assays are frequently performed on lysed lysosomes so that activities of the lysosomal enzymes may be more clearly separated from those present in the microsomal fraction. Marker enzymes frequently measured are the cathepsins A, B, C and D, acid phosphatase, aryl sulphatase, glycosidases, and acid RNAase.

X-ray microanalysis has been used by several investigators to demonstrate the presence of toxic trace metals within lysosomes following *in vivo* administration of the metal. Histochemical staining methods have also been used to demonstrate lysosomal uptake of metals in cells of metal-exposed animals.

In vitro exposure of lysosomes to agents such as toxic metals or mycotoxins has been found to alter the ability of lysosomes to perform the basic function of protein degradation. Protein degradation by lysosomes has been followed by monitoring the release of ^{125}I from labelled proteins following either *in vitro* or *in vivo* incubation. Alterations of lysosomal membrane stability has been shown to occur on exposure of lysosomes to chemicals such as the retenoids.

9.3.3.3   Endoplasmic reticulum

The main function of the endoplasmic reticulum is protein synthesis. The endoplasmic reticulum contains a series of flavoproteins and cytochromes that function in electron transport, ultimately resulting in the activation and reduction of molecular oxygen. The endoplasmic reticulum incorporates a number of oxidative (e.g. P-450 isoenzymes) and conjugative (e.g. glucuronyl transferases) drug metabolizing enzymes. Oxidative, reductive and occasionally conjugation reactions may lead to the formation of reactive electrophilic intermediates.

Viability of the endoplasmic reticulum can be assessed by measurement of malondialdehyde levels and the activity of glucose-6-phosphatase, P-450 or cytochrome P-450 reductase.

Toxicological interest in the endoplasmic reticulum relates particularly to the potential use of the proteins synthesized there as sensitive biochemical indicators of toxicity and the insight it may give into the mechanism of toxic actions of particular chemicals. A common approach is to inject radiolabelled amino acids into intact animals. The incorporation of the radiolabel into specific proteins is then determined. Subsequent protein purification is undertaken to assess synthesis/degradation of individual proteins.

Measurement of lipid peroxidation may be used as an index of oxygen or organic free-radical production. Malondialdehyde is the most widely measured index of lipid peroxidation, although it is insufficient on its own as an index of the peroxidation process.

Covalent binding of radiolabelled chemical to the microsomes themselves or to added macromolecules is an index of the reactivity of the chemical and/or its metabolites. In assessing covalent binding, it is most important to use exhaustive methods (e.g. solvent extraction) to distinguish accurately between true covalent binding and non-specific adsorption of the radiolabel.

9.3.3.4   *Reconstituted and purified subcellular systems*

The use of crude cell fractions allows only limited characterization of individual components. Research in respect of xenobiotics has focused particularly on the purification of the drug metabolizing enzymes. Studies have been or can be undertaken to assess substrate specificity of individual enzymes or identification of specific sites of covalent binding, for example. A variety of techniques have been used to purify individual components of the system and to reconstitute the electron transport chain.

The main methods to purify cell fractions are detergent extraction, column chromatography, and preparative electrophoresis. The success of the purification procedure can be assessed in a number of ways but no single technique is sufficient. Sodium dodecyl sulphate (SDS)-polyacrylamide gel electrophoresis is a powerful technique but has some limitations. Evidence has been presented that different microsomal enzymes cannot always be distinguished by this technique. Furthermore, the results obtained with this technique are rather dependent upon the exact procedure used.

Isoelectric focusing offers a great potential for resolution of enzymes and has been used in studying cytochrome P-450. However, a number of artefacts are related to the use of this methodology and, at the present time, one should view data obtained using isoelectric focusing of membrane proteins with caution.

Antibodies have been used to examine the homogeneity of isolated enzyme fractions, the multiplicity of enzymes in microsomes, and the amounts of individual enzyme forms in microsomal preparations. Other immunological techniques that can be used include double-diffusion analysis, radial diffusion quantitation, inhibition of enzyme activity complement fixation, radioimmune assay, crossed gel electrophoresis, immunoprecipitation, immunoaffinity column chromatography and immunohistochemical localization.

9.4   SUMMARY

No single test is now or is ever likely to be able to provide all the information that is required in order to assess the hepatotoxic properties of a chemical. Rather, a range of viable liver preparations is required from which can be selected the most appropriate model(s) for the particular question being asked. As yet, *in vitro* methods would not appear to be of much value in identifying delayed onset/idiosyncratic hepatotoxicity. Liver fractions and hepatocytes are presently most usefully employed once a hepatotoxic property of a chemical has been identified *in vivo*. These *in vitro* preparations are used to determine the contribution of reactive metabolites to the toxic process and ascertain the mechanism(s) of toxicity.

The rapid developments in methodology for handling isolated cells indicate that, in the near future, such *in vitro* preparations may also be suitable for the initial screening of chemicals for acute hepatotoxic properties and for obtaining information on the relative response to a chemical of human liver compared with other species.

9.5 RECOMMENDATIONS

In vitro methods to identify and characterize chemicals whose primary toxicity is to non-hepatocyte liver cells should be approached by the development of cell isolation and separation techniques which will enable such cells to be cultured in a viable state. This must be accompanied by improved liver perfusion methods in order to prolong the viability and reproducibility of perfusion systems. This work on techniques should be allied with detailed studies of the mechanisms of both acute and delayed cholestasis and portal hypertension.

Improvements are needed in the methods for producing and storing viable preparations of human liver cells so that they reflect the properties of these cells *in vivo*. Also required is standardization of criteria for reporting the purity, viability and reproducibility of *in vitro* preparations used in toxicology.

In view of the increasing evidence of large variations in human liver response due to genetic (interindividual) differences, the development of human liver bank(s) should be encouraged in order to identify likely types of susceptible individuals.

Extending the lifetime of cultures and the development of totally synthetic culture media is needed. Unless this is achieved, delayed onset hepatotoxicity cannot be investigated with confidence *in vitro*. There is also a need for incorporation of the hepatic drug metabolizing system into a rapidly dividing cell type in order to examine the effects of active metabolite generation on growth-related factors. Recent advances in genetic manipulation techniques should enable this to be achieved.

Improved monitoring techniques are required for both *in vivo* and *in vitro* systems. For *in vivo* systems, the principal requirement is for identifying the most appropriate indices of hepatic damage for each species which can be ascertained from blood. Also, whole body NMR offers great potential to detect hepatic and other tissue changes at an early stage. For *in vitro* systems, the development of quantitative cytochemical, immunochemical and lectin based identification methods merit priority because of their specificity and their facility to provide information at the individual cell level. Major progress here will depend on increasing understanding of mechanisms of hepatotoxicity.

Finally, effective training in *in vitro* methods is required for toxicologists who have been exclusively concerned with *in vivo* tests.

BIBLIOGRAPHY

Bein, H.J. (1963). Rational and irrational numbers in toxicology. *Proceedings of the European Society for the Study of Drug Toxicity*, **2**, 15–26.

Bridges, J.W. (1980). Monooxygenase reactions glucuronic acid sulphate conjugation in isolated hepatocytes. *Toxicology*, **18**, 195–204.

Bridges, J.W. (1981). The use of hepatocytes in toxicological investigations. In: Gorrod, J.W. (Ed.), *Testing for Toxicity*, Taylor and Francis, London, pp. 125–43.

Bridges, J.W., and Fry, J.R. (1978). Mammalian short-term tests for carcinogens. In: Dayan, A.D., and Brimblecombe, R.W. (Eds), *Carcinogenicity Testing: Principles and Problems*, Baltimore University Park Press, pp. 29–52.

Chayen, J., Bitensky, L., Johnstone, J.J., Gooding, P.E., and Slater, T.F. (1979). The application of microspectrophotometry to the measurement of cytochrome P-450. In: Pattison, J.R., Bitensky, L., and Chayen, J. (Eds) *Quantitative Cytochemistry and Its Applications*, Academic Press, London, pp. 129–37.

Elcombe, C. (1976). Ph.D. Thesis, University of Surrey.

Enderlin, F.E., and Honohan, T. (1977). Long term bile collection in the rat. *Lab. Anim. Sci.*, **27**, 490–93.

Fowler, B.A., Lucier, G.W., and Hayes, A.W. (1982). Organelles as tools in toxicology. In: Hayes, A.W. (Ed.), *Principles and Methods of Toxicology*, Raven Press, New York, pp. 509–60.

Horne, D.W., Briggs, W.T., and Wagner, C. (1976). A functional, active transport system for methotrexate in freshly isolated hepatocytes. *Biochem. Biophys. Res. Commun.*, **68**, 70–76.

Johnson, P., and Rising, P.A. (1978). Techniques for assessment of biliary excretion and enterohepatic circulation in the rat. *Xenobiotica*, **8**, 27–36.

Jones, D.P., Thor, H., Andersson, B., and Orrenius, S. (1978). Role of glutathione peroxidase, catalase and formaldehyde dehydrogenase in reactions relating to N-demethylation by the cytochrome P-450 system. *J. Biol. Chem.*, **253**, 6031.

Knook, D.L., and Sleyser, E.C. (1979). Liver sinusoidal cells: Isolation and purification by centrifugal elutriator. In: Reid, E. (Ed.), *Cell Populations*, Ellis Horwood, Chichester, pp. 47–52.

Lentz, P.E., and Di Luzio, N.R. (1971). Biochemical characterization of Kupffer and parenchymal cells isolated from rat liver. *Exptl. Cell Res.*, **67**, 17–26.

Lowing, R.K., Fry, J.R., Jones, C.A., Wiebkin, P., King, L.J., and Bridges, J.W. (1979). The early effects of chemical carcinogens on adult rat hepatocytes in primary culture: I. Quantitative changes in intracellular enzyme activities following a single dose of carcinogen. *Chem.-Biol. Interactions*, **24**, 121–31.

Lowing, R.K., Fry, J.R., King, L.J., and Bridges, J.W. (1979). The early effects of chemical carcinogens on adult rat hepatocytes in primary culture: II. Effects on unscheduled DNA synthesis, cell division and ∝-fetoprotein production. *Chem.-Biol. Interactions*, **25**, 303–19.

MacSween, R.N.M. (1980). Liver, biliary tract and exocrine pancreas. In: Anderson, J.R. (Ed.), *Muir's Textbook of Pathology*, Edward Arnold, London.

Mehendale, H.M. (1982). Application of isolated organ techniques in toxicology. In: Hayes, A.W. (Ed.), *Principles and Methods of Toxicology*, Raven Press, New York, pp. 509–59.

Miller, L.L., Bly, C.G., Watson, M.L., and Bale, W.F. (1951). The dominant role of the liver in lasma protein synthesis. A direct study of the isolated perfused rat liver with the aid of lysine-E-14-C. *J. Exp. Med.*, **94**, 431–53.

Plaa, G.L., and Hewitt, W.R. (1982). Detection and evaluation of chemically induced liver injury. In: Hayes, A.W. (Ed.), *Principles and Methods of Toxicology,* Raven Press, New York, pp. 407–45.

San, R.H.C., and Stich, H.F. (1975). DNA repair synthesis of cultured human cells as a rapid bioassay for chemical carcinogens. *Int. J. Cancer,* **16**, 284–91.

Schmidt, F.W. (1977). Enzymes in cholestasis. In: Bianchi, L., Gerok, W., and Sickinger, K. (Eds), *Liver and Bile*, Falk Symposium, vol. 23, Baltimore University Park Press, pp. 203–14.

Seglen, P.O. (1979). Separation approaches for liver and other cell sources. In: Reid, E. (Ed.), *Cell Populations,* Ellis Horwood, Chichester, pp. 25–46.

Thor, H., Moldeus, P., and Orrenius, S. (1979). Metabolic activation and hepatotoxicity: effect of cysteine, *n*-acetylcystein and methionine on glutathione biosynthesis and bromobenzene toxicity in isolated rat hepatocytes. *Arch. Biochem. Biophys.,* **192**, 405–13.

Tomlinson, P.W., Jeffery, D.J., and Filer, C.W. (1981). A novel technique for assessment of biliary secretion and enterohepatic circulation in the unrestrained conscious rat. *Xenobiotica,* **11**, 863–70.

Wiebkin, P., Fry, J.R., and Brĭdges, J.W. (1978). Metabolism-mediated cytotoxicity of chemical carcinogens and non-carcinogens. *Biochem. Pharmacol.,* **27**, 1849–51.

Woodman, D.D. (1981). Plasma enzymes in drug toxicity. In: Gorrod, J.W. (Ed.), *Testing for Toxicity,* Taylor and Francis, London, pp. 145–56.

Short-term Toxicity Tests for Non-genotoxic Effects
Edited by P. Bourdeau *et al.*
© 1990 SCOPE. Published by John Wiley & Sons Ltd

CHAPTER 10

The Developing Kidney in Toxicity Tests

Lauri Saxén

10.1 INTRODUCTION

The developing kidney offers several advantages for testing the harmful effects of genetic and non-genetic factors at the molecular, cellular, tissue and organism levels. The developmental stages of this organ are well understood, making toxic effects relatively easy to monitor. *In vivo*, the developing kidney is a sensitive target for harmful effects of biological, physical and chemical factors (see Monie, 1977). Recently, *in vitro* techniques have been elaborated to study the development and differentiation of the kidney and its components. These techniques have been devised primarily to explore normal kidney development, but they also provide a good basis for toxicological studies.

10.2 DEVELOPMENT OF THE METANEPHRIC KIDNEY

10.2.1 Early morphogenesis

Excellent accounts describing the histogenesis of the metanephric kidney have been published since the turn of the century by a number of scientists including Huber (1905) and Rienhoff (1922). These have been supplemented by observations using microdissection (Potter, 1965; Osthanondh and Potter, 1966), histochemistry (Vetter *et al.*, 1966; Kazimierczak, 1970), immunohistochemistry (Croisille *et al.*, 1971; Ekblom *et al.*, 1981a,b), and electronmicroscopy (Wartiovaara, 1966; Reeves *et al.*, 1978, 1980; Larsson and Maunsbach, 1980).

Three originally separate cell types contribute to the metanephric kidney: (1) the epithelium of the Wolffian duct; (2) the mesenchymal cells of the nephric blastema; and (3) the endothelial cells derived from an outside vasculature. The epithelial bud, the prospective collective system, invades the mesenchymal blastema where it branches repeatedly to form the ureteric tree. Mesenchymal cells around the tips of the ureteric tree differentiate to ultimately form the secretory portion of the nephron. In most mammalian species, the development of the nephron proceeds throughout the intra-uterine period. Therefore, it is possible to observe a whole repertoire of developing nephric tubules at various stages of development, an advantage in comparative studies.

The origin of the vascular component of the kidney, which includes the glomerular endothelium, has remained controversial until recent years. Some authors have regarded the mesenchymal cells of the nephric blastema as the progenitors of this important component of the kidney (Emura and Tanaka, 1972; Reeves *et al.*, 1980). Others have postulated that vascularization may have originated from outside vessels (Osthanondh and Potter, 1966; Kazimierczak, 1970).

Data from recent grafting experiments appears to support the hypothesis that the kidney's vascular component originates from outside vessels. The specific evidence for this hypothesis was acquired from an experiment which involved the grafting of mouse metanephric rudiments (prior to vascularization) onto the chorioallantoic membrane of the Japanese quail (Sariola *et al.*, 1983). These grafts regularly showed rich vascularization. The quail origin of these vessels could be verified by the quail-type nuclear structure of the endothelial cells and by monoclonal antibodies against quail endothelial (and haematopoietic) elements. The grafted kidneys developed rather advanced glomeruli showing a hybrid origin with mouse podocytes and avian endothelial cells. The same dual origin could be demonstrated in the glomerular basement membrane to which both mouse and quail cells had contributed (Sariola *et al.*, 1984a).

The initially separate mesenchyme also undergoes dramatic changes (Figure 10.1). In the early stages, it condenses around the epithelium where it forms a comma-shaped body. The mesenchyme then develops into an S-shaped structure which vascular elements invade. Growth continues centrifugally while the epithelium grows into deeper layers of the mesenchyme. New condensates are added and the more advanced tubules become established in the central portion of the anlage. As a result of this process, an arcade arrangement is created (Figure 10.2).

The early development of the kidney is preceded and accompanied by a variety of molecular changes. These changes can be detected by immunohistochemical staining using antibodies against the various components of the cells and their extracellular matrix (ECM).

Prior to any visible morphogenesis, the composition of the ECM of the tubule mesenchyme (around the epithelial tips) undergoes a change. The interstitial proteins (collagen type I and type III, fibronectin) are replaced by compounds which contribute to the basement membrane (collagen type IV, laminin, and heparin-sulphate proteoglycan) (Ekblom *et al.* 1981a).

The molecular changes in the ECM are accompanied by changes in the cytoskeleton indicating a transformation from a mesenchymal cell into an epithelial cell. The vimentin filaments of the mesenchymal cells are replaced by cytokeratin (Lehtonen *et al.*, 1984).

The subsequent segmentation of the nephron into a glomerular, proximal and

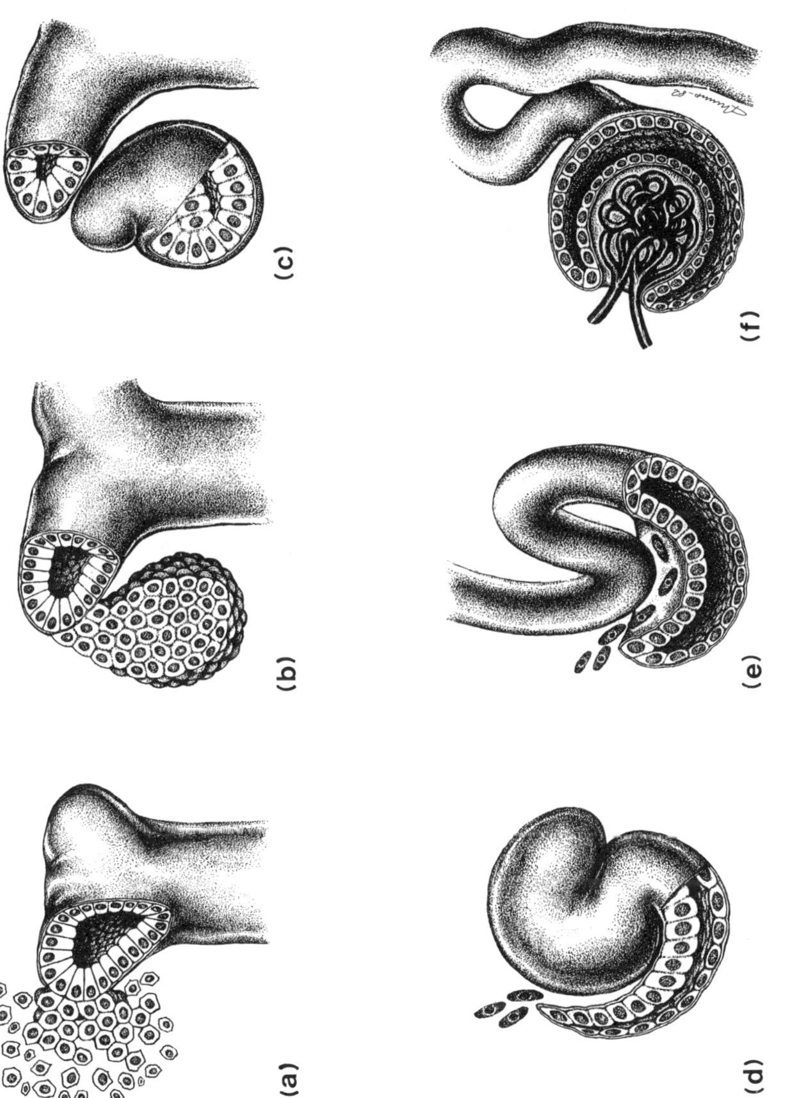

Figure 10.1   Early stages of morphogenesis of the metanephric nephron (Saxén, 1984).

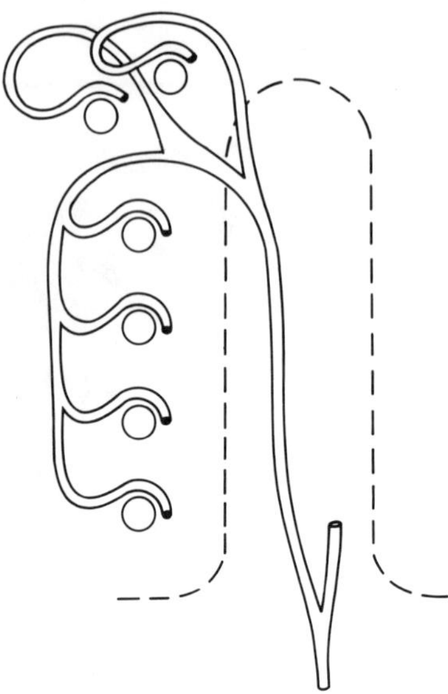

Figure 10.2   Arcade formation in the developing metanephric kidney (after Neiss, 1982).

distal portion can be studied with immunohistochemical, histochemical and electron microscopic techniques (Ekblom *et al.*, 1980; Lehtonen *et al.*, 1983). Also, important details of the ultra-structure of the nephron have been obtained by transmission, scanning and immunoelectron microscopy. These latter methods have focused on the glomerulus and its filtration barrier (Larsson and Maunsbach, 1980; Reeves *et al.*, 1980; Farquhar, 1981).

10.2.2   Control of early morphogenesis

Direct observations of certain urinary tract abnormalities (Gruenwald, 1939) and related studies of different kidney cell lineages demonstrates a significant morphogenetic relationship between cell lineages. This property has been observed in experiments involving the ureter bud and the mesenchyme. If separated by microdissection and cultured in isolation, neither the ureter bud nor the mesenchyme undergoes further differentiation. However, if recombined soon after separation, an almost normal morphogenesis is observed (Grobstein, 1953, 1955).

The inductive or morphogenetic tissue interaction which is frequently associated with embryonic organ formation has been analysed by the transfilter technique developed by Grobstein (1956).

The sequence of events during the epithelial transformation can be triggered by various heterotypic tissues through a filter membrane. This technique opens up various possibilities for the detailed analyses of morphogenetic tissue interaction. It also permits the use of different filter types and the separate analysis of two interacting tissues. More importantly, contact between the interacting cells can be broken at any time and the mesenchyme cultured separately for further study. This technique can also be used to study the temporal correlation of events at the molecular and structural levels.

The reader is referred to reviews by Grobstein (1967), Saxén *et al.* (1968, 1985), Lehtonen (1976) and Saxén (1987) for further information on morphogenesis. Some central conclusions about kidney morphogenesis are:

(1)   (i)   The nephrogenic mesenchyme is predetermined prior to the action of the ureter inductor;

     (ii)   various heterotypic tissues can trigger its differentiation (Grobstein, 1955);

    (iii)   no other embryonic mesenchyme will respond to the triggers by forming tubules (Saxén, 1970).

(2)   Induction requires actual cell-to-cell contact between the interacting tissues. Induction can be prevented by filters that do not allow close cell-to-cell appositions (Wartiovaara *et al.*, 1974; Lehtonen, 1976; Saxén *et al.*, 1976).

(3)   (i)   Induction is a time-related event. After 12 hours of contact, the first mesenchymal cells become irreversibly committed to become epithelial cells;

    (ii)   The process of induction is completed after some 24 to 28 hours of contact (Saxén and Lehtonen, 1978).

(4)   (i)   Immediately after the initial 24 hours of induction, no morphogenesis is detectable, but the mesenchymal cells have been programmed for differentiation;

    (ii)   After 24 hours, the cells begin to differentiate into specialized cell types such as glomerular podocytes, proximal tubule cells, and distal tubule cells;

    (iii)   These new phenotypes are expressed three to five days after the initial induction (Ekblom *et al.*, 1981b; Lehtonen *et al.*, 1983).

(5)   (i)   The first detectable change in the state of the cells is a decreased cell generation time (detected by increased uptake of tritiated thymidine);

    (ii)   This change coincides with the 'induction time' and occurs within 12 to 24 hours after the transfilter contact (Figure 10.3). Only an inductive situation leads to this change (Saxén *et al.*, 1983).

(6)   The changes in the protein composition of the extracellular matrix and in the cytoskeleton (described above) are regularly detected in the transfilter explants during early stages of differentiation but not in mesenchymes that are not exposed to an inductor (Ekblom *et al.*, 1981a; Lehtonen *et al.*, 1984).

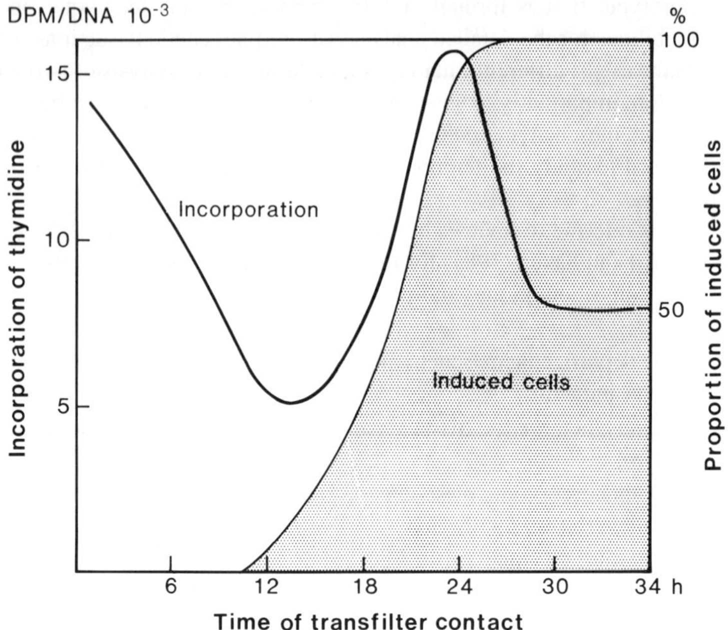

Figure 10.3   Correlation of the 'induction time' (shaded area) to the incorporation of thymidine into the induced mesenchyme after the onset of the transfilter contact (Saxén *et al.*, 1985).

Due to the technique used, the various events under (3) to (6) can be temporally correlated as in Figure 10.4. Speculations on their causal correlations have been presented (Lehtonen and Saxén, 1986), but final conclusions cannot yet be drawn about the mechanism of this complicated chain of events. The sequence of events and the kinetics described do, however, provide a useful background when the application of this model-system is considered for toxicological studies.

10.3   *IN VIVO* TOXICITY STUDIES

The urinary tract of murine embryos is a sensitive target for various exogenous factors. Wilson and Warkany (1948) found kidney malformations in the offspring of rats that were fed a diet which was deficient in vitamin A. Monie *et al.* (1954) reported malformations in rats following maternal pteroylglutamic acid deficiency (Monie *et al.*, 1954). Numerous other studies have been published (see Monie, 1977).

Sodium arsenate injected intraperitoneally into mice on days nine and ten of pregnancy caused various malformations and fetal death, but almost no effects if

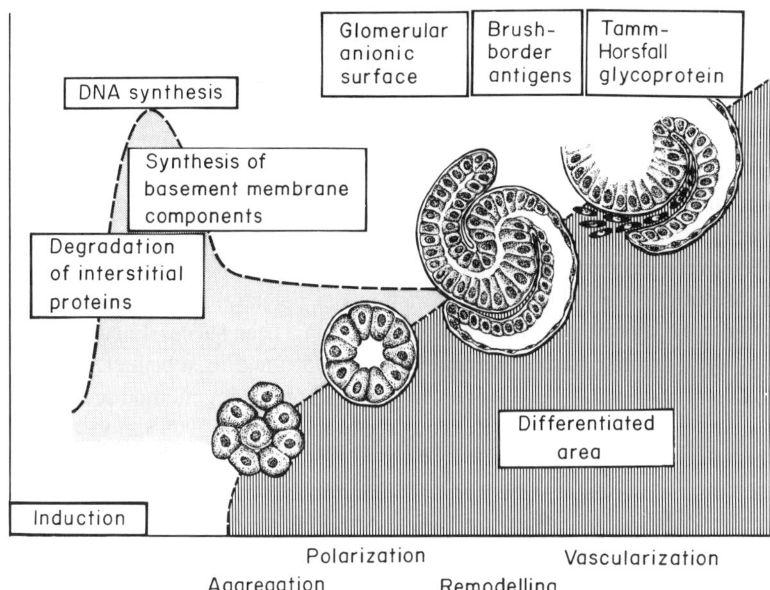

Figure 10.4   Summary of the differentiative events following the onset of transfilter contact between the metanephrogenic mesenchyme and its inductor (Lehtonen and Saxén, 1986).

injected after this time (Burk and Beaudoin, 1978). The primary defect caused by this exogenous factor was impaired growth of the ureteric bud (the inductor). This impaired growth prevented the ureteric bud from reaching the metanephric blastema, which subsequently failed to differentiate. A similar mechanism has been suggested for the genetically-determined renal agenesis in Sd-mutant mice (Gluecksohn-Waelsch and Rota, 1963).

Fetterman *et al.* (1974) provided an example of malformations caused by *in vivo* micromanipulation. Ligation of the ureter in fetal rabbits between days 19 and 24 of gestation proved successful in that a high percentage of fetuses developed cystic dilations in various portions of the nephron. The authors felt that this might be a good model for certain types of obstructive kidney cysts that occur in human subjects (see also Crocker and Vernier, 1970b; Crocker *et al.*, 1971).

Kavlock *et al.* (1982) have reported that the liver and kidney appear to be the most sensitive organs studied in tests involving the use of biochemical endpoints of organ differentiation as criteria for fetotoxicity. Various biochemical measurements were made to follow the growth and maturation of different organs in rat embryos on days 19 to 22 following maternal exposure to known fetotoxic chemicals. Some of the results reflected impaired kidney development (Figure 10.5). These authors have used a diuresis test (with and without anti-diuretic hormone on the third postnatal day) and a hydropenia test on the sixth postnatal day in addition to kidney weights, glomerular counts and renal alkaline phosphatase tests to assess the effects of toxicants (Kavlock and Gray, 1982, 1983).

An example of the use of newborn mice in toxicity tests is the work of Gresser *et al.* (1981). Purified interferon was injected into suckling mice daily for eight days. Light and electron microscopy revealed effects which included immature glomeruli, glomerulosclerosis, atrophy of the tubular epithelium and thickening of the glomerular basement membrane. These results confirmed an earlier study by Gresser *et al.* (1976) in which suckling mice treated with interferon at birth developed severe glomerulonephritis.

The use of current *in vivo* grafting methods as potential models for toxicological studies may hold promise. Embryonic kidneys have been successfully grafted in the anterior eye chamber (Grobstein and Parker, 1958) and in subcutaneous locations (Barakat and Harrison, 1971). However, the most promising method seems to be the chorioallantoic (CAM) grafting method (Preminger *et al.*, 1980; Sariola *et al.*, 1983, 1984b).

When mouse avascular kidney anlagen are grafted onto avian CAM, they quickly become vascularized by avian capillaries. Although this technique has not yet been adapted for toxicity tests, it may prove useful in the assessment of cell migration and circulation development.

This technique has been used to study abnormal kidney development in CAM-grafts with chick kidneys (Maizels and Simpson, 1983). These experiments succeeded in simulating human kidney dysplasia; however, it is not yet certain whether or not this is a true model-system for the human kidney defect.

10.4   *IN VITRO* METHODS AND TOXICITY STUDIES

Several *in vitro* techniques for the cultivation of kidney anlagen and the various cell types derived from it are now available. A number of these techniques have been developed for the study of normal kidney development, but they also have potential value for toxicity tests.

10.4.1   Cell cultures

In an experiment conducted by Taub *et al.* (1979), Nadin–Darby canine kidney cells were introduced to a chemically-defined medium supplemented with insulin, transferrin, prostaglandin E_1, hydrocortisone and tri-iodothyronine. Cell growth and survival were as good as in a serum-supplemented medium. Cells could be maintained in culture for a month. This technique allows detailed analysis of the effect and mode of action of various medium constituents on the growth and hemicyst formation of kidney epithelial cells.

Primary cultures can be prepared from mesenchyme explants derived by the transfilter technique (see Section 10.2.2). The mesenchyme, prior to overt

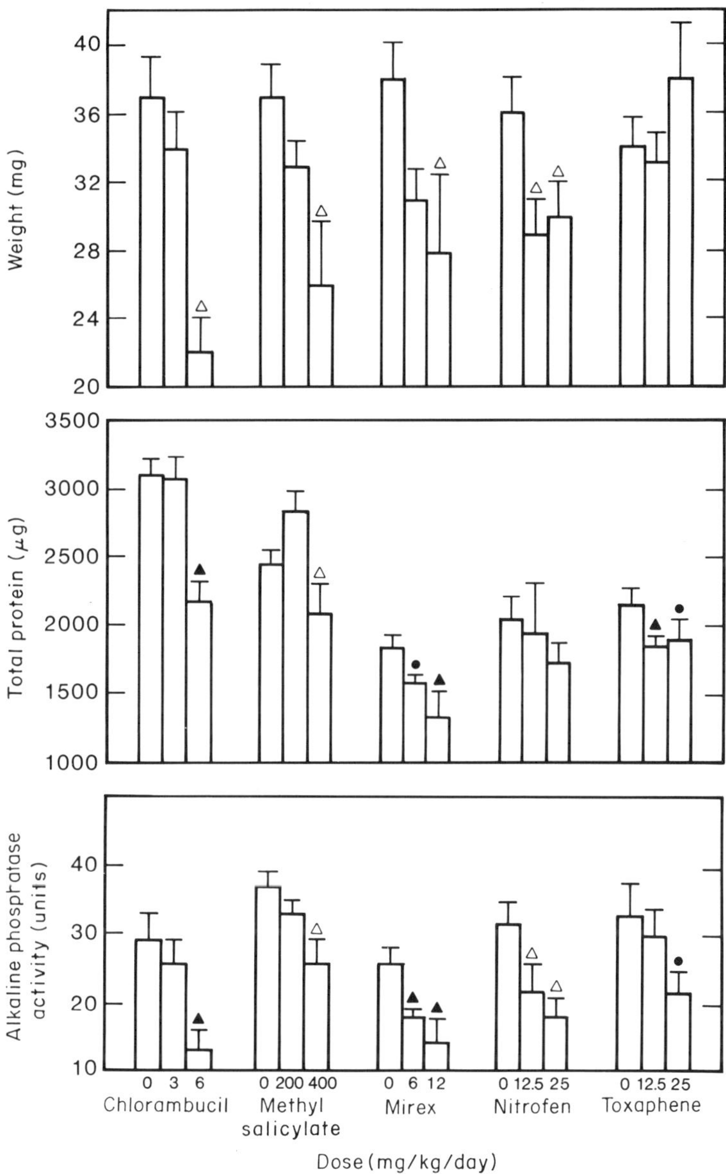

Figure 10.5 'Biochemical endpoint' measurement reflecting an impaired development of the kidney rudiment after treatment with various toxic compounds in different concentrations (after Kavlock *et al.*, 1982).

differentiation, can be cut into fragments which demonstrate good cell outgrowth in subculture. These outgrowths are known to contain both stroma, fibroblast-type and differentiating epithelial cells (Lehtonen *et al.*, 1985).

Minuth and Kriz (1982) developed an explanation technique for the study of kidney epithelial cells in their more advanced stages. Small cortical pieces were dissected from newborn rabbit kidneys. These pieces consisted of a fibrous capsule, collective duct fragments and immature, S-shaped tubule anlagen. Within 24 hours, these cortical pieces developed into globular bodies demonstrating epithelial outgrowth that apparently originated from the collecting ducts. The outgrowth also demonstrated a capacity to synthesize the renal glycoprotein $gp_{CD}I$ (Minuth *et al.*, 1984).

These cortical outgrowths may be useful in toxicological studies. Minuth (1983) has demonstrated that these are sensitive to various protein-inhibitors and cytoskeleton-blocking agents such as cycloheximide, actinomycin C, tunicamycin, 6-diazo-5-oxo-norleucine (DON), vinblastine, and cytochalasin B.

Minuth (1983) expressed the belief that cultures of this type could be employed for the direct testing of drug teratogenicity. Of special interest would be the effects of agents that interfere with cell attachment and cell locomotion. The method may have potential as a direct, rapid and convenient means of assessing toxicity.

10.4.2 Organ culture

Organ culture techniques developed in the 1920s make it possible to examine tissue fragments and whole organ rudiments in reproducible *in vitro* conditions. These techniques also have proven value in some toxicological studies (Saxén, 1983). Studies undertaken with the use of organ cultures offer distinct advantages over monolayer cell cultures since differentiation and certain physiological functions persist rather well.

Organ cultures of both murine and avian kidneys have been investigated *in vitro* since the early 1950s (Grobstein, 1953, 1955; Saxén *et al.* 1968; Bernstein *et al.*, 1981; Avner *et al.*, 1983a; Wolff and Haffen, 1952; Lash, 1963; Strudel and Pinot, 1965). The culture conditions of the different laboratories vary somewhat, and we have described ours in several contexts (Saxén *et al.*, 1968; Saxén and Saksela, 1971; Saxén and Karkinen-Jaaskelainen, 1975).

Recently, good growth and differentiation of kidney anlage has been reported in a chemically defined, serum-free medium. Using a transferrin-supplemented medium, it was possible to obtain good development of mouse kidney rudiments (Ekblom *et al.*, 1981b). Without transferrin, or in media with transferrin-depleted serum, culture survival was poor and differentiation did not proceed.

Avner *et al.* (1982) used a more complex medium where proteins were replaced with insulin, prostaglandin E_1, transferrin and hydrocortisone. This medium resulted in good differentiation of mouse embryonic kidneys with advanced proximal tubules, brush-border and avascular glomeruli and highly differentiated podocytes.

Although supplements added to synthetic media cannot fully compensate for the proteins present in serum-based organ culture media, the elimination of various serum factors from the culture medium (and their possible effects) is advantageous for experiments where additional factors are to be tested.

As *in vitro* microperfusion method to study the physiology and functional development of the nephron has been developed (Horster, 1978; Horster and Schmidt, 1978; Horster and Zink, 1982). Microperfusion of isolated tubular fragments, dissected from kidneys of embryonic and newborn rabbits, permitted the evaluation of fluid and ion transport by the epithelium during embryogenesis and postnatal development. Also, enzyme activities could be monitored in these nephron fragments. Horster and Zink (1982) used this method to study the effect of vasopressin on the functional maturation of the nephric epithelium. These experiments indicate that this system might be applicable to toxicological studies.

The use of human embryonic kidney tissues for organ culture analysis remains largely unexploited at this time. According to Lash and Saxén (1972), human embryonic kidneys grow well in organotypic culture. Studies by Crocker and Vernier (1970a) and Crocker (1973) provide further information on related experiments.

10.4.3 Effects of xenobiotics on *in vitro* systems

Some examples serve to illustrate the use of metanephric cultures in toxicological studies. Shabad *et al.* (1972) used kidney fragments obtained from mouse embryos in the third trimester. The embryos had been exposed to various carcinogens or their non-carcinogenic analogues as a result of maternal dosage and transplacental transport. In culture, the epithelium of kidneys taken from the embryos of mice exposed to carcinogens showed hyperplastic growth that was nodular, diffuse or that formed solid, compact zones. Occasional papillary outgrowth was also observed more frequently in the specimens from embryos exposed to carcinogens than in specimens from embryos in the control groups. Even though the assessment criteria were solely morphological and difficult to evaluate, the technique, nevertheless, merits further consideration for studies on transplacental exposure to chemical carcinogens.

By the addition of glycocorticoids to the culture medium, it has been possible to induce cystic maldevelopment in murine metanephric cultures (Avner *et al.*, 1983b, 1984). This defect is similar to that observed in the polycystic kidney disease, a condition well-known to both experimental teratologists and pediatric pathologists (Bernstein, 1968). Although the exact mechanisms involved in the occurrence of these maldevelopments remain unknown, this method does seem to allow new means for experimental studies involving the aetiology and pathogenesis of multicystic kidney disease and, possibly, a method to test certain drugs for side-effects.

The effects of interferon on development and differentiation in embryonic kidneys was recently tested in two types of metanephric cultures (Saxén, 1985). One culture type involved complete 11-day-old embryonic kidneys, while the other type consisted of a culture prepared by the transfilter technique. Kidneys were carefully dissected from pairs of mouse embryos, which were selected at random, and were cultured *in vitro*. Mouse interferon was added to the culture medium in final concentrations of 10^3 and 10^5 units/ml. The kidneys were harvested 24 or 48 hours later to measure growth and histogenesis, and five days later for immunohistology. The results were later compared with those obtained for control kidneys which were similarly cultivated. Proliferation was measured by incorporation of tritiated thymidine and by total DNA content (Table 10.1).

The results in Table 10.1 and other similar experiments suggest that interferon has no definite effect on DNA synthesis of the kidneys after 24 hours of cultivation but seems to interfere with thymidine incorporation following a prolonged cultivation period of 48 hours. The lower concentrations were without effect.

Histologically, the kidneys treated by the higher concentration of interferon showed a slightly delayed development. Similar symptoms appeared in transfilter cultures, subjected to the same treatment. Cultivation of these transfilter cultures for a period of five days, however, resulted in well differentiated tubules which expressed the various markers for the three main segments of the nephron: the glomerulus, the proximal tubule and the distal tubule (Saxén *et al.*, unpublished results).

Although some of the results on whole kidney rudiments are preliminary, they demonstrate the advantage of using paired organs. Even the most skilfully dissected kidney samples tend to show variations in size and growth rate. Therefore, pooled samples of such target tissues may render erroneous results. For this reason, the use of randomized pairs of kidney rudiments is favoured.

Induction and early differentiation of the metanephric nephron can be analysed in a simplified model-system by using transfilter induction. This model-system might prove useful in toxicity tests since the kinetics of this process are known and many of the first steps of differentiation have been characterized. Previous experience with this method can be found in Saxén and Ekblom (1981) and Saxén (1983). Figure 10.6 shows how various stages (and components) of the developing kidney can be

Table 10.1   The effect of interferon on the incorporation of thymidine into embryonic kidneys cultivated *in vitro* for 24 and 48 hours

| | Experiment | | | |
	Control		Interferon	
Number of kidneys	7	11	7	11
Time of cultivation (h)	24	48	24	48
Incorporation of thymidin (DPM/DNA)	5.900	10.200	4.500	6.400
Total DNA (ng)	294	320	283	337

Concentration of interferon was 10^5 u/ml in a medium supplemented with 10 per cent serum (Saxén 1985).

exposed to the compound in question. The whole inductor/mesenchyme explant can be exposed, or the inductor and the target mesenchyme might be pre-exposed and brought together after treatment. Exposure to exogenous compounds can be continuous, only during induction, or after induction. Criteria to be monitored in such experiments include survival of tissue(s), proliferation of the mesenchymal cells, incorporation of various radioactive precursors, as well as histochemical, immunohistochemical, and ultrastructural measures of differentiation.

Tests with compounds interfering with the synthesis of DNA, RNA, and proteins have shown that nephrogenesis is most sensitive during the initial induction period. At later stages, the mesenchyme is resistant to such chemicals (Nordling *et al.*, 1978).

To determine if nephrogenesis might be mediated by glycosylated surface-associated compounds, some inhibitors of glycosamine synthesis and protein glycosylation were tested. 6-diazo-5-oxo-norleucine (DON) is a glutamine analogue

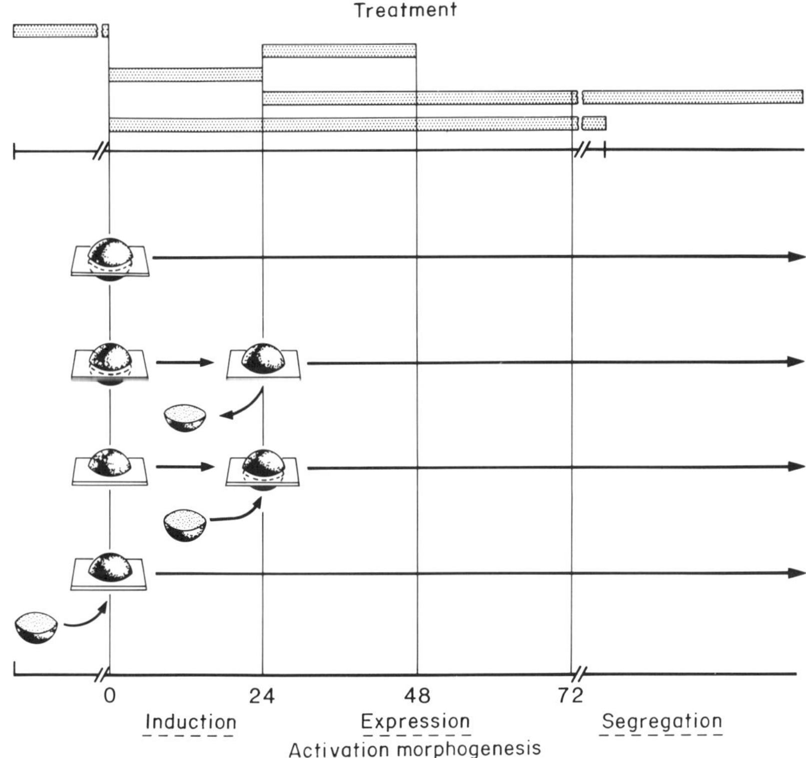

Figure 10.6   Experimental possibilities to expose the metanephrogenic mesenchyme and its inductor at various stages of determination and differentiation (Saxén, 1983).

which affects the synthesis of glycosaminoglycans as well as protein glycosylation. Tunicamycin is considered a rather selective inhibitor of protein glycosylation. When tested in transfilter explants of the metanephric mesenchyme, these compounds caused a dose-dependent inhibition of tubule formation during the early induction phase of kidney development (Figure 10.7) (Ekblom *et al.*, 1979a,b). However, if mesenchyme was induced for 24 hours before being exposed to DON or tunicamycin, no effect on morphogenesis was evident.

The mode of action of these two compounds is still open to speculation. If the inhibitors are removed after 24 hours of exposure, and the inductor kept in place, tubule formation will resume.

The transfilter model-system, although valuable, cannot fully simulate the kidney *in vivo* and must be used with caution. The procedures needed to prepare the system—enzymatic and microsurgical separation of components, transfer onto filters and into *in vitro* conditions, etc.—result in an adaptive phase of low metabolic activity (Vainio *et al.*, 1965; Saxén, 1983), and may cause sensitivity to some exogenous agents. The use of radioactive tracers, for instance, may cause direct toxicity instead of providing a method of monitoring the effects of other agents on kidney development. This high sensitivity of cultured organ rudiments to low levels of certain radiolabelled compounds (aminoacids) has been demonstrated by Minor (1982). Therefore, such experiments must be conducted and interpreted with care. This sensitivity might also be used to advantage for toxicity tests.

10.5 CONCLUSIONS

Analytical work over the past thirty years has elucidated many of the complex

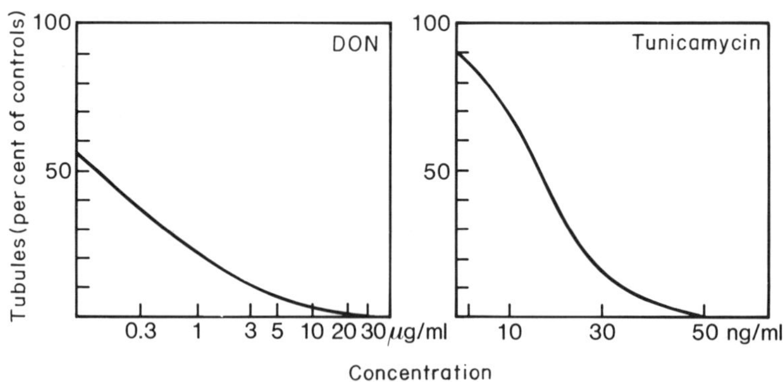

Figure 10.7 Graphs demonstrating the dose-dependent inhibitory action of DON and tunicamycin during the 24-hour induction period. The number of nephric tubules is given as percentage of that in untreated controls. The low number of DON-treated explants is partially due to the omission of glutamine from the medium (Ekblom *et al.*, 1979a, 1979b).

events and principles of kidney development. In addition to the classic *in vivo* tests, the kidney has proven to be a good object for various simplified grafting and *in vitro* methods. These techniques may be useful to toxicologists as they search for rapid and convenient tests for examining the effects of environmental chemicals. Effects that can be tested with these systems include direct toxic (lethal) effects on cells, interference with morphogenetic tissue interactions, inhibition of cell migration, aggregation and organization, and interference with known metabolic pathways (such as synthesis of macromolecules, protein glycosylation, energy metabolism and ion transfer).

REFERENCES

Avner, E.D., Ellis, D., Temple, T., and Jaffe, R. (1982). Metanephric development in serum-free organ culture. *In Vitro,* **18**, 675–82.

Avner, E.D., Villee, D.B., Schneeberger, E.S., and Grupe, W.E. (1983a). An organ culture model for the study of metanephric development. *J. Urol.,* **129**, 660–64.

Avner, E.D., Sweeney, W.E. Jr., and Ellis, D. (1983b). Cyst formation in metanephric organ culture induced by cis-dichlorodiamineplatinum (II). *Experientia,* **39**, 74–6.

Avner, E.D., Piesco, N.P., Sweeney, W.E. Jr., Stunicki, F.M., Fetterman, G.H., and Ellis, D. (1984). Hydrocortison-induced cystic metanephric maldevelopment in serum-free organ culture. *Lab. Invest.,* **50**, 208–18.

Barakat, T.I., and Harrison, R.G. (1971). The capacity of fetal and neonatal renal tissues to regenerate and differentiate in a heterotopic allogenic subcutaneous tissue site in the rat. *J. Anat.,* **110**, 393–407.

Bernstein, J. (1968). Developmental abnormalities of the renal parenchyma. Renal hypoplasia and dysplasia. In: Sommers, S.C. (Ed.), *Pathology Annual,* Appleton-Century-Crofts, New York, pp. 213–47.

Bernstein, J., Cheng, F., and Roszka, J. (1981). Glomerular differentiation in metanephric culture. *Lab. Invest.,* **45**, 183–90.

Burk, D., and Beaudoin, A.R. (1978). Arsenate-induced renal agenesis in rats. *Pathology,* **16**, 247–60.

Crocker, J.F.S. (1973). Human embryonic kidneys in organ culture: Abnormalities of development induced by decreased potassium. *Science,* **181**, 1178–9.

Crocker, J.F.S., and Vernier, R.L. (1970a). Fetal kidney in organ culture: Abnormalities of development induced by decreased amounts of potassium. *Science,* **169**, 485–7.

Crocker, J.F.S., and Vernier, R.L. (1970b). Chemically induced polycystic disease in the newborn. *Pediat. Res.,* **4**, 448.

Crocker, J.F.S., Brown, D.M., and Vernier, R. (1971). Developmental defects of the kidney. *Pediatr. Clin. North Am.,* **18**, 355–76.

Croisille, Y., Gumpel-Pinot, M., and Martin, C. (1971). Sur l'organogenèse du mésonéphros chez les oiseaux. Etude immunohistologique du tubule urinaire chez l'embryon de poulet. *C.R. Acad. Sc.,* Paris, **272**, 629–31.

Ekblom, P., Nordling, S., Saxén, L., Rasilo, M.L., and Renkonen, O. (1979a). Cell interactions leading to kidney tubule determination are tunicamycin sensitive. *Cell Differ.,* **8**, 347–52.

Ekblom, P., Lash, J.W., Lehtonen, E., Nordling, S., and Saxén, L. (1979b). Inhibition of morphogenetic cell interactions by 6-diazo-5-oxonorleucine (DON). *Exp. Cell Res.,* **121**, 121–6.

Ekblom, P., Lehtonen, E., Saxén, L., and Timpl, R. (1981a). Shift in collagen type as an early response to induction of the metanephric mesenchyme. *J. Cell Biol.,* **89**, 276–83.

Ekblom, P., Miettinen, A., and Saxén, L. (1980). Induction of brush border antigens of the proximal tubule in the developing kidney. *Dev. Biol.,* **74**, 263–74.

Ekblom, P., Thesleff, I., Miettinen, A., and Saxén, L. (1981b). Organogenesis in a defined medium supplemented with transferrin. *Cell Differ.,* **10**, 281–8.

Emura, M., and Tanaka, T. (1972). Development of endothelial and erythroid cells in mouse metanephric mesenchyme cultured with fetal liver. *Dev. Growth Differ.,* **14**, 237–46.

Farquhar, M.G. (1981). The glomerular basement membrane. A selective macromolecular filter. In: Hay, E.D. (Ed.), *Cell Biology of Extracellular Matrix,* Plenum Press, New York, pp. 335–78.

Fetterman, G.H., Ravitch, M.M., and Sherman, F.E. (1974). Cystic changes in fetal kidneys following uretal ligation: Studies by microdissection. *Kidney Int.,* **5**, 111–21.

Gluecksohn-Waelsch, S., and Rota, T.R. (1963). Development in organ tissue culture of kidney rudiments from mutant mouse embryos. *Dev. Biol.,* **7**, 432–44.

Gresser, I., Maury, C., Morel-Maroger, L., and Pontillon, F. (1976). Progressive glomerulonephritis in mice treated with interferon preparations at birth. *Nature,* **263**, 420–22.

Gresser, I., Aguet, M., Morel-Maroger, L., Woodrow, D., Puvion-Dutilleul, F., Guillon, J.-C., and Maury, C. (1981). Electrophoretically pure mouse interferon inhibits growth, induces liver and kidney lesions and kills suckling mice. *Am. J. Path.,* **102**, 396–402.

Grobstein, C. (1953). Inductive epithelio-mesenchymal interaction in cultured organ rudiments of the mouse. *Science,* **118**, 52–5.

Grobstein, C. (1955). Inductive interaction in the development of the mouse metanephros. *J. Exp. Zool.,* **130**, 319–40.

Grobstein, C. (1956). Trans-filter induction of tubules in metanephrogenic mesenchyme. *Exp. Cell Res.,* **10**, 424–40.

Grobstein, C. (1967). Mechanisms of organogenetic tissue interactions. *Nat. Cancer Inst. Monogr.,* **26**, 279–99.

Grobstein, C., and Parker, G. (1958). Epithelial tubule formation by mouse metanephrogenic mesenchyme transplanted *in vivo. J. Nat. Cancer Inst.,* **20**, 107–19.

Gruenwald, P. (1939). The mechanism of kidney development in human embryo as revealed by an early stage in the agenesis of the ureteric buds. *Anat. Record.,* **75**, 237–48.

Horster, M. (1978). Principles of nephron differentiation. *Am. J. Physiol.,* **235**, 387–93.

Horster, M., and Schmidt, U. (1978). *In vitro* electrolyte transport and enzyme activity of single dissected and perfused nephron segments during differentiation. In: *Current Problems in Clinical Biochemistry,* volume 7, Huber, Bern, pp. 98–106.

Horster, M., and Zink, H. (1982). Functional differentiation of the medullary collecting tubule: influence of vasopressin. *Kidney Int.,* **22**, 360–5.

Huber, G.G. (1905). On the development and shape of uriniferous tubules of certain higher mammals. *Am. J. Anat.,* **Suppl. 4**, 1–98.

Kavlock, R.J., and Gray, J.A. (1982). Evaluation of renal function in neonatal rats. *Biol. Neonat.,* **41**, 279–88.

Kavlock, R.J., and Gray, J.A. (1983). Morphologic biochemical and physiological assessment of perinatally induced renal dysfunction. *J. Toxicol. Environm. Health,* **22**, 1–13.

Kavlock, R.J., Chernoff, N., Rogers, E., Whitehouse, D., Carver, B., Gray, J., and Robinson, K. (1982). An analysis of fetotoxicity using biochemical endpoints of organ differentiation. *Teratology,* **26**, 183–94.

Kazimierczak, J. (1970). Histochemical observations of the developing glomerulus and juxtaglomerular apparatus. *Acta Pathol. Microbiol. Scand.,* A, **78**, 401–13.

Larsson, L., and Maunsbach, A.B. (1980). The ultrastructural development of the glomerular filtration barrier in the rat kidney: a morphometric analysis. *J. Ultrastruct. Res.,* **72**, 392–406.

Lash, J.W. (1963). Studies on the ability of embryonic mesenephros explants to form cartilage. *Dev. Biol.*, **6**, 219–232.

Lash, J.W., and Saxén, L. (1972). Human teratogenesis: *In vitro* studies on thalidomide inhibited chondrogenesis. *Dev. Biol.*, **28**, 61–70.

Lehtonen, E. (1976). Transmission of signals in embryonic induction. *Med. Biol.*, **54**, 108–28.

Lehtonen, E., and Saxén, L. (1985). Control of differentiation. In Falkner, F., and Tanner, J.M. (Eds), *Human Growth: A Comprehensive Treatise*, Plenum Press, New York, pp. 27–51.

Lehtonen, E., Jalanko, H., Laitinen, L., Miettinen, A., Ekblom, P., and Saxén, L. (1983). Differentiation of metanephric tubules following a short transfilter induction pulse. *Roux' Arch. Dev. Biol.*, **192**, 145–51.

Lehtonen, E., Saxén, L., and Virtanen, I. (1985). Reorganization of intermediate filament cytoskeleton in induced metanephric cells is independent of tubule morphogenesis. *Dev. Biol.*, **108**, 481–90.

Maizels, M., and Simon, S.B. Jr. (1983) Primitive ducts of renal dysplasia induced by culturing ureteral buds denuded of condensed renal mesenchyme. *Science*, **219**, 509–10.

Minor, R.R. (1982). Cytotoxic effects of low levels of ^{3}H-, ^{14}C-, and ^{35}S-labelled amino acids. *J. Biol. Chem.*, **257**, 10400–13.

Minuth, W.W. (1983). Induction and inhibition of outgrowth and development of renal collecting duct epithelium. *Lab Investig.*, **48**, 543–8.

Minuth, W.W., Lauer, G., and Kriz, W. (1984). Immunocytochemical localization of a renal glycoprotein ($gp_{CD}I$) synthesized by cultured collecting duct cells. *Histochemistry*, **18**, 171–82.

Minuth, W.W., and Kriz, W. (1982). Culturing of renal collecting duct epithelium as globular bodies. *Cell Tissue Res.*, **224**, 335–48.

Monie, I.W., Nelson, M.M., and Evans, H.M. (1954). Abnormalities of the urinary system of rat embryos resulting from maternal pteroylglutamic acid deficiency. *Anat. Rec.*, **120**, 119–36.

Monie, J.W. (1977). Abnormal organogenesis in the urinary tract. In: Wilson, J.F., and Fraser, F.C. (Eds), *Handbook of Teratology*, Plenum Press, New York, pp. 365–89.

Neiss, W.F. (1982). Morphogenesis and histogenesis of the connecting tubule in the rat kidney. *Anat. Embryol.*, **165**, 81–95.

Nordling, S., Ekblom, P., Lehtonen, E., Wartiovaara, J., and Saxén, L. (1978). Metabolic inhibitors and kidney tubule induction. *Med. Biol.*, **56**, 372–9.

Osthanondh, V., and Potter, E. (1966). Development of human kidney as shown by microdissection. V. Development of vascular pattern of glomerulus. *Arch. Pathol.*, **82**, 403–11.

Potter, E.L. (1965). Development of the human glomerulus. *Arch. Path.*, **80**, 241–55.

Preminger, G.M., Koch, W.E., Fried, F.A., and Mandell, J. (1980). Utilization of the chick chorioallantoic membrane for *in vitro* growth of the embryonic murine kidney. *Am. J. Anat.*, **159**, 17–24.

Reeves, W., Caulfield, J.P., and Farquhar, M.G. (1978). Differentiation of epithelial foot processes and filtration slits: sequential appearance of ocluding junctions, epithelial polyanion,and slit membrane in developing glomeruli. *Lab. Invest.*, **39**, 90–100.

Reeves, W.H., Kanwar, Y.P., and Farquhar, M.G. (1980). Assembly of glomerular filtration surface. Differentiation of anionic sites in glomerular capillaries of newborn rat kidney. *J. Cell Biol.*, **85**, 735–53.

Rienhoff, W.F. (1922). Development and growth of the metanephros or permanent kidney in chick embryos. *Johns Hopkins Hosp. Bull.*, **33**, 392–406.

Sariola, H., Ekblom, P., Lehtonen, E., and Saxén, L. (1983). Differentiation and vascularization of the metanephric kidney grafted on the chorioallantoic membrane. *Dev. Biol.*, **96**, 427–35.

Sariola, H., Timpl, R., von der Mark, K., Mayne, R. Fitch, J.M., Linsenmayer, T.F., and Ekblom, P. (1984a). Dual origin of glomerular basement membrane. *Dev. Biol.*, **101**, 86–96.

Sariola, H., Saxén, L., Dieterlen, F., and LeDouarin, N. (1984b). Extracellular matrix and capillary ingrowth in interspecies chimeric kidneys. *Cell Diff.* (in press).

Saxén, L. (1970). Failure to demonstrate tubule induction in a heterologous mesenchyme. *Dev. Biol.*, **23**, 511–23.

Saxén, L. (1983). *In vitro* model-systems for chemical teratogenesis. In: Kolber, A.R., Wong, T.K., Grant, L.D., DeWoskin, R.S., and Hughes, T.J. (Eds), *In Vitro Testing of Teratological Agents: Current and Future Possibilities* Plenum Press, New York, pp. 173–190.

Saxén, L. (1984). Implementation of a developmental programme. In: Chagas, C. (Ed.), *Modern Biological Experimentation, Pontificia Academia Scientiarum*, Città del Vaticano, pp. 155–63.

Saxén, L. (1985). Effect of interferon tested in a model-system for organogenesis. *J. Interferon Res.*, **5**, 355–9.

Saxén, L. (1987). *Organogenesis of the Kidney*. Cambridge University Press, Cambridge, 173 pp.

Saxén, L., and Ekblom, P. (1981). The developing kidney as a model system for normal and impaired organogenesis. In: Neubert, D., and Merker, H.-J. (Eds), *Culture Techniques*, Walter de Gruyter and Co., Berlin–New York, pp. 291–300.

Saxén, L., and Karkinen-Jääskeläinen, M. (1975). Inductive interactions in morphogenesis. In: Balls, M., and Wild, A. (Eds) *The Early Development of Mammals*, Cambridge University Press, Cambridge, pp. 319–34.

Saxén, L., and Lehtonen, E. (1978). Transfilter induction of kidney tubules as a function of the extent and duration of intercellular contacts. *J. Embryol. Exp. Morphol.*, **47**, 97–109.

Saxén, L., and Saksela, E. (1971). Transmission and spread of embryonic induction. II. Exclusion of an assimilatory transmission mechanism in kidney tubule induction. *Exp. Cell Res.*, **66**, 369–77.

Saxén, L., Koskimies, O., Lahti, A., Miettinen, H., Rapola, J., and Wartiovaara, J. (1968). Differentiation of kidney mesenchyme in an experimental model system. In: Abercrombie, M., Brachet, J., and King, T.J. (Eds), *Adv. Morphog.*, volume 7, Academic Press, London, pp. 251–93.

Saxén, L., Lehtonen, E., Karkinen-Jääskeläinen, M., Nordling, S., and Wartiovaara, J. (1976). Are morphogenetic tissue interactions mediated by transmissible signal substances or through cell contacts? *Nature*, **259**, 662–3.

Saxén, L., Salonen, J., Ekblom, P., and Nordling, S. (1983). DNA synthesis and cell generation cycle during determination and differentiation of the metanephric mesenchyme. *Dev. Biol.*, **98**, 130–38.

Saxén, L., Ekblom, P., and Sariola, H. (1985). Organogenesis. In: Marios, M. (Ed.), *Prevention of Physical and Mental Congenital Defects, Part A: The Scope of the Problem*, Progress in Clinical and Biological Research, volume 163A, Alan R. Liss, New York, pp. 41–53.

Shabad, L.M., Sorokina, J.D., Golub, N.I., and Bogovski, S.P. (1972). Transplacental effect of some chemical compounds on organ cultures of embryonic kidney tissue. *Cancer Res.*, **32**, 617–27.

Strudel, G., and Pinot, M. (1965). Differenciation en culture *in vitro* du mesonephros de l'embryon de poulet. *Dev. Biol.*, **11**, 284–99.

Taub, M., Chuman, L., Saier, M.H. Jr., and Sato, G. (1979). Growth of Madin-Darby canine kidney epithelial cell (MDCK) line in hormone-supplemented, serum-free medium. *Proc. Nat. Acad. Sci.*, USA, **76**, 3338–42.

Vetter, M.R. and Gibley, C.W. Jr. (1966). Morphogenesis and histo-chemistry of the developing mouse kidney. *J. Morphol.*, **120**, 135–56.

Vainio, T., Jainchill, J., Clement, K., and Saxén, L. (1965). Studies on kidney tubulogenesis. VI. Survival and nucleic acid metabolism of differentiating mouse metanephrogenic mesenchyme *in vitro. J. Cell. Comp. Physiol.*, **66**, 311–18.

Wartiovaara, J. (1966). Cell contacts in relation to cytodifferentiation in metanephrogenic mesenchyme *in vitro. Ann. Med. Exp. Fenn.*, **44**, 469–503.

Wartiovaara, J., Nordling, S., Lehtonen, E., and Saxén, L. (1974). Transfilter induction of kidney tubules: correlation with cytoplasmic penetration into Nuclepore filters. *J. Embryol. Exp. Morphol.*, **31**, 667–86.

Wilson, J.G., and Warkany, J. (1948). Malformations in the genito-urinary tract induced by vitamin A deficiency in the rat. *Am. J. Anat.*, **83**, 357–407.

Wolff, E., and Haffen, K. (1952). Sur une méthode de culture d'organes embryonnaires *in vitro. Texas Rept. Biol. Med.*, **10**, 463–72.

Short-term Toxicity Tests for Non-genotoxic Effects
Edited by P. Bourdeau *et al.*
© 1990 SCOPE. Published by John Wiley & Sons Ltd

CHAPTER 11

The Skin: Predictive Value of Short-term Toxicity Tests

Raymond R. Suskind

11.1 INTRODUCTION

The skin is an important interface between man and his environment. It is a significant portal of entry of hazardous agents and a vulnerable target organ system. It is also a uniquely accessible model system for detecting hazards and for studying mechanisms of a wide variety of biological functions. It is a target organ, not only for xenobiotics absorbed through the skin itself, but also for those absorbed through the respiratory and gastrointestinal tracts (Occupational Safety and Health Administration, 1978; Suskind, 1977).

The skin is endowed with a versatile group of adaptive and defence mechanisms. These include multiple defences against penetration, fluid loss, solar radiation, physical trauma, penetration and thermal stress (Suskind, 1977).

Epidemiologic information regarding cutaneous involvement in environmentally-induced disease is limited. Disease frequency information, obtained from occupational skin disease statistics, varies considerably in quality and accuracy. Roughly 20 per cent of occupational skin disease involves allergic responses; the remainder consists of non-allergic inflammatory responses to irritants, or involves other cutaneous features (such as pigmentation, pilosebaceous structures and eccrine sweat glands) or skin cancer. Eczematous dermatoses constitute the largest group of skin problems induced by xenobiotic agents. The majority of these involve primary irritant dermatitis, allergic eczematous contact dermatitis and atopic dermatitis. Those of atopic origin are influenced considerably by multiple environmental factors as well. Of irritant problems, the most common and difficult to manage are those induced by marginal irritants to which the human skin responds only after multiple exposure (Occupational Safety and Health Administration, 1978; Suskind, 1977).

11.2 PERCUTANEOUS ABSORPTION

The normal barrier to the passage of water and other chemical penetrants is the stratum corneum. This is composed of bonded, interdigitating keratinized cells. It is a compact structure except for the outermost layers, which are shed continuously. It is not a uniform membrane but a composite made up of at least ten distinct cell layers. The basal cells are characterized by an 80 Å unit membrane while the stratum corneum cell membrane is about 200 Å in thickness. It is likely that the thickened cell membrane contributes significantly to the defensive properties of the strateum corneum.

Skin penetration is generally considered to be a process of passive diffusion. The factors which influence the rate of penetration or flux include the lipid partition coefficient, concentration gradients, molecular size of the penetrant, thickness of the horny layer, ambient and skin temperature, ambient humidity, chemical or physical damage to the barrier, pH, duration of exposure, skin area exposed, blood flow in the skin and rate of metabolic transformation within the skin (Malkinson and Rothman, 1963; Rothman, 1954; Scheuplein, 1978; Tregear, 1966).

11.3   CLINICAL AND PATHOLOGICAL PATTERNS OF ADVERSE REACTIONS

Xenobiotics may affect a single tissue component (such as the epidermis, dermis, blood vessels, pilosebaceous unit, melanocytes or eccrine sweat glands), or they may affect several components. Therefore, the type of pathological pattern may vary with the particular stimulus. In order to appreciate the current state of scientific methodologies for hazard assessment and the need for short-term tests, it is essential to identify those pathological patterns which characterize specific clinical reactions to xenobiotics (Occupational Safety and Health Administration, 1978; Suskind, 1977).

11.3.1   Inflammatory responses

The most common pathological pattern is that of an inflammatory response which, except for infection, is of an eczematous nature. The latter is the characteristic response to non-allergic, primary irritants and in antigen-induced cell-mediated hypersensitivity reactions.

11.3.1.1   Primary irritation

There is a lack of scientific information regarding mechanisms of damage to the skin characterized by inflammatory reactions having no immunological basis. These reactions are commonly lumped into the category of primary irritation. McCreesh and Steinberg (1977) distinguish between the following types for which there are predictive short-term animal tests:

(1)   Acute primary irritation, which is a local inflammatory response to a single

exposure that does not ostensibly produce cell death and is completely reversible;
(2)   A local inflammatory reaction produced after repeated exposure; this group includes the marginal irritant;
(3)   Chemical damage leading to irreversible destruction of skin tissue (ulceration) which may result in scarring; this category includes corrosive substances;
(4)   Phototoxic reactions, which are characterized by irritation induced by a chemical agent in the presence of ultraviolet light.

11.3.1.2   Allergic reactions

Cutaneous reactions with an immunologic basis can be classified into three types using the criteria of Coombs and Gell (1975):

(1)   Type I—anaphylactic reactions. Humoral antibodies are produced with the participation of B cells. The reactions are reagin dependent and the antibody is an IGE protein bound to the cell surface. The urticarial response in the skin is a vascular response to a vasoactive amine, such as histamine, which is present in mast cells and basophils. In the respiratory tract, clinical signs include allergic rhinitis and asthma. In this type of skin reaction, the xenobiotics enter via the respiratory or gastrointestinal tract, but rarely percutaneously. Diagnostic tests, through which hypersensitivity states can be determined, elicit an immediate wheal and flare response from intradermal or scratch tests to the antigen (Coombs and Gell, 1975). There are sufficient incidents to verify the infrequent but definite occurrence of contact uriticaria. This syndrome has been classified into three types (Maibach and Johnson, 1975): (i) non-immunologic or primary urticaria, (ii) immunologic urticaria, and (iii) urticaria of uncertain mechanism. Non-immunologic urticariogens provoke release of vasoactive agents, such as histamine, SRS-A and bradykinin. Known non-immunologic urticariogens include DMSO, a variety of plants such as nettles, the heirs of caterpillars and moths, esters of nicotinic acid, and cobalt chloride. Case studies of immunologic urticaria are often unclear about the major route of absorption involved. This is especially true when cutaneous as well as respiratory reactions—urticaria as well as asthma—are involved. Nevertheless, there are some cases in which cutaneous absorption of a chemical agent alone has induced a wheal-flare type of reaction, along with other anaphylactoid symptoms.

Vasoactive agents which elicit wheal-flare reactions in human skin include the following (in addition to histamine and the kinins): prostaglandins, PGE_1 and PGE_2 and several complement factors including C3a, C5a and C2 peptide.

Urticaria from workplace hazards is rare and usually occurs following respiratory exposure. Chemical agents that have been implicated in this way include drugs (e.g. penicillin), pesticides (e.g. lindane), ammonia, sulphur dioxide, formaldehyde, aminothiazole and sodium sulphide (Key and Withers, 1969).

(2)   Type IV—Allergic contact dermatitis. This is the most common skin response; it involves an immunologic mechanism. Simple chemical compounds (e.g. nickel, chromium salts, *p*-phenylenediamine, poison ivy resin) are initially absorbed through the skin and conjugate with protein. This protein antigen is presented by macrophages, which interact with T cells leading to the recognition of the protein antigen by T lymphocytes. Recent studies have demonstrated that Langerhans' cells, which are dendritic cells located above the basal cell layer of the epidermis, bear receptors for the F_c portion of IgG and for C_3 (Stingl *et al.*, 1978; Stingl *et al.*, 1977). The Langerhans' cells subserve the function of macrophages by processing and presenting antigens to T lymphocytes in lymph nodes. The recognition process, on continuous exposure or re-exposure to the allergen, provokes the eczematous response in the skin (allergic contact dermatitis). Allergic eczematous responses are characterized by erythema, swelling and vesiculation, and delayed reaction occurring twelve to forty-eight hours after re-exposure (i.e. challenge). Much new knowledge has been developed recently regarding the interaction between the antigen and the several cell types involved in delayed hypersensitivity (viz. T lymphocytes, B lymphocytes and macrophages (Katz, 1980). This includes interaction between T and B cells in antibody production, in antibody suppression and tolerance; interaction of B cells with other B cells and T cells, where the B cells influence the response of other lymphocytes via a secreted antibody; T cell synergy in graft versus host reaction, and in the suppression of contact dermatitis in the tolerant host. Suppression of hypersensitivity reactions of the delayed type will also occur with B–T cell interaction. Poulter and Turk (1972) have proposed a theory that, under normal circumstances, B cells modulate the effective function of T cells in allergic contact dermatitis.

(3)   Type III reactions. These are cutaneous reactions to xenobiotics which involve damage by antigen–antibody complexes (Coombs and Gell, 1975). The antibodies designated are IgG, IgM and, perhaps, even IgA. In the skin, one of the reaction types is known as the Arthus phenomenon; it is seen in reactions to drugs such as penicillin. In this type of reaction, the antigen reacts with precipitating antibodies in and around small blood vessels or in basement membranes. This causes severe local inflammation.

11.3.1.3   Photosensitization

Chemical agents may cause cutaneous reactions in the presence of ultraviolet light (Epstein, 1974). There are two types of such reactions:

(1)   Phototoxic reactions induced by coal tar products, essential oils such as bergamot, angelica root, cumin, psoralens, and photoinitiators such as amyl *p*-aminobenzoates. Phototoxic reactions may be accompanied by residual hyperpigmentation. No immunological mechanism is involved.

(2)   Photoallergic reactions are allergic contact reactions, the induction of which require exposure to ultraviolet light and a chemical agent. These are usually responses to long-wave ultraviolet light (above 320 nm). Examples of photo-allergens are tetrachlorosalicylanilide, tribromosalicylanilide, and bithional. Ultraviolet light may enhance conjugation with polypeptides or may induce photoproducts or photometabolites which are allergenic following conjugation.

11.3.1.4   Pigment changes

Xenobiotics may lead to pigmentary disturbances in the skin, such as localized hypopigmentation or leukoderma, or conversely hyper-pigmentation, as in the case of post-inflammatory reactions. In most instances, the pathologic process can be explained on the basis of changes in the biochemical synthesis of melanin (Fitzpatrick, 1965; Fitzpatrick *et al.*, 1950; Fitzpatrick *et al.*, 1979).

The biochemistry of melanin and the pigmentation system have been studied in great detail (Seiji, 1963; Seiji and Iwashita, 1963; Seiji *et al.*, 1963). In the human epidermis, each melanocyte is associated with about thirty-six viable keratinocytes that transport and, in some cases, degrade the melanin received from the melanocyte. The melanocytes, in association with the keratinocytes, form the epidermal-melanin unit. Human skin contains a very large number of these units, and skin colour is the visual impact of melanin within them. The coloured polymer, melanin, is formed from tyrosine in the presence of the enzyme tyrosinase with the production of dopa, which in turn is converted to dopaquinone. Through a series of subsequent steps, 5,6-dihydroxyindole is formed which is polymerized into melanin. The work of Nicolaus (1962) indicated that melanin is a heteropolymer or a random polymer derived from the linkage of many different indoles.

The range in skin colour among negroids and caucasoids may be accounted for by the interaction of three to four additive gene pairs. The regional frequency distribu tion of melanocytes are similar in skin of all races. The racial colour differences in man are related to the fine structure of the melanocyte, variation in area are occupied by the rough endoplasmic reticulum and in the development of the Golgi zone, as well as in the relative proportions of melanosomes in the four developmental stages of cutaneous differentiation.

Ultraviolet light may increase pigmentation in several different ways: (1) by catalysing the oxidation of tyrosine to dopa, (2) by decreasing the redox potential of the skin, (3) by thermal enhancement of melanin formation following exposure to actinic radiation, and (4) by darkening of melanin granules already present.

11.3.1.5   Pilosebaceous reactions

Reactions involving the pilosebaceous structure may elicit a variety of damage patterns. They include damage to the hair shaft, damage to the matrix cells which produce the hair, acneform eruptions and folliculitis. Petroleum and cutting oils may induce a folliculitis (an inflammatory reaction). Occupational and cosmetic acne are common skin problems. Workplace chemicals that are able to induce acne include: petroleum-based cutting oils, coal tar fractions, chlorinated hydrocarbons (e.g. chlorinated naphthalenes, chlorinated biphenyls), and chlorinated phenoxy contaminants such as tetrachlorodibenzo-*p*-dioxin (TCDD) and polychorinated dibenzofurans (PCDF). In the case of chlorinated hydrocarbons, the acneform eruption is the clinical manifestation of changes in the differentiation process of sebaceous cells. The latter are replaced by keratinocytes. Hence, instead of the differentiated acinar cells forming lipid secretions, which is their normal function, the acinar cells become keratin-producing cells. These modifications in differentiation and function may persist for more than thirty years following initial exposure to the acnegenic agent (Suskind and Hertzberg, 1984).

Hair shaft breakage can be induced by exposure to alkaline substances which break the disulphide linkages in keratin. Inorganic agents such as thallium and organic molecules such as chloroprene dimers and a number of therapeutic agents interfere with the metabolism of the hair-forming matrix cells; hair loss may ensue as the result of such exposures.

11.3.1.6   *Eccrine sweat gland reactions*

Changes in the skin involving eccrine sweat glands are most frequently associated with a combination of high temperature environments and cutaneous irritation. The most common outcome is miliaria, in which epidermal injury produces abnormal keratinization and plugging of the eccrine duct orifices. When the sweat glands are subsequently stimulated thermally, sweat is trapped in a plugged duct. With increased pressure, the duct wall breaks and the collected sweat extravasates in the skin, producing the inflammatory response of miliaria (Suskind, 1977).

11.3.1.7   *Other tissue components*

Collagen and elastic tissue components of the skin are primarily damaged through the direct effects of radiation, both ultraviolet and ionizing, and only rarely through association with chemical absorption. Blood vessels in the skin are involved in inflammatory reactions. However, they are singularly damaged in prolonged low temperature exposures. Ionizing radiation will also produce irreversible dilatation of capillaries and fibrotic changes in vessels leading to ischaemia, atrophy, necrosis and ulceration.

While cutaneous sensation is informative as well as protective, potential and actual damage may be signalled by several sensory modalities, including itching and pain. Both modalities of sensation are subserved by the same receptors and nerve fibres. Inflammatory reactions provoked by primary irritants as well as allergic sensitizers are characterized by pruritis, which may precede the objective signs of inflammation (Suskind, 1977).

11.4 TESTS FOR THE ASSESSMENT OF CUTANEOUS TOXICITY AND REACTIONS

11.4.1 Dermal toxicity

Following the determination of an oral LD50 on the chemical agent in question, it is appropriate to determine the LD50 using the skin as the route of exposure. This may be carried out in one of several species of animals (rat, guinea-pig or rabbit); ten or more animals are exposed to three dose levels up to 2 g/kg applied for a period of two to 24 hours duration inside a rubber or plastic dam to assure absorption. The necropsy should include gross observations on all vital organs.

For most chemical agents that are absorbed through the skin, subacute percutaneous toxicity can be determined in either the rat, guinea-pig or rabbit. Ten or more animals are exposed daily or every other day for 90 days, using three concentrations up to a minimal effective dose of the dermal LD50. These are applied under a plastic or rubber dam for a period of four to 24 hours duration. Necropsy should include gross observations of the skin and all vital organs, as well as microscopic examinations.

Anderson and Keller (1984) have described the toxicokinetic parameters which determine dose delivered to the skin. They believe that the extrapolation of kinetic data derived from other routes of administration, using *in vitro* permeability constants to predict cutaneous hazard, seems to be a promising application for toxicokinetic simulation.

11.4.2 Methods of assessment of skin penetration

While extensive literature reports *in vivo* and *in vitro* techniques to determine rates of penetration, there is no single method which is standardized for a particular family of chemical agents. One report (Bronaugh and Maibach, 1985) claims good correlation between *in vitro* and *in vivo* human results for several compounds.

The factors involved in cutaneous penetration have been described by Dugard (1977) who indicates that the assessment of hazard in relation to absorption rate must consider the release of the chemical agent from the skin as well as its detoxification and/or elimination. Thus, consideration of the 'dynamic parameters permits an estimate of whether a toxic material accumulates in the body in sufficient quantity to produce adverse effects—measurement of absorption from different formulations may indicate which is the safest'. Dugard also states: 'the comparison of absorption properties of different chemical substances does not indicate the relative safety unless relative potencies and preferably detoxification and elimination kinetics are known'. At least one new *in vitro* method considers rate of penetration in relation to metabolism and biotransformation. This technique uses a multisample apparatus for the kinetic evaluation of skin penetration in relation to viability and metabolic status (Holland *et al.*, 1984; Kao *et al.*, 1984).

The most useful method for the assessment of xenobiotics is the model recently developed by Wojciechowski and Krueger at the University of Utah. It employs a rat/human skin flap served by a defined and accessible vasculature on a congenitally athymic (nude) rat (Krueger *et al.*, 1985; Wojciechowski *et al.*, 1987). It has been used successfully to quantify transdermal fluxes of drugs such as benzoic acid (Burton *et al.*, 1984), and caffiene and is now being used to study polycyclic aromatic carcinogens and chlorinated dioxins.

Factors which influence passive diffusion through the rate-limiting barrier—the stratum corneum—have already been discussed. Although the stratum corneum is the rate-limiting membrane, other structures of the skin such as the pilosebaceous and eccrine sweat structures are also involved. The relative role of the stratum corneum in relation to these two structures is difficult to measure. The pilosebaceous structure provides a shunt or transient state route of absorption. Other factors which complicate penetration rate measurement methods include the quantity of the penetrant used, the absorption from a solid milieu or whether the penetrant is a liquid, a vapour or a gas (Dugard, 1977).

Recent comparative studies of the absorption of several hydrophobic compounds using *in vivo* and *in vitro* techniques indicate poor correlation between the results using the two types of assessment methods (Bronaugh *et al.*, 1982a and b; Bronaugh and Stewart, 1984).

11.4.3   Primary irritation

A standard irritation test specified by the Federal Hazardous Substances Act (USEPA, 1975) has been in use since 1944 (Draize *et al.*, 1944). It is a simple test in which clipped albino rabbits with intact and abraded skin are exposed to 0.5 ml (in the case of liquids) or 0.5 g (in the case of solids or semi-solids) of the test substance placed under a rubber or plastic dam for a period of 24 hours. Skin reactions are scored after 24 hours of exposure based on the degree of erythema, eschar formation and oedema; reactions are graded again 72 hours subsequently. Modifications of this method have been proposed and the National Institute for Occupational Safety and Health has published interpretations of the skin reaction values with respect to safety for contact with intact human skin (Campbell *et al.*, 1975). Problems encountered with the standard test have been reviewed by McCreesh and Steinberg (1977).

In order to determine the cumulative effect of repeated exposure to a chemical agent, either rabbit or guinea-pig is usually employed, using several concentration levels of the test agent at and below the minimal irritant level. To determine threshold levels, preliminary tests are carried out using six to ten rabbits or guinea-pigs at four concentration levels. The exposure time is 24 hours and the reactions observed after 24 and 48 hours. To assess cumulative effects, animals are exposed daily or every other day for a period of up to three months. Repeated exposures also provide information about accommodation, a phenomenon in which repeated exposure to an irritant (e.g. fatty acids and aliphatic alcohols) results in initial irritation followed by decreased response even to the point of non-responsiveness. Accommodation has been observed in both guinea-pigs and man but the mechanisms have yet to be determined.

Rabbit skin is more readily irritated by chemical agents than human skin but the reliability of the rabbit model is very limited for predicting the effects of weak irritants in man. Steinberg *et al.* (1975) compared a series of chemicals that were tested for their irritancy in both rabbit and man; the correlation was weak. A useful parameter is the threshold for irritation or the concentration which, after one exposure or a repeated daily 21 day exposure, produces no response in the rabbit. This achieves particular significance where the concentration of a chemical agent intended for topical use is known. It is generally believed that substances which elicit no irritant response or a minimal response in rabbits are unlikely to cause irritation in man.

For chemicals which are likely to contact human skin extensively, either because of intentional contact (e.g. toiletries and cosmetics) or because of inadvertent exposure (such as may occur in certain occupational situations), it is useful to investigate whether the concentration used will produce a reaction in a small panel of human subjects after single or repeated exposures. This is determined by means of the single patch test using a range of concentrations up to ten times the intended use concentration for a period of four to 24 hours. The substance may be applied at the same site daily or every other day for a period of three weeks in order to determine if cumulative effects occur.

No *in vitro* method for irritancy has yet been developed that is a satisfactory substitute for the whole animal. Although the models using intact animals are relatively short-term, the potential for developing an *in vitro* method is promising since the methods of growing human and animal whole skin in culture have improved significantly. Leighton *et al.* (1983) have recently demonstrated that a method using the chorioallantoic membrane of the chick egg can be considered as a substitute for the Draize eye irritancy test for a limited number of chemicals.

11.4.4 Immunologic reactions

The test model for inducing Type I reactions in animals was first described in 1940 (Jacobs, 1940; Jacobs *et al.*, 1940). In the original investigation, both an immediate urticarial reaction and a delayed reaction were elicited in guinea-pigs. The guinea-pig model for assessing potential urticariogenic agents has not been standardized. A major problem is that some substances which induce urticaria-like reactions in the guinea-pig are known not to be hazardous to man.

Predictive tests in laboratory animals for investigating the delayed hypersensitivity (Type IV) potential of chemical agents have been studied extensively. Using the research model designed by Landsteiner and Jacobs (1935), Draize *et al.* (1944) proposed a so-called predictive test which for many years was the recommended procedure by federal regulatory agencies in the USA. A summary of procedures for identification of contact allergens in guinea-pig is presented in Table 11.1. The original Draize method employs 40 albino guinea-pigs—20 in an experiment group and 20 in a control group. The test substance is injected intradermally as a 0.1 per

Table 11.1   Predictive tests for contact allergenicity in guinea-pigs

Test	Year published	Induction			Challenge	
		Route	Skin	No. of exposures	Route of exposure	Test days (total)
Landsteiner and Jacobs	1935	Intradermal		10	Intradermal	39
Draize *et al.*	1944	Intradermal		10	Intradermal	39
Buehler Griffith and Buehler	1965 1969	Topical	Occluded	1–9	Closed	16–44
Magnusson and Kligman	1970	Intradermal, + topical	Occluded	1	Closed	24
Maguire	1975	Topical	Occluded	4	Closed	23
Klecak *et al.*	1977	Topical	Open	20	Open × 2	40

cent solution, suspension or emulsion in 0.85 per cent NaCl, paraffin oil or poly-ethylene glycol. The test group receives a series of ten intradermal injections given every other day in the anterior flank over an area of 3×4 cm. The initial injection is 0.05 ml and the remaining nine are 0.1 ml, all injected at different sites. The test animals are challenged on the contralateral flank, corresponding to the site of the first injection, with 0.05 ml of 0.1 per cent of the test solution. Challenges are performed 35 days after the initial induction injection and the challenge sites are observed for reaction 24 and 48 hours after the challenge exposure. Reactions are graded on the basis of the intensity of the erythema and size of the edema. While this is a relatively simple test, the induction concentration is fixed and no consideration is given to the use concentration. The original method is not sensitive enough to identify many allergenic materials.

The most sensitive method using guinea-pigs is the 'maximization' test (Magnuson and Kligman, 1970). In this procedure, the experimental group receives three pairs of simultaneous intradermal injections in the shoulder region, followed by an application of a closed patch over the injection site one week afterwards. The injection consists of : (1) 0.1 ml of Freund's complete adjuvant (FCA), (2) 0.1 ml of the test material, and (3) 0.1 ml of the test material in FCA. Injections 1 and 2 are made close to each other and injection 3 caudal to the first two. The control group also receives three pairs of injections: (1) 0.1 ml of FCA, (2) 0.1 ml of the vehicle alone, and (3) 0.1 ml of the vehicle in FCA. Three weeks after the initial exposure, the experimental control animals receive occlusive applied patches with the test agent as well as the vehicle alone. This test will identify all allergenic agents. It is more sensitive than the 'maximization' test using human subjects and it has been noted that there are chemical substances which are not known to be sensitizing to humans which will sensitize guinea-pigs. For example, humans are not sensitized by several alkyl derivatives of cinnamic aldehyde that induce sensitization in the guinea-pig 'maximization' test.

Buehler (1965) introduced a relatively simple procedure that is used for cosmetic components as well as drug products, fragrances and household products. According to the author, this predictive procedure, when compared with the human repeated insult patch test, missed less than 3 per cent of the materials found to be sensitizing by the latter test.

In the United States, panels of human subjects are still used to test chemical materials for their irritancy as well as sensitizing potential. Methods used include the repeated insult test (Draize, 1959), the Kligman 'maximization' test (Kligman, 1966), as well as the methods of Shelanski and Shelanski (1953) and Schwartz (1957). In the repeated insult test, as well as the 'maximization' test, the concentrations of chemicals applied can be related to intended use concentrations. In the case of fragrances and flavours, for example, the human 'maximization' test is carried out with a concentration of ten times the expected maximum use concentration.

It should be noted that all of the animal or human tests for determining potential allergenicity require a minimum five to six weeks. It is not possible to shorten the induction period.

So far, no standardized method has been developed to sensitize cultured cells *in vitro* so that the sensitization potential of a chemical agent can be measured. However, several cellular phenomena have been used to determine the possible antigenic potential of chemical agents. These include the blastogenic effect to leukocytes of such agents as tuberculin-purified protein, phytohaemaglutinin and antiserum. The lymphocyte transformation phenomenon has been used as an *in vitro* method to determine whether or not an animal or a human has been sensitized. Sensitized T cells can be identified *in vitro* by the use of a test for a migration inhibiting factor (MIF) (Unanue and Benacerraf, 1984). In theory, all antigens which induce delayed hypersensitivity reactions should sensitize T lymphocytes, and peritoneal exudates from a sensitized animal inhibit the migration of macrophages in a capilloary tube. This is the basis of a test which provides a highly specific *in vitro* correlate of delayed hypersensitivity in the intact animal. However, the MIF test cannot be used itself to predict the sensitizing potential of a chemical since the whole animal is necessary to produce MIF-containing lymphocytes.

11.4.5 Assay methods for phototoxicity and photoallergenicity

Tests have been developed to determine potential phototoxic effects of chemical agents absorbed through one of several routes and these have been used to assess the activity of drugs, fragrances, flavours and some industrial materials. The effectiveness of some of the models is summarized in Table 11.2. Phototoxic reactions are probably the best understood drug photosensitivity reactions (Harber, 1981). Responses are dose-related, both with respect to the drug and with respect to the ultraviolet light. Harber (1981) has reviewed the status of mammalian and human models for predicting drug photosensitivity. The development of a simple and effective *in vitro* predictive test to assess phototoxicity remains an ideal goal. The work of Schothorst *et al.* (1973) describing biochemical alterations in aminoacids, glutathione and unsaturated fatty acids indicates promise but currently is not standardized for predictive purposes. The use of cell cultures (Freeman, 1970), red blood cells (Blum, 1941), paramecia (Raab, 1900), fungi (Daniels, 1965) and viral systems (Fowlks, 1959) have been described for assaying phototoxicity. Each of these assays is dependent on the detection of a chemical or biological change in the system when the photoabsorbing and phototoxic agent is introduced and exposed to ultraviolet light. Results obtained with these models do not correlate well with photosensitivity reactions in man. The factors which are responsible for the poor correlation include: (1) failure to account for the variations in percutaneous absorption; (2) failure to account for variations in gastrointestinal absorption, cutaneous storage, and excretion of the photosensitizer; (3) failure to account for the metabolic transformation of the sensitizer in liver and in skin; and (4) failure to account for the inactivation of the photosensitizer by metabolism and detoxification following absorption. Mammalian models have better predictive value than those using non-mammalian species but they still have limitations. As is noted in Table 11.2, several animal models have been used effectively for the assessment of

Table 11.2   Summary of findings in some animal models used for detection of agents with phototoxicity

Author(s) reference	Animal	UV-source	Positive	Negative
Stott *et al.* (1970)	Guinea-pig ears (DMSO vehicle)	Fluorescent blacklights (UV-A)	8-methoxypsoralen chloropromazine prochlorperazine demeclocyclin3	Sulphanilamide Chlorothiazide Griseofulvin Chlortetracycline
Gloxhuber (1970)	Hairless mouse	Filtered Osram (UV-A)	8-methoxypsoralen certain essential oils	Chlorpromazine Chlorothiazide
Morikawa *et al.* (1974)	Rabbit, guinea-pig	Blacklights (UV-A)	Phenothiazine coal tar derivatives acridine, etc.	Sulphanilamide Demeclocycline Griseofulvin
Forbes *et al.* (1977)	Hairless mouse, miniature swine	Xenon arc solar simulator blacklights (UV-A)	Certain fragrance materials 8-methoxypsoralen	

From Kaidbey and Kligman (1980).

phototoxicity including mice, mouse ears, hairless mice, rats, rabbits, miniature pigs and guinea-pigs. Phototoxic reactions used as critera for phototoxicity in mice include cutaneous oedema, erythema and necrosis, observed on the ears and tail. However, the mouse epidermis is relatively thin compared with that in man resulting in greater penetration of UVB to the basal cell layer and connective tissue. Rat skin resembles the mouse in this respect (rat tail is the part of the body that is often exposed). The albino Hartley strain guinea-pig is widely used for assessing topical phototoxicity. Some investigators believe that the rabbit is superior to the rat, the mouse and the guinea-pig with respect to both sensitivity and quantitative inflammatory response. In a comparison study with 21 phototoxic agents applied to rabbits and guinea-pigs, it was found that rabbits were more sensitive qualitatively and quantitatively than guinea-pigs (Morikawa *et al.*, 1974).

Human volunteers can be used for the assessment of phototoxic agents. The procedures used include scotch tape stripping and exposure to a solar simulator. Human subjects can also be exposed by intradermal injections of a 0.1 ml aliquot of the photosensitizer in saline, followed by a ten to 30-minute exposure to UVA or UVB radiation. The simplest technique for assessing topical phototoxic agents requires application of fixed amounts to lumbar or scrotal skin, followed by irradiation with known doses of UV light. A 'simulated-use' test can be employed to assess the phototoxicity of drugs (e.g. methacycline). Volunteers are given a therapeutic dose of the drug in question on a double blind basis, followed by exposure to natural sunlight for up to six hours.

Chemical agents which are known to produce photoallergic reactions in the skin include sulphonamides, halogenated salicylanalides, griseofulvin, Fentichlor, promethazine, blankophores, thiazides, chlorpromazine, cyclamates and chlordiazepoxide (Librium). A very potent sensitizing agent is tetrachlorosalicylanalide. It is now used as a positive control substance when materials are being tested in a guinea-pig model.

The photosensitizing and photoeliciting techniques in guinea-pigs (Buehler, 1984; Harber, 1981; Morikawa *et al.*, 1974) involve topical application of the potential photosensitizer to the shaved nuchal area of guinea-pigs 30 minutes prior to irradiation. Two types of UV radiation are employed: (1) a sunlamp with an emission spectrum of 285 nm to 350 nm, and (2) a blacklight fluorescent tube with an emission of 320 nm to 450 nm. Cutaneous exposure followed by irradiation is repeated three times during a seven-day period. Three weeks after the last sensitizing exposure, three concentration levels of the test material are applied to areas not previously exposed, followed by irradiation with non-erythemogenic doses of UVA or blacklight. The response is scored and interpreted on the basis of degree of erythema, comparing the irradiated sites to the non-irradiated sites. Almost all contact photoallergens appear to require wavelengths greater than 320 nm (Kaidbey and Kligman, 1980).

11.4.6   Methods for assessing the effects of xenobiotics on melanin in the skin

Research methods have been developed to determine the effects of xenobiotics on melanin pigment. These are short-term tests requiring from one to three hours. They include:

(1) The effect of the xenobiotic on tyrosinase activity *in vitro*. Mushroom tyrosinase is incubated with radio-labelled tyrosine; tyrosinase activity is measured by determining the amount of radio-labelled tyrosine that is oxidized.
(2) Interference with the transformation of tyrosine to dopa and dopaquinone *in vitro* in the presence of tyrosinase. The amount of dopa, dopaquinone and the polymer itself can be measured quantitatively.
(3) The effect of different concentrations of a chemical on a culture of murine melanoma cells.

The whole animal can be used to determine the effect of the xenobiotics on pigmented skin. The DBA or C3H strain of mouse is preferred. The site of exposure is the ear. Three to five days after the animals are first exposed, the increase or decrease in pigmentation is observed and the number of melanocytes per mm^2 is determined microscopically.

In assessing a number of human depigmenting agents using black guinea-pigs and black mice as test animals, Gellen *et al.* (1979) noted various confounding factors which needed to be controlled. These included the choice of vehicle, irritation, and false positive reactions produced by either the vehicle or the test material itself as well as false negative responses to known depigmenting agents.

11.4.7   Assessment of toxic effects on the pilosebaceous structures

Although there are no recognized standard methods for measuring the effects of chemical agents on the keratin of the hair shaft or on the matrix cells which produce the hair itself, relatively simple methods are available to screen both topical agents and agents such as drugs intended for systemic administration.

For effects on the hair shaft keratin, segments of human or experimental animal hair can be immersed in solutions of the test agent for specified periods of time, rinsed with water and examined for structural and chemical changes. Components of cosmetics such as hair straightening or waving agents, hair colouring process components, shampoos and pomades are routinely subjected to such examinations.

Protocols can be designed to determine toxic effects on matrix cells (which result in reversible or irreversible hair loss depending upon the extent of the damage to the matrix cells). Thallium, chloroprene, thyroid antagonists, anticoagulants (heparin, heparinoids, coumarin), antimitotic agents (e.g. colchicine), immunosuppressive agents (e.g. folic acid antagonists), purine antagonists, alkylating agents, antipsychotic drugs (e.g. triparanol), antiepileptic agents (e.g. trimethadione) and vinca alkyloids are known to affect the matrix cells. The test protocol can include the administration of graded doses to rodents with known hair growth cycles (e.g. mice with a cycle of 30 days). The test group includes animals whose hair has been plucked and a group with intact hair. Following administration of graded doses, the plucked group of animals (test and controls) is observed for dose-related differences in rate of growth of hair and hair structure. The unplucked animals are observed for differences in onset of hair loss.

11.4.8   Chemically-induced acne

The first standardized test, published by Adams *et al.* (1941), is still the most widely used. The material to be tested is applied repeatedly (undiluted and in several concentrations) to the pinna of the inner surface of the rabbit ear using an appropriate solvent (olive oil, paraffin oil, ethanol, propylene glycol, etc.). Applications are repeated daily for four weeks or until a reaction is noted. Assessment is made both by clinical examination as well as histologic examination for epidermal hyperplasia, comedones and epithelial cysts. Further modifications of this technique were made by Shelley and Kligman (1957), and Hambrick (1957). Hambrick and Blank (1956) found that the external canal of the rabbit ear, rather than the pinna, is richest in sebaceous structures. The Hambrick technique requires a minor surgical procedure in order to lay open the ear canal surfaces for testing.

Inagami *et al.* (1969) applied rice oil contaminated with chlorinated biphenyls (that was responsible for the Yusho epidemic in Japan) to the skin of hairless mice. He reported follicular hyperkeratotic changes in the sebaceous follicle. More recently, the use of hairless mice has been explored as a model for testing potential acnegens (Puhvel *et al.*, 1982). The strains used were Skh-HR-1 and the HRS/J strains and the materials were applied to the dorsal skin in volumes of 0.1 ml in different vehicles. The response to known human acnegens was not constant. Polychlorinated naphthalenes, such as Halowax 1014, produced hyperkeratosis, epidermal hyperplasia, sebaceous gland involution and keratin cysts within fourteen days. Polychlorinated biphenyls such as Arochlor 1254, in sublethal concentrations, induced no observable changes either grossly or histologically; however, Phenclor 54 produced the same changes as the polychlorinated naphthalenes. 2,3,4,8-TCDD caused hyper-keratinization of the stratum corneum, epidermal hyperplasia, disappearance of sebaceous glands and follicles and numerous keratin cysts. All of the animals treated with these materials and which developed the cutaneous changes, also developed large intraabdominal fat deposits. The authors commented that it was only the 2,3,4,8-TCDD which produced the changes which were close to human chloracne, and only in one of the strains of mice (Skh-HR-1).

A potentially useful model for the short-term study of human acnegens is human skin which has been transplanted to the skin of athymic rats (Brungger *et al.*, 1984; Krueger *et al.*, 1985; Wojciechowski *et al.*, 1987). These transplants have been successfully grown and they completely retain the characteristics of human skin. Laboratory experience with this model has been limited to studies of percutaneous absorption and metabolism. Its usefulness as a bioassay model for xenobiotics, especially acnegens, deserves further exploration.

11.5   DISCUSSION AND STRATEGY FOR TESTING

The development of a strategy for testing a xenobiotic (or combination of chemicals, as in a product) requires knowledge at the outset about its intended uses and background information on its chemical structure, physical properties and known biological activity. If basic toxicological properties are not known, information on the acute toxicity, oral and dermal, should be obtained.

Studies of skin penetration may be of some value, but there are no *in vitro* models which provide data directly applicable to human beings demonstrated to be useful over a wide range of chemicals. Cutaneous exposure of rodent species or rabbit to the penetrant in an appropriate vehicle can provide estimates of the rate of penetration as measured by amount of material (or its metabolite) transferred per unit time into the dermis blood, or that is excreted. Alternatively, the rate of disappearance from the skin surface can be measured. The Wojciechowski/Krueger model is useful in determining rates of absorption and metabolism of xenobiotics.

The most common clinical consequence of xenobiotic exposure is inflammatory skin reactions that are caused by irritants and by antigens. Similar reactions may be enhanced by ultraviolet radiation. Model test systems to assess potential for irritancy require biologically responsive living tissue. Rabbit and guinea-pig are appropriate test subjects for both single and repeated exposure tests. Both are used to determine the threshold and subthreshold irritant dose(s) as well as for classification of irritants as strong, moderate, or weak. For some substances, there is poor correlation between results obtained in rabbits and in humans after repeated exposure; therefore, tests on panels of human subjects may be indicated. This can be carried out on panels used to appraise the sensitizing capacity using 'maximization' (Kligman, 1966) and repeated insult (Draize, 1959) protocols. Repeated exposure of animals to irritant concentrations of a chemical can provide information regarding accommodation or 'hardening'. The *in vitro* model using the chlorioallantoic membrane of the chick egg shows considerable promise as a substitute for the rabbit eye irritancy test and it may have promise as a substitute for the hole animal skin irritancy test.

Many agents or products intended for skin exposure require assessment for potential immunologic reactions, particularly cell-mediated hypersensitivity. Other agents which may be absorbed from the gastrointestinal tract or respiratory tract may be assessed for humoral antibody-associated reactions (Coombs-Gell Type I) in the guinea-pig. Standardized systems for detecting and measuring potency of antigenic agents which induce cell-mediated hypersensitivity reactions should involve panels of guinea-pigs or humans. The most sensitive involves 'maximizing' induction in guinea-pigs with FCA. The minimum duration of tests is four to five weeks. Assessment for allergenic potential requires the living organism. No *in vitro* tests have been developed which correlate with sensitizing capacity determinations in man.

While *in vitro* models using single cell organisms have been described for measuring phototoxic activity, the results of these tests do not correlate well with tests in man. Photoallergic potential can be determined with a relatively simple guinea-pig model. The minimum time required is four weeks.

Very simple short-term and useful tests are available for detecting effects of a xenobiotic on melanin synthesis using *in vitro* models. They include measuring effect of tyrosinase activity, the transformation of tyrosine to melanin, and the effect on mouse melanoma cells.

The tests for effects on pilosebaceous structures include simple *in vitro* methods of determining damage to hair shaft and whole animal (mouse) models for determining effects on hair-producing cells in which the end-points are: interruption of hair cycle; loss of hair; change in rate of hair growth; damage to matrix cells; and changes in hair structure.

In tests for acnegenic potential, the xenobiotic can be screened with the rabbit ear model. New procedures have been described using hairless mice which show potential for measuring acnegenicity. The use of human skin transplants to athymic rats may provide a fertile method for assaying agents for acnegenicity.

REFERENCES

Adams, E.M., Irish, D.D., Spencer, H.C., and Rowe, V.K. (1941). The response of rabbit skin to compounds reported to have caused acneform dermatitis. *Ind. Med.*, **10**, Industrial Hygiene Section, 2(1), 1–4.

Anderson, M.E., and Keller, W.C. (1984). Toxicokinetic principles in relation to percutaneous absorption and cutaneous toxicity. In: Drill, V.A., and Lazar, P. (Eds), *Cutaneous Toxicity*, Raven Press, New York, pp. 9–27.

Blum, H. (1941). *Photodynamic Action and Diseases Caused by Light,* Rheinhold, Princeton.

Bronaugh, R.L., and Maibach, H.I. (1985). Percutaneous absorption of nitroaromatic compounds: *In vivo* and *in vitro* studies in the monkey *J. Invest. Dermato.*, **84**, 180–83.

Bronaugh, R.L., and Stewart, R.F. (1984). Methods for *in vitro* percutaneous absorption studies. III. Hydrophobic compounds. *J. Pharm. Sci.*, **73**(9), 1255–8.

Bronaugh, R.L., Stewart, R.F., Congdon, E.R., and Giles, A.L. Jr. (1982a). Methods for *in vitro* percutaneous absorption studies. I. Comparison with *in vivo* results. *Toxicol. Appl. Pharmacol.*, **62**, 474–80.

Bronaugh, R.L., Stewart, R.F., and Congdon, E.R. (1982b). Methods for *in vitro* percutaneous absorption studies. II. Animal models for human skin. *Toxicol. Appl. Pharmacol.*, **62**, 481–8.

Brungger, A., Hubler, M., and Rohr, H.P. (1984). Human skin grafts on athymic nude rats. An experimental model for dermatological research. *Exper. Cell Biol.*, **52**, 122–4.

Buehler, E.V. (1965). Delayed contact hypersensitivity in the guinea pig. *Arch. Dermatol.*, **91**, 171–7.

Buehler, E. (January 1984). Personal communication.

Burton, S.A., Wojciechowski, Z.J., Krueger, G.G., and Huether, S. E. (1984). Transcutaneous absorption of benzoic acid in a unique isolated skin flat model. *Clinical Research*, **37**, 574.

Campbell, K.I., George, E.L., Hall, L.L., and Stara, J.F. (1975). Dermal irritancy of metal compounds. *Arch. Environ. Health*, **30**, 168–70.

Coombs, R.R.A., and Gell, P.G.H. (1975). Classification of allergic reactions responsible for clinical hypersensitivity and disease. In: Gell, P.G.H., Coombs, R.R.A., and Lachmann, P.J. (Eds), *Clinical Aspects of Immunology,* 3rd Edn, Blackwell Scientific Publications, Oxford, Chapter 25.

Daniels, R. (1965). A simple microbiological method for demonstrating phototoxic compounds. *J. Invest. Dermatol.*, **44**, 259.

Draize, J.H. (1959). Dermal toxicity. Appraisal of the safety of chemicals in foods, drugs and cosmetics. The Assoc. of Food and Drug Officials of the United States. Texas State Dept. of Health, Austin, TX, p. 46.

Draize, J.H., Woodgard, G., and Calvery, H.O. (1944). Methods for the study of irritation and toxicity of substances applied topically to the skin and mucous membranes. *J. Pharmacol. Exp. Ther.*, **82**, 377–90.

Dugard, P.H. (1977). Skin permeability theory in relation to measurements of percutaneous absorption in toxicology. In: Marzulli, F.N., and Maibach, H.I. (Eds), *Advances in Modern Toxicology*, volume 4, Dermatotoxicology and Pharmacology, Hemisphere Publishing Corp., Washington, D.C., Chapter 22.

Epstein, J.H. (1974). Phototoxicity and photoallergy: Clinical syndromes. In: Fitzpatrick, T.B., Pathak, M.A., Harber, L.C., Seiji, M., and Kukita, A. (Eds). *Sunlight and Man*, University of Tokyo Press, Tokyo, Chapter 9.

Fitzpatrick, T.B. (1965). Mammalian melanin biosynthesis. *Trans. St. John's Hosp. Dermatol. Soc.*, **52**(1), 1–26.

Fitzpatrick, T.B., Becker, S.W. Jr., Lerner, A.B., and Montgomery, H. (1950). Tyrosinase in human skin: demonstration of its presence and of its role in human melanin formation. *Science*, **112**, 223–5.

Fitzpatrick, T.B., Szabo, G., Seiji, M., and Quevedo, W.C. (1979). The biology of the melanin pigmentary system. In: Fitzpatrick, T.B., Arndt, K.A., Clark, W.H., Eisen, A.Z., Van Scott, E.J., and Vaughan, J.H. (Eds), *Dermatology in General Medicine*, 2nd Edition, McGraw-Hill Book Co., New York, Chapter 14.

Forbes, P.D., Urbach, F., and Davies, R.E. (1977). Phototoxicity testing of fragrance raw materials. *Food Cosmet. Toxicol.*, **15**, 55.

Fowlks, W.L. (1959). The mechanisms of photodynamic effect. *J. Invest. Dermat.*, **32**, 233.

Freeman, R.G. (1970). Interaction of phototoxic compounds with cells in tissue culture. *Arch. Dermat.*, **102**, 521–6.

Gellen, G.A., Maibach, I.H., Misiaszek, M.H., and Ring, M. (1979). Detection of environmental depigmenting substances. *Contact Dermatitis*, **5**, 201–13.

Gloxhuber, C. (1970). Prufung Von Kosmetik—grundstoffen auf fototoxische wirkung. *J. Soc. Cosmet. Chem.*, **21**, 825.

Griffith, J.F., and Buehler, E.V. (1969). Experimental skin sensitization in the guinea pig and man. Procter and Gamble Co., Cincinnati, Ohio.

Hambrick, G.W. Jr. (1957). The effect of substituted naphthalenes on the pilosebaceous apparatus of rabbit and man. *J. Invest. Dermatol.*, **29**: 89–103.

Hambrick, G.W. Jr., and Blank, H. (1956). A microanatomical study of the response of the pilosebaceous apparatus of the rabbit's ear canal. *J. Invest. Dermatol.*, **26**, 185–200.

Harber, L.C. (1981). Current status of mammalian and human models for predicting drug photosensitivity. *J. Invest. Dermatol.*, **77**, 65–70.

Holland, J.M., Kao, J.Y., and Whitaker, M.J. (1984). A multisample apparatus for kinetic evaluation of skin penetration *in vitro*: the influence of viability and metabolic status of the skin. *Toxicol. Appl. Pharmacol.*, **72**, 272–80.

Inagami, K., Koga, T., Kibuchi, M., Hashimoto, M., Takahashi, H., and Wada, K. (1969). Experimental study of hairless mice following administration of rice oil used by a 'Yusho' patient. *Fukuoka Igaku Zasshi*, **60**, 548–53.

Jacobs, J.L. (1940). Immediate generalized skin reactions in hypersensitive guinea pigs. *Proc. Soc. Exp. Biol. Med.*, **43**, 641–3.

Jacobs, J.L., Golden, T., and Kelley, J. (1940). Immediate reactions to anhydride, of wheal and erythema type. *Proc. Soc. Exp. Biol. Med.*, **44**, 74–7.

Kaidbey, K.H., and Kligman, A.M. (1980). Identification of contact photosensitizers by human assay. In: Drill, V., and Lazar, P. (Eds), *Current Concepts in Cutaneous Toxicity*, Academic Press, New York, pp. 55–68.

Kao, J., Hall, J., Shugart, L.R., and Holland, J.M. (1984). An *in vitro* approach to studying cutaneous metabolism and disposition of topically applied xenobiotics. *Toxicol. Appl. Pharmacol.*, **75**(2), 289–98.

Katz, S.I. (1980). New aspects of delayed hypersensitivity. In Drill, V.A., and Lazar, P. (Eds), *Current Concepts of Cutaneous Toxicity*, Academic Press, New York, pp. 11–23.

Key, M.M., and Withers, A. (1969). Anaphylaxis to streptomycin and hyposensitization. *Trans. St. John's Hosp. Dermatol. Soc.*, **55**, 184–8.

Klecak, G., Geleick, H., and Frey, J.R. (1977). Screening of fragrance materials for allergenicity in the guinea pig. I. Comparison of four testing methods. *J. Soc. Cosmet. Chem.*, **28**(2), 53–64.

Kligman, A.M. (1966). The identification of contact allergens by human assay. III. The maximization test: A procedure for screening and rating contact sensitizers. *J. Invest. Dermatol.*, **47**, 393–409.

Krueger, G.G., Wojciechowski, Z.J., Burton, S.A., Gilhar, A., Huether, S.E., Leonard, L.G., Rohr, U.D., Petelenz, T.J., Higuchi, W.I., and Pershing, L.K. (1985). The development of a rat/human skin flap served by a defined and accessible vasculature on a congenitally athymic (nude) rat. *Fund. Appl. Toxicol.*, **5**, S112–S121.

Landsteiner, K., and Jacobs, J. (1935). Studies on sensitization of animals with simple chemical compounds. *J. Exp. Med.* **61**, 643–56.

Leighton, J., Nassauer, J., Tchao, R., and Verdone, J. (1983). Development of a procedure using the chick egg as an alternative to the Draize rabbit test. In: Goldberg, A.M. (Ed.), *Alternative Methods for Toxicology, Volume 1: Product Safety Evaluation*, Mary Ann Liebert Inc., New York, pp. 163–77.

Magnusson, B., and Kligman, A.M. (1970). *Allergic Contact Dermatitis in the Guinea Pig: Identification of contact allergens*. Charles C. Thomas, Springfield, Illinois.

Maguire, H.C. Jr. (1975). Estimation of the allergenicity of prospective human contact sensitizers in the guinea pig. In: Maibach, H. (Ed.), *Animal Models in Dermatology*, Churchill Livingstone, Edinburgh, Chapter 7.

Maibach, H.I., and Johnson, H.L. (1975). Contact urticaria syndrome. *Arch. Dermatol.*, **111**, 726–30.

Malkinson, F.D., and Rothman, S. (1963). Percutaneous absorption. In Judassohn, J. (Ed.), *Handbuch der Haut- und Geschlechtskrankheiten, Normale und Pathologische Physiologie der Haut*, volume 1, Part 3, Springer, Berlin, pp. 90–156.

McCreesh, A.H., and Steinberg, M. (1977). Skin irritation testing in animals. In: Marzulli, F.N., and Maibach, H.I. (Eds), *Advances in Modern Toxicology*, volume 4. *Dermatotoxicology and Pharmacology*, Hemisphere Publishing Corp., Washington, D.C., Chapter 5.

Morikawa, F., Nakayama, Y., Fukuda, M., Hamano, M., Yokoyama, Y., Nagura, T., Ishihara, M., and Toda, K. (1974). Techniques for evaluation of phototoxicity and photoallergy in laboratory animals and man. In: Fitzpatrick, T.B., Pathak, M.A., Harber, L.C., Seiji, M., and Kukita, A. (Eds), *Sunlight and Man*, University of Tokyo Press, Tokyo, Chapter 34.

Nicolaus, R.A. (1962). Biogenesis of melanins. *Rass. Med. Sper.*, **9** (Suppl. 1), 1–32.

Occupational Safety and Health Administration (1978). *Report of the Advisory Committee on Cutaneous Hazards*. Standards Advisory Committee on Cutaneous Hazards, Washington, D.C.

Poulter, L.W., and Turk, J.L. (1972). Proportional increase in the g-carrying lymphocytes in peripheral lymphoid tissue following treatment with cyclophosphamide. *Nature (London) New Biol.*, **238**, 17–18.

Puhvel, S.M., Sakamoto, M., Ertl, D.C., and Reisner, R.M. (1982). Hairless mice as models for chloracne: A study of cutaneous changes induced by topical application of established chloracnegens. *Toxicol. Appl. Pharmacol.*, **64**, 422–503.

Raab, O. (1900). Uber die wirkung fluorescierender stoffe auf infusorien. *Z. Biol.*, **39**, 524.

Rothman, S. (1954). *Physiology and Biochemistry of the Skin*, University of Chicago Press, Chicago, Chapter 3.

Scheuplein, R.J. (1978). Permeability of the skin: A review of major concepts. In: Simon, G.A., Paster, Z., Klingberg, M.A., and Kaye, M. (Eds), *Current Problems in Dermatology. Skin: Drug Application and Evaluation of Environmental Hazards*, volume 7, S. Karger, Basel, pp. 172–86.

Schothorst, A.A., Suurmond, D., and deLuster, A. (1973). A biochemical screening test for the photosensitizing potential of drugs and disinfectants. *Photochem. Photobiol.*, **29**, 531–7.

Schwartz, L. (1957). The prophetic patch test. In Schwartz, L., Tulipan, L., and Birmingham, D.J. *Occupational Diseases of the Skin*. Lee and Febiger, Philadelphia, pp. 64–5, 386–7.

Seiji, M. (1963). Formation of mammalian melanin, *Jpn. J. Dermatol.*, *Series B*, **73**(1), 4–6.

Seiji, M., and Iwashita, S. (1963). On the site of melanin formation in melanocytes. *J. Biochem. (Tokyo)*, **54**(5), 465–7.

Seiji, M., Shimao, K., Birdeck, M.S.C., and Fitzpatrick, T.B. (1963). Subcellular localization of melanin biosynthesis. *Ann. N.Y. Acad. Sci.*, **100** (Part II), 497–533.

Shelanski, H.A., and Shelanski, M.V. (1953). A new technique of human patch tests. *Proc. Sci. Sect. Toilet Goods Assoc.*, **19**, 46.

Shelley, W.B., and Kligman, A.M. (1957). The experimental production of acne by penta- and hexachloronaphthalenes. *AMA Arch. Dermatol.*, **75**, 689–95.

Steinberg, M., Akers, W.A., Weeks, M.H., McCreesh, A.H., and Maibach, H.I. (1975). A comparison of test techniques based on rabbit and human skin responses to irritants with recommendations regarding the evaluation of mildly or moderately irritating compounds. In: Maibach, H. (Ed.), *Animal Models in Dermatology*, Churchill Livingstone, Edinburgh, pp. 1–11.

Stingl, G., Katz., S.I., Shevach, E.M., Wolff-Schreiner, E.C., and Green, I. (1978). Detection of Ia antigens on Langerhan's cells in guinea pig skin. *J. Immunol.*, **120**, 570–78.

Stingl, G., Wolff-Schreiner, E.C., Pichler, W.J., Gschnait, F., Knapp, W., and Wolff, K. (1977). Epidermal Langerhan's cells bear F_c and C3 receptors. *Nature (London)*, **268**, 245–6.

Stott, C.W., Stasse, J., Bonomo, R., and Camphell, A.H. (1970). Evaluation of the phototoxic potential of topcially applied agents using long-wave ultraviolet light. *J. Invest. Dermatol.*, **55**: 335.

Suskind, R.R. (1977). Environment and the skin. *Environ. Health Perspect.*, **20**, 27–37.

Suskind, R.R., and Hertzberg, V.S. (1984). Human health effects of 2,4,5-T and its toxic contaminants. *J. Am. Med. Assoc.*, **251**, 2372–80.

Tregear, R. (1966). *Physical Functions of Skin*, Academic Press, New York, pp. 1–52.

Unanue, E.R., and Benacerraf, B. (1984). *Textbook of Immunology*, 2nd Edition, Williams and Wilkins, Baltimore, p. 154.

U.S. Environmental Protection Agency (1975). Title 40—Protection of Environment, Chapter 1—Environmental Protection Agency, Subchapter E—Pesticide Programs, Part 162—Regulations for the Enforcement of the Federal Insecticide, Fungicide and Rodenticide Act, Subpart A—Registration. Reregistration and Classification Procedures. *Fed. Regist.*, **40** (July 3), 28242–86.

Wojciechowski, Z., Pershing, L.K., Huether, S., Leonard, L., Burton, S.A., Higuchi, W.I., and Krueger, G.G. (1987). An experimental skin sandwich flap on an independent vascular supply for the study of percutaneous absorption. *J. Invest. Dermatol.*, **88**(4), 439–46.

Short-term Toxicity Tests for Non-genotoxic Effects
Edited by P. Bourdeau *et al.*
© 1990 SCOPE. Published by John Wiley & Sons Ltd.

CHAPTER 12

Evaluation and Prediction of Chemical Toxicity using Haematopoietic Cell Renewal Systems

T.M. FLIEDNER, H. HEIT AND G. PABST

12.1 INTRODUCTION

Some 200 billion red cells, 120 billion granulocytes, 20 billion lymphocytes and 150 billion platelets are lost from the blood stream every day by migration and/or removal (Fliedner *et al.*, 1976). For each cell lost, another will enter the blood stream from extravascular storage and/or production sites to maintain a steady state equilibrium. Under these circumstances, health is maintained; if the balance between cell production and removal is disturbed, health is impaired. A reduction in the red cell concentration in the blood affects the oxygen supply to the brain, the heart, and other vital organs. If granulocytes and/or lymphocytes reach critically low levels, or if their quality is impaired, then specific or non-specific defence mechanisms will fail, leading to an increased risk from infectious diseases. In the case of thrombocytopenia (low platelet count), bleeding episodes may occur as well as other haemostatic problems. Thus, it is evident that blood cell renewal and the maintenance of a steady state equilibrium is of vital importance for health.

The haematopoietic organs are readily affected by a wide variety of chemicals. Wintrobe (1981) listed 317 drugs and other chemicals that have been reported to cause blood dyscrasias. It is expected that there are many more chemicals that could affect the haematopoietic cell renewal system. It is, therefore, understandable that examination of the 'blood picture' is one of the routine procedures performed in the health surveillance of workers exposed to infectious, chemical, or physical agents (including ionizing radiation) and that haematological studies form an essential part of the testing of chemicals which are to be used in industry and by the public.

The aim of this chapter is to review present knowledge on the functional structure and regulation of haematopoietic cell renewal systems and to examine various testing strategies using these systems for the safety assessment of chemicals.

12.2   HAEMATOPOIETIC CELL RENEWAL SYSTEMS

The elements of a haematopoietic cell renewal system are shown schematically in Figure 12.1. This scheme is relevant for the erythrocytic, granulocytic, and, to a certain extent, the megakaryocytic series. In lymphopoiesis, there are distinct differences due to the fact that lymphocytes do not represent a homogeneous population of cells either functionally or kinetically (Stutman and Good, 1972). Furthermore, lymphocytes in blood are by no means 'end cells' but represent only a stage in the life cycle of this cell type and are on their way to recirculate and to eventually start a new proliferative cycle under appropriate conditions.

Bone marrow is a major site of haematopoiesis but other organs are also involved; for example, the spleen is an important site of haematopoiesis in mice, but less so in rats and hardly at all in dogs. Replacement of cells lost from the blood depends on the active function of a pool of precursor cells that undergo a series of catenated cell divisions thereby multiplying their numbers. The erythrocyte originates from what one may describe as a proerythroblast, passing through the stages of makroblast, a basophilic, polychromatic, and orthochromic normoblast which then discards its nucleus to became a reticulocyte. The ganulocytic series of white blood cells originates from a myeloblast and passes through the stages of a large and small myelocyte which undergoes a final mitosis and becomes a metamyelocyte which matures into a band and segmented cell capable of entering the peripheral blood. In the case of blood platelets, proliferation and maturation of the precursors occur within one cell, the megakaryocyte. This so-called 'giant cell' is polyploid and may contain up to 32 cell nuclei depending on its state of maturity. The platelets are cytoplasmic extrusions of a megakaryocyte. Each megakaryocyte may produce up to 4000 platelets in this manner.

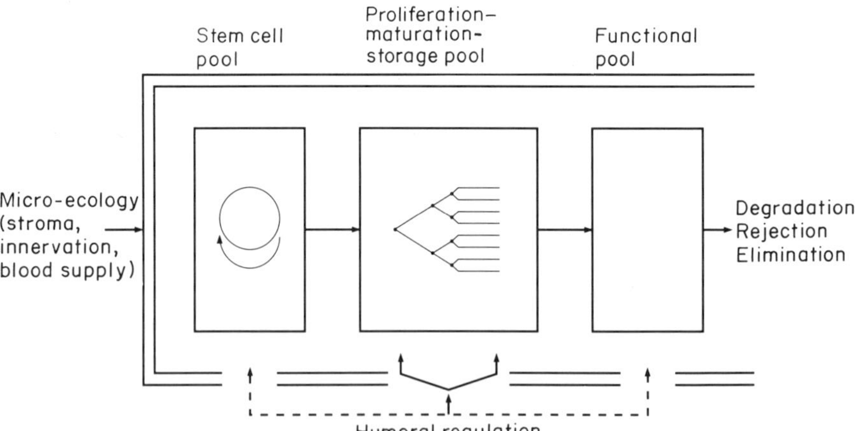

Figure 12.1   Elements of a cell renewal system (schematic representation).

Information concerning the average life-span of major blood cell types and their precursors are given for some laboratory animals in Table 12.1. Clearly there are species differences which one must be aware of in order to interpret toxicity data correctly. For details of species differences, the reader is referred to other texts (Jacobson and Doyle, 1962; Whipple, 1964; Bond *et al.*, 1965; Paulus, 1971; Pietschmann, 1972; Gordon *et al.*, 1972; Schalm *et al.*, 1975; Theml and Begemann, 1975; Quesenberry and Levitt, 1979).

The balance between the production and destruction of blood cells depends upon the functioning of the stem-cell pool. Stem cells possess an unlimited, self-replicative potential and are susceptible at the same time to respond to specific stimuli with cellular differentiation. According to the model represented in Figure 12.1, the various cellular elements in blood originate from a common pluripotent stem cell. The stem cells have the capacity to differentiate — after specific hormonal stimulation — into cells capable of producing erythrocytic, granulocytic or megakaryocytic cells. Erythropoietin is accepted to represent the stimulus that will trigger haemoglobin synthesis in a stem cell and thus convert it to a morphologically identifiable red cell precursor. Along the same line of thinking, one can predict the existence of a 'granulopoietin' and a 'thrombopoietin' which cause stem cells to develop into granulocytic or megakaryocytic precursor cells, respectively.

Stem cells cannot be identified morphologically in cell smears, histological sections, or by cell membrane markers. They are indistinguishable from cells usually identified in cell suspensions as 'lymphocytes'. Stutman and Good (1972) pointed

Table 12.1   Main parameters of haemopoietic systems

	Man	Dog	Rat	Mouse
(a) Granulocytopoiesis:				
marrow transit time	8–13 d	4–5 d	4 d	
$t_>$ in blood	6–7 h	6 h		8–12 h
numbers (10^3/mm^3 blood)	4.4	8.8	3.5	1.6
(b) Erythropoiesis:				
marrow transit time	4–7 d			2 d
life-span in blood	120 d	110 d	65 d	45 d
numbers (10^6/mm^3 blood)	5.1	6.3	8.0	9.6
(c) Thrombopoiesis:				
marrow transit time	4–10 d		2 d	
$t_>$ in blood	9.5 d		4 d	
numbers (10^3/mm^3 blood)	260	320	1000	1100
(d) Blood volume (ml/kg)	74	94	64	78

Commentary: Approximate numbers only. for more information see Bond *et al.* (1965), Shalm *et al.* (1975).

out that some of their 16 sub-types of lymphocytes seem to possess stem-cell characteristics.

The microecology of the haematopoietic cell systems is also important. It is well appreciated that the day-to-day maintenance of a constant blood cell number by life-long replication and differentiation of stem and/or progenitor cells in the haematopoietic tissue is the result of a functioning interaction between haematopoietic cells and their 'microenvironment'.

The microenvironment is of great importance in the regulation of the homeostatic mechanisms that guarantee the physiological steady state of haematopoietic cell renewal. During embryogenesis, haematopoiesis is initiated by the seeding of appropriate stem cells into a cellular microenvironment capable of inducing, maintaining, and regulating haematopoietic cell replication, differentiation, proliferation, and maturation (Kelemen *et al.*, 1979). All haematopoietic organs are, in essence, composed of two cell types: the stem cells and their progeny and the mesenchymal cells and their progeny. The main cellular elements of the haematopoietic environment are so-called reticular and endothelial cells. In addition, the microenvironment is influenced by myelinated and unmyelinated nerve fibres and by intercellular substances (Fliedner and Calvo, 1978). It should be pointed out, however, that details of the mechanisms that govern haematopoietic renewal are still largely unknown.

12.3   *IN VIVO* HAEMATOPOIETIC TEST METHODS

12.3.1   General considerations

There are a large number of end-points that can be used to determine the effects of chemicals, *in vivo*, on the haematopoietic systems. These include changes in the number of cells per unit blood volume, changes in the cellular composition of the bone marrow, and changes in the number and characteristics of stem cells in marrow or in the spleen of rodents. Metabolic changes (e.g. iron metabolism of erythrocytes) are amenable to investigation, as are changes in the humoral factors in the blood.

Toxic effects that result in changes in the blood picture can affect it through several different mechanisms. It is important, therefore, to consider how the ultimate target is affected when interpreting the significance of the observation. A chemical may affect only circulating red cells by inducing haemolysis. This is the case for benzene, for example, which is known to shorten the life-span of red cells by inducing increased haemolysis. Were this the sole effect (which it certainly is not), increased haemolysis would result in an increased erythropoiesis, would stimulate the stem-cell turnover and affect a variety of end-points commonly used (e.g. bone marrow cell composition, 'suicidal fraction' of CFU-S, etc.).

Other compounds influence the release of mature granulocytes from the bone marrow into the blood. When this occurs in rodents, granulocytosis is seen within hours resulting in changes in the bone marrow precursor population. This has been termed the 'stress reaction' of the bone marrow because it is a specific reaction of the bone marrow cell release mechanism that can be triggered by many factors including ionizing radiation, corticosteroids, and cytotoxic agents.

Other substances, such as lead, mainly affect cell production or cell differentiation/maturation in the bone marrow. Lead is known to interfere with haemoglobin synthesis causing porphyria and also a haemolytic and sideroblastic anaemia. Other compounds affect cellular proliferation. In the case of alkylating agents, mitotically connected cell abnormalities may become evident in cell smears and histological sections or in chromosomal preparations. This inefficient cell production results in an increased recruitment of haematopoietic stem cells.

The 'microenvironment' that guarantees the maintenance of haematopoietic cell renewal may also be the target of chemicals and thereby cause haematopoietic effects. Very little systematic research has been done as yet to explore the usefulness of 'microenvironmental targets' as end-points for the prediction of chemical toxicity. However, there is evidence that certain cytotoxic drugs not only affect cells capable of proliferation but also the microenvironment (Haen *et al.*, 1980).

Methods for testing chemicals in the whole animal with respect to its haematological consequences require careful consideration of the choice of animal species. The use of any one animal species requires a full knowledge and consideration of the physiological haematopoietic parameters of the species; these can be found in a variety of reference works (Farris and Griffith; 1949; Spiegel, 1973; Schalm *et al.*, 1975; Green, 1975; Benirschke *et al.*, 1978; Shifrine and Wilson, 1980).

12.3.2 Blood cell counts and smears

The simplest approach to testing chemical toxicity in laboratory animals is to evaluate the effects on the circulating blood cells. An important decision to be made is when to collect blood with respect to the time of administration of the chemical compound. The time intervals of study depend on the life-span of the cells under consideration. In mice, for example, the life-span of a red cell is about 44 days; of a platelet, about four days; and of a granulocyte, about two days. If one wants to carefully evaluate chemical toxicity to the granulocytic series, most of the blood examinations should lie within the first three days. If longer intervals are chosen, one may miss valuable information on cell changes that are of great importance for analysing possible mechanisms of chemical toxicity. To study effects on erythropoiesis, on the other hand, the time intervals may need to be longer if the red cell concentrations are used as end-points. If, however, the number of reticulocytes is used as an indicator of toxicity, then short time intervals of no more than 1–2 days are necessary due to the short life-span of these cells.

While blood cell counting by ordinary methods is still the simplest and most reliable way to evaluate the effects of chemicals on the haematopoietic system, it requires the full knowledge of the relevant haematopoietic cell systems to understand the meaning of observed effects and to interpret them. It is essential to express the results of blood cell counting in absolute terms; one needs the absolute number of erythrocytes, reticulocytes, granulocytes, monocytes, lymphocytes and platelets per mm^3 blood.

Any systematic changes in cell numbers in the peripheral blood indicate the need to examine the underlying pathophysiological mechanisms. This requires further tests such as the examination of the bone marrow, or functional studies.

The morphological evaluation (and possibly cytochemical evaluation) of blood cells in stained smears may be quite helpful. In the case of red cells, a classical sign of increased cellular turnover is the 'basophilic stippling', as seen in lead poisoning as a result of aggregation of ribosomes (Jensen *et al.*, 1965; Albahary, 1972). In addition, the shape of the red cell may indicate disturbances in red cell production, maturation or turnover. In the case of granulocytes, cytological abnormalities such as 'giant cells', 'pyknotic cells', or cells with mitotically connected abnormalities (such as karyomeres or micronuclei) may be indicative of effects on granulo-cytopoiesis. In the case of monocytes and lymphocytes, the trained observer will be able to judge whether the cells are normal. If they are abnormal, additional tests to investigate the underlying pathophysiological mechanisms may be required. Occasionally, platelets may show abnormal form (giant platelets) in blood smears. Again, in such a case, further studies are needed, directed towards the bone marrow.

In all cases, it is insufficient to rely on a single blood count; several, performed over a period of time, are necessary. The number required depends on the end-point used and should allow the investigator to observe the course of blood cell changes during a period of 3–4 weeks following a single dose of a chemical. If a chemical is administered continuously, a longer period of blood sampling is necessary and blood counts should be continued until 3–4 weeks after the last dose of the chemical.

12.3.3   Bone marrow studies

Haematological studies need not be confined to the peripheral blood cells. In all laboratory animals used for toxicity testing, effects on bone marrow can be easily studied serially. Two basic approaches are in common use: (1) examination of bone marrow smears; and (2) histological examination of bone marrow sections. Long experience and skill is required to procure bone marrow samples of high quality (aspirates or preparations using marrow from the shaft of long rodent bones) and to prepare smears that can be evaluated reproducibly. Stained smears allow identification of cell types and, in particular, cytological abnormalities characteristic of cytotoxic effects (such as giant cells, bi- or multi-nucleated cells, cells with micronuclei or karyomeres), or that allow one to predict metabolic alterations (disturbances or nuclear-cytoplasmic relationships such as 'megaloblasts'). If systematic blood cell changes are observed after the administration of a chemical, the bone marrow smear gives information as to the possible mechanisms. Increased haemolysis in the peripheral blood will result in a definite shift in the ratio of granulocytic to erythrocytic precursors and there will be a high degree of erythropoietic proliferation. A granulocytopenia of the blood may be indicative of haematopoietic failure that would be reflected in a hypocellular marrow smear with a relative lack of haematopoietic cells and an over-representation of lymphocytic/plasmacytic elements.

Parameters to be measured include 'bone marrow differential cell count' (based on at least 1000 cells), the relative distribution of erythropoietic cells capable of division (stages E1–E4 cells) compared with those not capable of further division and of myelocytic cells that may still divide (stages M1–M4) in relation to non-dividing, maturing cells (stages M5–M8). Changes in these relations are indicative of increased or decreased proliferative activity and may point out cases of increased inefficient cell production seen after exposure of the marrow to some chemicals.

It should be noted that the different mammalian species have their own specific bone marrow cytology. For example, granulocytic precursor cells in mice and rats are characterized by 'ring-shaped' nuclei; dog marrow shows round-shaped or sausage-shaped nuclei. Thus, the use of bone marrow smears to judge chemical toxicity requires special training in the evaluation of preparations of a particular animal species.

Histological techniques are particularly valuable to study the toxic effects of chemicals to the bone marrow. However, only the examination of 'semi-thin-sections' (prepared from marrow embedded in plastic (e.g. methacrylate) and cut with special microtomes) give sufficiently useful information. With such 'special histology', it is possible to now examine the haematopoietic precursor cells in relation to the microarchitecture of the marrow.

One can observe the condition of the sinusoidal structure and the integrity of the bone marrow microcirculation. Chemicals such as hydroxyurea produce, within hours of exposure, severe alteration of the sinusoidal structure in mice, resulting in a severe marrow haemorrhage. Then, after several days, it is possible to observe the regeneration of the marrow commencing with normalization of the structure and proliferation of very early precursor cells (stem cells). The bone marrow cellularity is easily quantified although bone marrow cellularity is not necessarily indicative of the picture in the whole animal since, under stress situations, haematopoiesis may shift to bones usually not haematopoietically active or even to other organs like the spleen or liver.

Electron microscopy is valuable in evaluation of the pathophysiological mechanisms involved in the action of cytotoxic or metabolically active chemicals. However, this technique is time-consuming and requires special methods and experience; it does not lend itself to routine toxicity testing.

12.3.4 Functional test systems

For screening purposes, examination of blood cell changes and bone marrow cell changes is sufficient to rapidly and easily detect the effects of chemicals on haematopoietic cell renewal. In certain circumstances, however, it may be necessary to evaluate the haematopoietic potentialities in more detail after single or chronic exposure to chemical compounds. The use of functional test systems aims at obtaining information on the kinetic parameters of haematopoietic cell renewal systems. These methods can also be used to estimate the degree of functional impairment after exposure to chemicals has been discontinued or during continuous low level exposure.

The life-span of circulating red cells can be studied by *in vitro* labelling with a suitable radioactive marker (e.g., ^{51}Cr) and determination of their disappearance rate after reinfusion. Increased haemolysis can be investigated quantitatively with this approach. Similarly, granulocyte and lymphocyte life-spans can be measured by collection of cells from the blood and *in vitro* labelling by means of DF^{32}P or ^{3}H-cytidine, respectively, prior to reinfusion and measurement of the disappearance rate from the blood stream. The survival of blood platelets can be measured by use of ^{35}S as a marker.

With such methods, subtle alterations in cell function can be demonstrated and quantified. Because blood has to be collected repeatedly from the same animal, large animals are usually used in applying these methods.

Several methods are available and useful for specific pathophysiological investigations into bone marrow cell function. One widely used test uses radioactive iron to label red cells. Radioactive iron is readily taken up by erythroblasts of the bone marrow during the formation of globin. The rate of increase of radioactively labelled red cells in blood is used as a measure of the turnover rate. This technique was used by Lee *et al.* (1974) to study the effects of benzene exposure in mice. In haemolytic conditions, the rate of uptake is increased due to a more rapid cell turnover. The use of radioactive iron has also proved useful in investigations of altered iron metabolism (e.g. Colli Franzone *et al.*, 1979).

Tritiated thymidine has been used to study cell renewal characteristics of haematopoietic bone marrow cells. In the study of chemical toxicity to bone marrow, one may evaluate the fraction of DNA-synthesizing cells, the generation times of different blood cell precursors, as well as transit times of cells through the different compartments of cell renewal systems before, during and after chemical exposure. It is, however, a time-consuming technique requiring autoradiography.

The fraction of DNA-synthesizing cells, as a measure of cellular toxicity of chemical compounds, can be more easily determined by flow-cytophotometric techniques as used in the study of leukaemia patients after cytoreductive therapy. As a consequence of this therapy, the relative number of remaining cells in the 'S-phrase' may well be increased (Buchner, 1974).

Evaluation of the influence of chemicals on the stem-cell pool is of considerable importance in chemical toxicity studies. Stem-cell assay systems have been developed for many laboratory animal species. Till and McCulloch (1961) first developed the spleen colony assay system in mice which allowed the study of 'CFU-S' (colony forming units in spleen) that were shown to be proportional to the number of pluripotent stem cells in a given suspension of haematopoietic cells. Today, the

'CFU-S' assay system is probably the most widely used short-term *in vivo* toxicity test system for predicting haematological effects.

This basic method—the so-called 'Till and McCulloch Spleen Colony Assay'—can and has been successfully employed to study stem-cell toxicity of chemicals. Bruce *et al.* (1966) demonstrated clearly that there are some chemical compounds, such as some of the alkylating agents, that injure even resting stem cells while other compounds, such as hydroxyurea, harm only stem cells that are in cell cycle. These authors demonstrated a significant depletion of bone marrow colony forming units (CFC) after exposure of mice to benzene via inhalation. Thus, it is evident that the Till and McCulloch assay may well be applicable to the demonstration and study of chemical toxicity to the most vulnerable elements of haematopoiesis, the stem cells. Care must be taken, however, to distinguish between toxic effects on the stem cells and those attributable to chemical impairment of the function of the haematopoietic microenvironment. Frash *et al.* (1976) provided evidence that the exposure of mice to benzene impairs the microenvironment of the haematopoietic stem cells and may not affect the stem cells directly.

Nevertheless, examination of stem-cell function after exposure of animals to toxic chemicals is a very powerful tool to study haematotoxicity.

12.4   *IN VITRO* TEST SYSTEMS

In the past 20 years, enormous efforts have been put into the characterization of the 'committed' progenitor cells in *in vitro* culture systems. Bradley and Metcalf (1966) and Pluznik and Sachs (1965) pioneered the concept that one can 'plate' haematopoietic cells in a petri-dish containing agar or methylcellulose semi-solid medium, add certain stimulating factors to them, and incubate the culture under appropriate conditions for 1–2 weeks. Depending on the culture conditions these cells develop into cell line specific 'colonies' of erythroblasts (CFU-E, BFU-E), granulocytic/monocytic cells (CFU-GM), or megakaryocyte cells (CFU-MEG). More recently, it has been possible to grow 'mixed colonies' containing erythrocytic, granulocytic as well as megakaryocytic cells. Such colonies are believed to originate from very immature stem cells, perhaps from pluripotent stem cells (the cells of origin for all haematopoietic cell lineages). Dexter and Lajtha (1974) showed that pluripotent stem cells of mice could be maintained *in vitro* for several weeks by plating them on to an appropriate 'feeder layer' that was designed to simulate the haematopoietic microenvironment of the blood cell-forming organs.

The reader is referred to Smith (1975) for a detailed review of *in vitro* test systems that may be or have proved to be relevant for predicting certain types of chemical toxicity.

There are two primary approaches to *in vitro* testing for chemical haematotoxicity. One approach is to test blood-derived cells (such as red cells, granulocytes, or platelets) for certain functions (osmotic fragility of red cells; metabolism of red cells; mobility or phagocytosis of granulocytes; spreading properties of platelets).

These *in vitro* tests of cell metabolism and function were originally developed to characterize metabolic properties of blood cell types and should prove useful for monitoring certain types of chemical toxicity. They allow conclusions to be drawn with respect to chemicals causing metabolic or functional changes and their dose–response relationships.

The second approach is to examine chemicals for their ability to impair the proliferative potentialities of cells or to alter the differentiation properties of progenitor cells. The basic *in vitro* technique to study the various progenitor cell populations from mice and other animals (including man) has been described by Metcalf (1977). In essence, bone marrow cell suspensions of mice exposed to toxic chemicals are prepared and cultured *in vitro* at various times after onset of exposure using appropriate conditions for stimulation. Thus, after some days, the culture dishes may be scored for colonies comprised of haematopoietic precursor cells of various types (erythropoietic, granulopoietic, megakaryocytic or mixed).

Substances such as benzene influence the growth of haematopoietic cells *in vitro* when they are added to the culture medium. Frash *et al.* (1976), for example, incubated mouse bone marrow cells in a homologous serum to which benzene was added. These authors found that the efficiency of colony formation was not altered and concluded that any effect of benzene on stem cells is probably due to an effect on the haematopoietic microenvironment of the marrow. This approach may well be useful in the future to detect effects caused by chemical agents on the replication and differentiation of multi- or pluripotent stem cells.

The effects of chemicals on chromosomes and the observation of chromosomal aberrations can also be studied *in vitro*. These tests were originally developed to study the effects on cell proliferation *in vitro* using irradiated cells. Lymphocytes from the peripheral blood, stimulated *in vitro* by means of phytohaemaglutinine, undergo mitosis within 48 to 72 hours. If these cells are exposed to ionizing radiation before being placed in culture, they exhibit chromosomal aberrations and/or 'micronuclei' (Bajerska and Liniecki, 1969; Countryman and Heddle, 1976; Virsik *et al.*, 1977; Hori and Nakai, 1978). In a similar way, one may use the *in vitro* growth characteristics of lymphocytes in culture to examine the sensitivity of this growth to chemicals. Possible end-points are the number of cell progeny produced within a fixed time period, the development of micronuclei, or the development of chromosomal aberrations.

12.5 EXAMPLES OF HAEMATOTOXIC COMPOUNDS

12.5.1 Benzene

Benzene interferes with cell division and maturation. Speck and co-workers showed that DNA synthesis is impaired at the maturation levels of E3 and E4 cells (basophilic and polychromatophilic erythroblasts) (Speck *et al.*, 1966). The ^{59}Fe incorporation method was used by Lee *et al.* (1974) following subcutaneous injection of benzene to show direct effects on all nucleated erythropoietic cells (E1 to E5). Pollini and Columbi (1964) described chromosomal aberrations which are another expression of the damage this substance does to nucleic acids. It is also known that benzene damages the haematopoietic stem cells (Frash *et al.*, 1976, Uyeki *et al.*, 1977).

It may be that the decrease of erythrocytic and granulocytic progenitor cells in rabbit blood observed by Speck *et al.* (1966) was due to microecological effects of benzene, liberating inhibitor substances from 'adherent' cells (see also Frash *et al.*, 1976). One day following benzene inhalation by mice, Uyeki *et al.* (1977) observed a decrease of granulocytically-committed progenitor cells without an effect on the total marrow cellularity. This finding could be explained as a direct cytotoxic effect of benzene on stem cells; equally, it can be explained with the assumption that there is an influence on the stem-cell microenvironment promoting inhibition of stem-cell replication.

12.5.2 Lead

Lead affects the haematopoietic system in a different way to benzene. In this case, neither the stem cells nor the synthesis of nucleic acids are affected *per se*. However, there is ample evidence that the membranes of circulating red cells are injured and that their life-span is shortened. The resulting haemolysis provokes an increase in the proliferative activity of the immature red cell precursors in the bone marrow (i.e. erythroblasts E1–E5), but lead also affects haem synthesis as well as globin synthesis so that premature death of nucleated red cell precursors in the bone marrow also occurs. In turn, this triggers an increase in stem-cell replication and differentiation in order to compensate for the decreased effectiveness of erythropoiesis. Brookfield (1928) showed that the administration of lead to human beings resulted in an initial decrease of erythrocytes in the blood (increased haemolysis) followed by reticulocytosis as well as basophilic stippling of red cells, a sign of ineffective erythropoiesis. Griggs (1964) published data on the appearance and disappearance of coproporphyrins and 5-amino-levulinic acid in the urine after oral lead administration; it takes about 5–6 days in man before these biochemical parameters start to increase. This may be taken as an indication that lead accumulates in the marrow before haemoglobin synthesis is disturbed.

12.6 SIMULATION MODELS

Simulation models are useful for predicting the potential influence of single or chronic exposures either to a single chemical, or to a mixture of chemicals. It is assumed that the haematopoietic system will attempt to compensate for injury to any one component by changes that will result in the number of cells in the functional pool (usually blood) being maintained. Except in those cases where the dose is sufficiently high that the primary toxic effect (e.g. haemolysis) causes death, the ability of the stem cell pool to compensate for cell loss by increased production becomes the limiting factor. This is, in turn, dependent upon the number of unaffected stem cells and their ability to function through replication and differentiation; this may be affected also by the influence of chemicals on the microenvironment.

A simulation model of erythropoiesis in a mouse, using all known cell parameters of the mouse, has been developed (Fliedner *et al.*, 1982; Pabst, 1984). In this model it is assumed that a defined number of red cells is lost (and needs to be replaced) per unit time. It is then possible to assume increased cell loss rates in the different compartments of the cell renewal system and to compare the simulated effects with biological observations. In Figure 12.2 (upper panel) it is assumed that a substance A (for instance, lead) primarily damages the circulating red cells resulting in increased demands on the proliferation and maturation pools. After a time, a second substance B (for instance, benzene), which has different targets, is added. In the lower panel of Figure 12.2, substance B is given first followed by substance A.

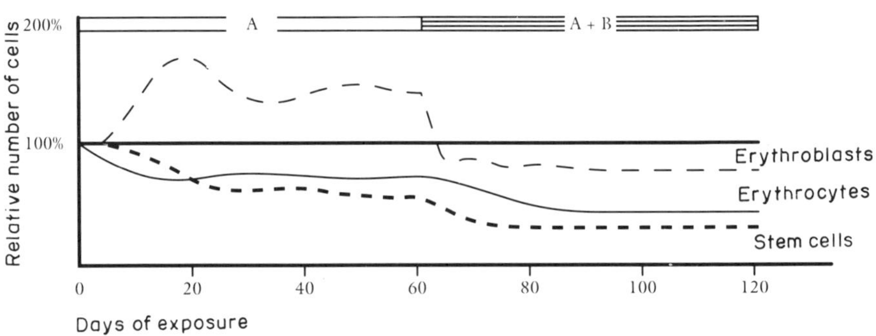

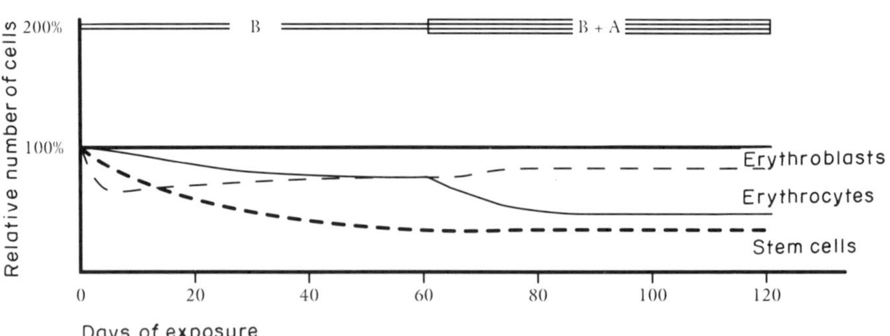

Figure 12.2   Changes in erythroid cell numbers provoked by noxious substances (model simulation). *Upper panel:* exposure to substance A followed by substance A + B; *lower panel:*exposure to substance B followed by substance B + A.

Exposure to substance A results first in a decline of red cells as a consequence of increased haemolysis. This causes an increase in erythroblasts of the bone marrow and a decrease of the stem cell flux. The erythroblasts are then damaged by interference with haemoglobin metabolism and this causes a further increase in erythroblast turnover. If substance B is added (affecting proliferation of erythroblasts and stem cells) then there is a sudden decrease of stem cells and erythroblasts, causing the red blood cells to decrease further. If one reverses the experiment (see Figure 12.2, lower panel), then there is first an effect on stem cells and erythroblasts, causing a decline of the mature red cells in the blood. If substance A is added— causing an increase in haemolysis—then there is a further decline of red cells, but the erythroblasts cannot respond with increased proliferation, nor can the stem cells make up for the increased cell loss.

Each chemical, in so far as haematopoietic effects are concerned, must be considered in relation to its action on the different elements of cell renewal systems. Direct effects on cells or their metabolism will result in compensatory feedback causing other parts of the system to respond (indirect action). Simulation models based on these principles are useful in predicting the ability of haematopoietic cell systems to tolerate single or chronic exposure to one or more chemicals.

12.7 SUMMARY

Different chemicals affect haematopoietic cell renewal systems in different ways. The cause of the resulting disease state depends on which cells of the system are affected and how they are altered. It is important to realize also that haematopoietic cell renewal systems may tolerate cytotoxic injury provided the stem-cell pool is not reduced to a level from which a spontaneous recovery becomes impossible. If the life-span of cells is shortened, if the rate of destruction of cells is increased, or if qualitative changes of cell function occur, then these effects cause an increase in cell production in order to compensate for overall cell loss to assure a sufficient level of circulating blood cells. However, irreversible injury to stem cells eventually results in a breakdown of the haematopoietic systems.

In most toxicity studies, mice or rats are used to provide initial information concerning the toxicity of a chemical, including effects on haematopoietic end-points. Mice are preferred because of the possibility to study all end-points from the mature blood cells to the most immature, but, nevertheless, highly sensitive pluripotent stem cells. If larger animals are used, they have many advantages (large blood volume for sampling, haematopoiesis more comparable to that of man, etc.) but they are much more expensive.

Results from haematological studies in laboratory animals may be used to predict possible chemical toxicity in human beings because human haematopoietic cell renewal systems are similar in their principal structure and function to those of laboratory animals. However, care must be taken in the interpretation of observed changes; for example, it would be misleading to predict the time of maximum depression of the white cell count in man based on a study of this effect in mouse in response to administration of a certain chemical. The basic mechanisms that are operative in each species must be considered. However, if such factors are taken into consideration, a predictive analysis is possible.

The study of circulating blood cells will reflect direct chemical effects on these cells—at least during the initial period after exposure. In this sense, the relatively long-lived red cells should receive the highest degree of attention. Haemolysis is a well-known effect; on the other hand, the oxygen-carrying capacity of red cells is also very sensitive (e.g. following exposure to carbon monoxide). In contrast, changes in granulocytes or platelets more probably reflect effects on the bone marrow precursor pool.

To be most useful, all blood cell changes (increase or decrease or metabolic differences) that occur within four weeks of the administration of the chemical should be observed. Cytological and histological examinations of bone marrow may be considered a second step in chemical toxicity evaluation. This step might have to be followed by a third step involving the use of functional studies. These are much more expensive, time-consuming and require sophisticated methods. Studies using radionuclides may be necessary to characterize metabolic effects (e.g. iron metabolism, nucleic acid metabolism).

In vitro test systems are useful but have severe limitations. One can expect that blood or bone marrow cells will be injured or damaged by almost any chemical if it is given in a sufficiently high dose. Nevertheless, the end-points available for *in vitro* studies (specific cell suspensions of red cells, granulocytes, platelets, etc.) can be used to test certain types of toxicity (metabolic, functional, etc.). In addition, modern haematological cell culture systems (for stem as well as for progenitor cells) will help to identify certain detrimental effects of the chemical on proliferation and differentiation, as well as their mechanisms.

More research is needed in the field of haematotoxicology. Systematic investigations should be carried out in order to evaluate which haematological end-points may be most relevant. But, in general, it may be concluded that haematology offers a wide range of suitable test systems to predict the type of cellular damage that may be inflicted by chemicals.

REFERENCES

Albahary, C. (1972). Lead and haematopoieses. *Ann. J. Med.*, **52**, 369.

Benirschke, K., Garner, F.M., and Jones, T.C. (Eds) (1978). *Pathology of Laboratory Animals*, Springer, New York.

Bajerska, A., and Liniecki, J. (1969). The influence of x-ray dose and time of its delivery *in vitro* on the yield of chromosomal aberrations in the peripheral blood lymphocytes. *Int. J. Radiat. Biol.*, **16**, 467–81.

Bond, V.P., Fliedner, T.M., and Archambeau, J.O. (1965). *Mammalian Radiation Lethality*, Academic Press, New York.

Bradley, T.R., and Metcalf, D. (1966). The growth of mouse bone marrow cells *in vitro*. *Austr. J. Exp. Biol Sci.*, **44**, 287.

Brookfield, R.W. (1928). Blood changes occurring during the course of treatment of malignant disease by lead with special reference to punctate basophilia and the platelets. *J. Path.*, **31**, 277–301.

Bruce, W.R., Mecker, B.E., and Valeriote, F.A. (1966). Comparison of the sensitivity of normal haematopoietic and transplanted lymphoma colony-forming cells to chemotherapeutic agents administered *in vivo*. *J. Natl. Cancer Inst.*, **37**, 233.

Buchner, T. (1974). Impulscytophotometrie in der Hamatologie: Diagnostische Wertigkeit. *Diagnostik*, **7**, 284–6.

Colli Franzone, P., Stefanelli, M., and Viganotti, C. (1979). A distributed model of iron kinetics for clinical assessment of normal-abnormal erythropoietic activity. *IEEE Trans. Biomed. Eng.*, **26**, 586–96.

Countryman, P.I., and Heddle, A. (1976). The production of micronuclei from chromosome aberrations in irradiated cultures of human lymphocytes. *Mutat. Res.*, **41**, 321–32.

Dexter, T.M., and Lajtha, L.G. (1974). Proliferation of haematopoietic stem cells *in vitro*. *Br. J. Haemat.*, **28**, 525–30.

Farris, E.J., and Griffith, J.Q. (Eds) (1949). *The Rat in Laboratory Investigation*, Lippincott, New York, 2nd Edn (reprinted 1967; Hafner, New York).

Fliedner, T.M., and Calvo, W. (1978). Haematopoietic stem-cell seeding of a cellular matrix: A principle of initiation and regeneration of haematopoiesis. In: Clarkson, B., Marks, P.A. and Till, J.E. (Eds), *Differentiation of Normal and Neoplastic Haematopoietic Cells*, Cold Spring Harbor Laboratory, Cold Spring Harbor, p. 757.

Fleidner, T.M., Pabst, G., and Wandl, U. (1982). Pathophysiologie der Mehrfachbelastungen von Zellsystemen. In: Fliedner, T.M. (Ed.), *Kombinierte Belastungen am Arbeitsplatz*, Gentner, Stuttgart, pp. 85–98.

Fliedner, T.M., Steinbach, K.H., and Hoelzer, D. (1976). Adaptation to environmental changes: The role of cell-renewal systems. In: Finckh, E.S., and Clayton-Jones, E. (Eds), *The Effects of Environment on Cells and Tissues*, Excerpta Medica, Amsterdam, pp. 20–38.

Frash, V.N., Yushkov, B.G., Karaulov, A.V., and Skuratov, V.L. (1976). Mechanisms of action of benzene on haematopoiesis (Investigation of haematopoietic stem cells). *Bull. Exp. Biol. Med.*, **87**, 985–7.

Gordon, A.S., Gondorelli, M., and Peschle, C. (Eds) (1972). *Regulation of Erythropoiesis*, II Ponte, Milano.

Green, E.L. (Ed.) (1975). *Biology of the Laboratory Mouse*, Dover, New York, 2nd Edn.

Griggs, R.C. (1964). Lead poisoning. Haematopoietic aspects. *Progr. Haemat.*, **4**, 117–37.

Haen, M., Grilli, G., Nothdurft, W., and Fliedner, T.M. (1980). Studies on the repopulating ability of blood stem cells of dogs given a single high dose of cyclophosphamide. *Exp. Hameatol.*, **8**, Suppl. **7**, 26.

Hori, T.-A., and Nakai, S. (1978). Unusual dose–response of chromosome aberrations induced in human lymphocytes by very low dose exposures to tritium. *Mutat. Res.*, **50**, 101–10.

Jacobson, L.O., and Doyle, M. (Eds) (1962). *Erythropoiesis*, Grune & Stratton, New York.

Jensen, W.N., Moreno, G.D., and Bessis, M.C. (1965). An electron microscopic description of basophilic stippling in red cells. *Blood*, **25**, 933–43.

Kelemen, E., Calvo, W., and Fliedner, T.M. (1979). *Atlas of Human Haemopoietic Development*, Springer, Berlin.

Lee, E.W., Kocisis, J.J., and Snyder, R. (1974). Acute effect of benzene on ^{59}Fe-incorporation into circulating erythrocytes. *Tox. and Appl. Pharmacology*, **27**, 431–6.

Metcalf, D. (1977). *Haemopoietic Colonies*, Springer, Berlin.

Pabst, G. (1984). A simulation model of murine erythropoiesis. In Breitenecker, F., and Kleinert, W. (Eds), *Simulationstechnik*, Springer, Heidelberg.

Paulus, J.M. (Ed.) (1971). *Platelet Kinetics*, North-Holland, Amsterdam.

Pietschmann, H. (Ed.) (1972). *Der Lymphozyt*, Verlag Wiener Med. Akad., Wien.

Pluznik, D.H., and Sachs, J. (1965). The cloning of normal mast cells in tissue culture. *J. Cell. Comp. Physiol.*, **66**, 319–24.

Pollini, G., and Columbi, R. (1964). Il danno cromosomico del lin tociti nell 'emopatia benzenica. *Med. Lavoro*, **55**, 641–54.

Quesenberry, P., and Levitt, L. (1979). Haematopoietic stem cells. *N. Eng. J. Med.*, **301**, 755–60, 819–23, 868–72.

Schalm, O.W., Jain, N.C., and Carroll, E.J. (Eds) (1975). *Veterinary Haematology*. 3rd Edn. Lea and Febinger, Philadelphia.

Shifrine, M., and Wilson, F.D. (Eds) (1980). The canine as a biomecidal research model: immunological, haematological and oncological aspects. Technical Information Center/U.S. Department of Energy, Springfield.

Smith, Th. P. (1975). Toxicology of the formed elements of the blood. In: Casarett, L.J., and Doull, J. (Eds), *Toxicology: The Basic Science of Poisons*, MacMillan, New York.

Speck, B., Schnider, Th., Gerber, U., and Moeschlin, S. (1966). Experimentelle Untersuchungen uber den Wirkungsmechanismus des Benzols auf das Knockenmark. *Schweiz. Med. Wschr.*, **96**, 1274–6.

Spiegel, A. (Ed.) (1973). *The Laboratory Animal in Drug Testing*. Fischer, Stuttgart.

Stutman, O., and Good, R.A. (1972). Heterogeneity of lymphocyte populations. *Rev. Europ. Etudes Clin. Biol.*, **17**, 11.

Theml, H., and Begemann, H. (1975). *Lymphozyt und klinische immunologie*, Springer, Berlin.

Till, J.E., and McCulloch, E.A. (1961). A direct measurement of the radiation sensitivity of normal bone marrow cells. *Rad. Res.*, **14**, 213.

Uyeki, E.M., Ashkar, A.E., Shoeman, D.W., and Bisle, T.V. (1977). Acute toxicity of benzene inhalation of haematopoietic precursor cells. *Toxicol. Appl. Pharmacol.*, **40**, 49–57.

Virsik, R.P., Harder, D., and Hansmann, I. (1977). The RBE of 30 kV x-rays for the induction of dicentric chromosomes in human lymphocytes. *Rad. Environm. Biophys.*, **14**, 109–121.

Whipple, H.E. (Ed.) (1964). Leukopoiesis in health and disease. *Ann. N.Y. Acad. Sci.*, **113**, 513–1092.

Wintrobe, M.M. (Ed.) (1981). *Clinical Haematology*, 8th Edn. Lea and Febiger, Philadelphia.

Short-term Toxicity Tests for Non-genotoxic Effects
Edited by P. Bourdeau *et al.*
© 1990 SCOPE. Published by John Wiley & Sons Ltd

CHAPTER 13

Short-term Tests for Neurotoxicity

Silvio Garattini

13.1   INTRODUCTION

A neurotoxic event may be defined as any change in the morphology, biochemistry or function of the nervous system, peripheral or central. Psychotropic drugs are neurotoxic chemicals according to this definition because, although they are intended to relieve mental illness, they certainly alter biochemical and functional activities of the central nervous system and, at high doses, even the morphology. However, this definition of a neurotoxic event, though broad, includes chemical contaminants in the environment.

Although it is outside the scope of this review to discuss the general problems of neurotoxicity, it should be recalled that in an evaluation of neurotoxicity, at least four aspects must be considered separately: the neurotoxic *potential*, which is a substance's ability to cause neurotoxic effects; the neurotoxic *potency*, which includes concepts of dose-range and duration of the neurotoxic effect; the neurotoxic *hazard* which is the specificity of a chemical to cause neurotoxic effects in relation to other toxic actions; and the neurotoxic *risk* which is the likelihood that a given neurotoxic effect will be produced in real life.

This review is restricted to the various ways of detecting the neurotoxic potential of chemicals that affect the central nervous system. Short-term tests will be taken to include both *in vitro* and *in vivo* tests. Frequent reference will be made to drug neurotoxicity because studies in this field are more advanced than for environmental contaminants.

13.1.1   The role of the blood/brain barrier

The brain is protected against the entry of many chemicals by the blood/brain barrier cells (Saunders, 1977). Chemicals can enter the brain by at least two mechanisms: (i) passive diffusion, which applies mostly to small lipophylic compounds and (ii) active transport of compounds of physiological importance. It is important to recognize that a chemical that is a potent neurotoxic agent *in vitro* is not necessarily neurotoxic *in vivo* if it does not enter the brain because of the blood/brain barrier.

The blood/brain barrier is not equally effective in all parts of the brain. For example, this barrier is less efficient in the so-called circumventricular organs (CVO) (Weindl, 1973). The capillaries of the CVO have large interendothelial pores (and exhibit active pinocytosis) instead of tight junctions (Brightman, 1977; Partridge, 1979). This is well demonstrated by glutamic acid, an excitatory aminoacid and a putative chemical transmitter in the brain (Shank and Aprison, 1979; Curtis, 1979; Johnston, 1979), which is neurotoxic when injected intracerebrally (Simson *et al.*, 1977; Olney *et al.*, 1975). When administered systemically, even at high doses, it does not accumulate in the brain (Garattini, 1979) although, under certain conditions, it accumulates (Perez *et al.*, 1973) in the nucleus arcuatus of the hypothalamus (Perez and Olney, 1972) where it may cause rather selective degeneration of some neurones (Olney, 1969). It has been suggested that this is probably responsible for late onset of obesity (Matsuyama, 1970) and endocrine disturbances (Lamperti and Blaha, 1976; Pizzi *et al.* 1977). This sequence of events has been best demonstrated by the use of newborn mice (Olney, 1969) receiving glutamate by parenteral injection (Garattini, 1979) at high doses capable of increasing osmolarity (Airoldi *et al.*, 1979).

It can be argued that some chemicals exert profound effects on the central nervous system without entering the brain; in fact, brain composition and/or function may change in relation to stimulation of peripheral inputs. For instance, stimulation of prolactin secretion from the hypophysis results in feed-back mechanisms on dopaminergic functions in the hypothalamus (Höhn and Wuttke, 1978; Perkins and Westfall, 1978). This mechanism has been suggested as an explanation for why domperidone, an anti-emetic drug, increases dopamine metabolites in the striatum even though it does not cross the blood/brain barrier (Ferretti *et al.*, 1983).

13.1.2 The role of metabolism

If a chemical is metabolized rapidly, very little may be available to the brain. Since, in several cases, the metabolic products are more polar and less lipophylic than the parent compound, metabolism may represent a detoxifying mechanism with respect to the brain. However, sometimes the metabolic products are still sufficiently lipophylic to cross the blood/brain barrier; in such cases, the metabolites may contribute to the neurotoxicity of the parent compound , or even be more toxic than the parent compound.

It is highly advisable to measure metabolites directly in the central nervous system. As is exemplified by the data summarized in Table 13.1, some metabolites may occur in significant concentrations in brain whereas they are present only in trace quantities (or undetectable) in the blood. Hence, analyses in readily available body fluids such as blood or urine may be unreliable indicators of the presence or absence of neurotoxic metabolites.

The capacity of nervous tissue to metabolize xenobiotics is largely unknown. In some cases, metabolic activity in the brain may result in short-lived, unstable

Table 13.1   Examples of relationship between levels of metabolites in blood and in brain as measured by the area under the curve (AUC) of cencentration–time curves of 1-aryl-piperazines after oral administration of various drugs (Caccia *et al.*, 1985)

| | | | AUC (nmoles/ml × min) | | Brain to |
Parent drug	Dose (mg/kg)	Metabolite	Plasma	Brain	plasma ratio
Trazodone	25	mClPP	51	1 336	26
Etoperidone	25	mClPP	163	4 978	27
Mepiprazole	23	mClPP	27	657	24
Enpiprazole	100	oClPP	N.D.	567	N.D.
Niaprazine	25	pFPP	681	11 442	16
Antrafenine	25	mCF$_3$PP	6	445	16
Millipertine	25	oOCH$_3$PP	156	841	5
Oxypertine	25	PP	210	1 920	8
Azaperone	25	Pdp	123	1 331	10
S-3608	100	TzP	N.D.	83	N.D.
Piribedil	100	PmP	N.D.	474	4
Buspirone	10	PmP	350	1 525	4

* N.D., Plasma concentrations below the sensitivity of the analytical procedure; mClPP, 1-(*m*-chlorophenyl-piperazine; oClPP, 1-(*o*-chlorophenyl-piperazine; pFPP, 1-(*p*-fluorophenyl-piperazine; mCF$_3$PP, 1-(*m*-trifluoromethylphenyl)--piperazine; oOCH$_3$PP, 1-(*o*methoxyphenyl)-piperazine; PP, 1-phenyl-piperazine; PdP, 1-(2-pyridyl)-piperazine; TzP, 1-(2-thiazolyl)-piperazine; PmP, 1-(2-pyrimidinyl)-piperazine.

metabolites which can covalently bind to macromolecules (proteins or nucleic acids) of the brain. Alkylation and carbomylation of some nitrosoureas which accumulate in the brain is a typical example. Another case is the neurotoxin, 6-hydroxydopamine, which enters catecholaminergic nerve terminals quite selectively by means of the uptake mechanism for dopamine and noradrenaline (Iversen, 1970) where it gives rise to unstable radicals which denature proteins (Garattini and Samanin, 1977; Heikkila and Cohen, 1971; Heikkila and Cohen, 1972).

13.1.3   Compensatory mechanisms

Within limits, the central nervous system can regenerate nerve terminals and compensate for neuronal damage. Furthermore, several nervous functions are *protected* by redundant mechanisms. Therefore, especially *in vivo*, it may be difficult to detect neuronal damage because morphological damage may not result in readily demonstrable behavioural effects.

Intracerebral administration of neurotoxins (such as 6-hydroxydopamine, 5,7-dihydroxytryptamine and kainic acid) may not elicit signs of neurotoxicity even though their ability to cause lesions in specific neurones is well documented. This makes it especially difficult to detect neurotoxicity; furthermore, there are biochemical mechanisms such as changes in turnover of certain neurochemicals or modulators of receptors which compensate for neurotoxic effects. One consequence of this is the fact that major degeneration of the dopaminergic system is necessary before disturbances such as Parkinson's disease appear.

13.1.4   Difficulties in establishing short-term tests for neurotoxicity

If the definition of a neurotoxic event provided at the outset of this chapter is accepted, it is apparent that the detection of neurotoxic effects caused by certain chemicals may be extremely difficult. The brain has such a variety of cells with specialized functions, different chemical mediators and innumerable connections with other cells that it is difficult to analyse the individual and cumulative effects of a chemical on all these variables systematically. Even if it were possible to obtain neurones in culture representative of all the brain neurones (i.e. containing all the known chemical mediators), only very marginal information could be gathered because such a system will lack the network of interneuronal connections which may be important sites for toxic effects. More importantly, the functional or degenerative effects of chemicals on neurones may be age-dependent; the balance between formation and connection of axons and dendrites compared with the 'spontaneous' degeneration of neurones is known to be quite different in newborn and aged organisms. This difference in vulnerability of neurones in relation to age would hardly be seen *in vitro*.

Despite these difficulties, the field of neurotoxicity is expanding, utilizing a multidisciplinary approach. For several chemicals, there is now a body of knowledge describing the site of action and in some cases also the mechanism of action. This information is extremely important as a reference point for new chemicals which may share chemical or functional analogies.

In this chapter, the various approaches and methods to detect neurotoxic effects will be briefly described. To avoid repetition, it is stressed here that investigators must always consider a number of variables that may substantially influence the possibility of detecting neurotoxicity of chemicals including animal species, strain, sex, age, diet, concomitant pathology and interactions with other chemicals present in the environment.

13.2   NERVOUS SYSTEM CULTURE TYPES

Rapid advances in the use of cell culture systems to detect mutagenesis and carcinogenesis has aroused interest in the possibility of using more or less complex elements of nervous tissue *in vitro* as targets for neurotoxicological studies. The necessary techniques have been available for some time and have received fresh impetus from modern knowledge of cell biology. Some of these techniques have been recently carefully described by Yonezawa *et al.* (1980).

Schrier (1982) described six types of nervous system cultures for toxicologic testing; the advantages and disadvantages of each type are shown in Table 13.2.

Table 13.2 Nervous system culture types used for toxicologic testing (Schrier, 1982)

Culture type	Advantages	Disadvantages
Whole embryo	(a) Fetal metabolism probably intact but isolated from maternal metabolites (b) Normal or near-normal development and cellular and tissue interactions (c) Cultures may be initiated at a very early fetal age and toxicity tests done at any time in culture development; therefore, a wide range of development and differentiation is available	(a) Difficult to visualise toxicity at cellular and molecular levels (b) Complexity of presence of other organs and tissues (c) Reproducibility for biochemistry
Whole organ (e.g. DRG, SCG, etc.)	(a) Most neurone–neurone, neurone–glia, and glia–glia spatial relationships maintained (b) Cultures may be initiated from more mature (e.g. newborn or older) animals. Animal may be treated with potential toxins in advance or organ removal	(a) Some difficulties with hypoxia, cell death at centre of organs (b) Complex and poorly visualized intercellular interactions and communications
Explant (organo-typic cultures)	(a) Most cytoarchitecture maintained (b) Usually some flattening to allow morphologic evaluation (c) Myelination occurs reliably and is readily detected by light microscopy (d) Extracellular recording of 'organotypic' electrical activity is possible	(a) Poor morphology in living state (b) Poor visualization of individual cells and accessibility to them for intracellular recording (c) Suboptimal reproducibility for biochemistry

Table 13.2   *(continued)*

Reaggregation (of primary dispersed cell cultures)	(a) Glial multiplication limited (see also dispersed cell cultures) (b) Three-dimensional cytoarchitecture partially restored (c) Reproducibility of biochemical parameters probably better than explants (d) Maturation more complete than dispersal cell cultures	(a) Embryonic timing and dissociation procedures very crucial (b) Completely normal cytoarchitecture never restored, and degree of restoration varies among aggregates (c) Poor accessibility for electrophysiology
Dispersed cell cultures (a) Primary dispersed (b) Outgrown from explants (c) Secondary dispersed (cells obtained from primary dispersed)	(a) Increased reproducibility for biochemical studies (b) Good visualization with phase or Nomarski optics (c) Some neurohistochemical characters maintained (d) Capacity to use intracellular microelectrodes under direct microscopic observation (e) Analysis of individual synapsis possible (f) Electrophysiology, morphology and biochemistry may be done on single identified cells.	(a) Two-dimensional rather than three (b) Little or no myelination (c) Most normal cytoarchitecture lost (d) Some cell types may not survive
Cell lines (neuroblastomas, Schwannomas, hybrid lines, phaeochromocytomas, gliomas)	(a) Can obtain large quantities of single cell types for biochemical studies (b) Usually good single cell visualization (c) Ease of electrophysiologic studies (d) Provide both undifferentiated and 'differentiated' cells	(a) Near-total loss of normal cytoarchitecture (b) Cell lines may not accurately represent their counterparts *in vivo*

These six types are amenable to all possible kinds of observations—morphological, electrophysiological, biochemical, etc. The use of nervous tissue from different species including man (Buravlev, 1978) means that *in vitro* and *in vivo* data can be compared. Several cell lines are neoplastic cells such as neuroblastomas (Walum and Peterson, 1983); this may complicate the evaluation of neurotoxicity because a chemical that is cytotoxic for a neuroblastoma may not necessarily be neurotoxic for normal cells.

Although it would be impractical to summarize all studies that have been carried out with various chemicals, particularly significant results have been obtained in studies of the effects of heavy metals such as mercury (Saida, 1984; Kim, 1971), thallium (Hendelman, 1969; Spencer *et al.*, 1973) and tellurium (Lampert *et al.*, 1970). Obviously, these are areas with the best potential for correlation between *in vitro* and *in vivo* effects due to the lack of metabolism for these neurotoxic agents. It is more difficult to establish a correlation with organic compounds which undergo complex metabolic processes and have relatively selective effects. For instance, the tardive dyskinesia arising after repeated treatment with chlorpromazine or other phenothiazines seems difficult to reconcile with the morphological changes in lysosomes observed *in vitro* (Brosnan *et al.*, 1970). In order to simulate *in vivo* metabolic processes, techniques have been developed recently in which neuroblastoma cells are co-cultured with liver cells. Using this technique, cyclophosphamide (a non-reactive alkylating agent *in vitro*) becomes cytotoxic under these experimental conditions (Ericsson and Walum, 1984). However, it should be stressed that the metabolism of liver cells is not identical *in vivo* and *in vitro*.

Despite growing interest in tissue culture techniques, there is still no basis for standardization of such tests involving the nervous system because there are no reports to date concerning quality control or validation of these techniques using a number of agents to assess false positive or false negative compounds. In a recent comprehensive review, Dewar (1983) states:

As yet, however, there has been relatively little experience of the application of tissue culture techniques in what may be termed routine neurotoxicology. Most of the neurotoxicological studies where they have been applied have been primarily concerned with mechanisms of pathogenesis using known toxicants—a task for which these techniques are particularly suited.

13.3 ELECTROPHYSIOLOGICAL METHODS

Several techniques are available to measure the electric activity of single cells (Jacques *et al.*, 1980), isolated nerves or slices from different brain areas *in vitro*. However, these techniques have not been used systematically as testing procedures for neurotoxicants although they may be potentially useful (Fox *et al.*, 1982; Johnson, 1980).

Electrophysiological methods *in vivo* have been more widely used. An account of the results obtained with the available methods has been reported by Johnson (1980) and by Fox *et al.* (1982). Table 13.3, from the review of Dewar (1983), summarizes current uses of electrophysiological techniques in neurotoxicity. Most of these techniques have the advantage that measurement can be repeated in the same animal over a period of time so that the onset and duration of neurotoxic effects can be followed. Computerized systems have enabled electrophysiology to become more quantitative and, therefore, more suitable for evaluating effects of chemicals. However, so far, electrophysiological methods have been used mainly for studies on the mechanisms of neurotoxic action of drugs. The high cost of the equipment and skill required limit the application of electrophysiological techniques in routine neurotoxicology. Lower vertebrates, such as Xenopus or Aplisia, have been used but, because of their relatively limited neuronal network, they should be used only when there is already an indication of the putative mechanism of neurotoxicity. In this respect, it has been shown that pyrethroids have no blocking activity in the peripheral nerves of frogs or rats while they are quite active on arthroprod nerve fibres (Van den Bercken *et al.*, 1973).

13.4   BIOCHEMICAL METHODS

Knowledge of the role of chemical agents in neurotransmission makes it possible to devise important experimental conditions for neurotoxicity tests. An effect of a chemical agent on a well established molecular mechanism can be extrapolated to man with more confidence than any other kinds of functional activity. The correlation between the neurotoxic action of organophosphates and their effects on acetylcholinesterase gives rise to great hopes for the evaluation of other toxic agents. In fact, Lotti and Johnson (1978) found that the inhibitory power of organophosphates against hen brain neurotoxic esterase (NTE) correlates with the effect obtained on human post mortem brain acetylcholinesterase and with the ability to produce neuropathy *in vivo*. Unfortunately, similar examples have not been found with other classes of neurotoxins.

13.4.1   Neurochemical mapping

Descriptions of all the possible biochemical points of attack for neurotoxic agents is beyond the scope of this chapter (see Damstra and Bondy, 1982). Only some aspects of the various biochemical pathways and their influence of chemical agents in brain are considered here. However, biochemical techniques, linked with morphological studies, have been used effectively to plot a map of the brain.

Horseradish peroxidase (HRP), when injected in discrete brain areas is taken up mainly by nerve terminals and is transported throughout the neurones. The location of HRP can be determined on serial sections by various histochemical procedures

Table 13.3 Electrophysiological methods in neurotoxicity testing (Dewar, 1983)

Test	Function tested	Comments	References
Maximum motor nerve conduction velocity (MCV)	Function of large diameter motor fibres in peripheral nerve	Relatively widely used as an indication of peripheral nerve damage but relatively insensitive	Fullerton, 1966; Fullerton and Barnes, 1966
Partial antidromic block-conduction velocity of slower fibres (CVSF)	Function of slower (smaller diameter) motor fibres in peripheral nerve	At present not used to any significant extent in neurotoxicology	Seppaläinen and Hernberg, 1972
Sensory nerve conduction (SNV)	Function of sensory fibres in peripheral nerve	At present relatively under-utilized in neurotoxicology. Technique is more difficult than MCV measurement but potentially more useful	Le Quesne, 1978a, b; De Jesus *et al.*, 1978
Electromyography (EMG)	Neuromuscular function	Extensively used in clinical studies but as yet not widely used in animal studies	Goodgold and Eberstein, 1977; Mendell *et al.*, 1974
Stimulus strength duration testing (S–D curves)	Detects denervation of muscles (innervated and denervated muscles differ in their thresholds to excitation)	Little used in neurotoxicology at present	Johnson, 1980
Electroence-phalography (EEG)	Spontaneous electrical activity of the brain	Particularly useful for study of effects of sleep	Takeuchi and Hisanaga, 1977
Electroretinography (ERG)	Retinal function, susceptibility of rods and cones to toxic effects	Feasible to include ERG measurements in chronic studies in dogs	Liverani and Schaeppi, 1979
Sensory evoked potentials, average evoked potentials (AEP)	Function of different sensory modalities. The AEP indicates the neural activity of the brain involved in processing sensory input	Techniques are available for use in rodents	Niemeyer, 1979

(Llamas *et al.*, 1975). It is, therefore, possible to compare distribution of HRP in normal and treated animals, revealing damage in the morphology of the nervous tissue.

To study the proximo-distal migration of proteins, labelled aminoacids can be injected in discrete brain areas. Autoradiographic methods, coupled with the light or electron microscopy, enable a map to be plotted of where the axons from a collection of neurones terminate (Wiesel *et al.*, 1974; Pickel *et al.*, 1974; Jones and Moore, 1977). Another way to map those neurones containing monoamines (such as dopamine (DA), noradrenaline (NA) and serotonin (5HT) involves the use of procedures which result in specific fluorescence (Falck *et al.*, 1962; Lindvall and Bjorkland, 1974).

Immunochemical methods have been utilized to locate a variety of enzymes and proteins within the central nervous system. The principle consists of producing specific antibodies which are then linked to fluorescent dyes. Incubation of these complexes with brain slices results in fluorescence at sites where the enzyme or the protein binds to the specific antibodies (Bock, 1978).

Labelled 2-deoxyglucose (2-DG), injected intravenously, is taken up into the neurones by an active process with an intensity related to the rate of glucose oxidation. Autoradiographic techniques can be used to detect 2-DG-6-phosphate which is formed from the phosphorylation of 2-DG but it cannot be further metabolized (Sokoloff *et al.*, 1977). Computerized imaging procedures permit quantitation of autoradiography thus enabling a 'metabolic' map of the brain to be constructed. This technique is widely used. For instance, d-amphetamine which stimulates dopamine release in the synapses increases glucose consumption and, therefore, 2-DG uptake in brain areas rich in dopaminergic terminals such as the striatum (Wolfson and Brown, 1976). This technique has a great potential for the detection of neurotoxic effects in the brain that are related not only to blockade of glucose metabolism but also to activation or inhibition of neuronal activity related to glucose metabolism.

Protein synthesis can also be measured in brain by the incorporation of various aminoacids into the protein macro-molecules. The turnover of proteins differ widely in brain (Lajtha and Marks, 1971) and, therefore, appropriate times must be carefully selected in order to study the effect of neurotoxic agents. Acrylamide (Schotman *et al.*, 1978), methylmercury (Omata *et al.*, 1978) and carbondisulphide (Savolainen and Jarvisalo, 1977) affect protein synthesis in brain but interpretation of the results is difficult because these agents may affect protein synthesis only by impairment of factors which modulate it (hormones, diet, cofactors, transport of aminoacids, etc.).

Proteins are transported along the axons at different rates; this axoplasmic flow can now be measured by various techniques. This may provide a means for further study of agents that induce peripheral neuropathies (Bondy and Madsen, 1974; Schechter *et al.*, 1979; Starkey and Brimijoin, 1979).

13.4.2 Neurotransmitter biochemistry

The functional aspects of chemical neurotransmitters as communicators among neurones has been extensively studied in recent years. From the large amount of information now available, it is clear that all stages of the neurotransmission process may be influenced by neurotoxic agents. This is exemplified by considering the monoamines.

Precursors of monoamines (e.g. tryptophan for 5HT and tyrosine for catecholamines) must enter the brain; this occurs as a consequence of active transport across the blood/brain barrier. Transport of monoamine precursors competes with the transport of other aminoacids, for example, the transport of tryptophan depends on the concentrations of the neutral aminoacids present in the blood (Osborne, 1982). After gaining access to the neurones, precursors are involved in one or more enzymic steps that result in the synthesis of specific chemical neurotransmitters. In the case of tryptophan, it is transformed by tryptophan hydroxylase to 5-hydroxytryptophan which is then decarboxylated by a *l*-aromatic aminoacid decarboxylase to form 5HT (Osborne, 1982); tyrosine is hydroxylated (tyrosine hydroxylase) to form dopa that in turn is decarboxylated to dopamine; dopamine-beta-hydroxylase catalyses the formation of noradrenaline from dopamine (Iversen and Callingham, 1971).

Once the monamine is formed, it is stored in vesicles from which it can be released into the synaptic cleft. Many chemical agents (e.g. reserpine) affect storage (Shore and Giachetti, 1978) or induce release of the monoamine (e.g. *d*-amphetamine for catecholamines (Paton, 1979), *d*-fenfluramine for 5HT (Garattini *et al.*, 1979). Once released, the monoamine is metabolized to an inactive chemical species. In the case of 5HT, it is transformed into 5-hydroxyindole acetic acid in the presence of monoamine oxidase A (Osborne, 1982); catecholamines are also subjected to the action of *O*-methylcatechol-transferase (COMT) (Iversen and Callingham, 1971). However, the principal mechanism of inactivation of monoamine is uptake inside the nerve terminals (Fonnum *et al.*, 1980). This process requires energy, is specific for given nerve terminals and is probably modulated by endogenous inhibitors of uptake. Monoamine which is not subject to metabolism or uptake interacts with postsynaptic receptors.

Recently developed methods to measure quantitatively the density (B_{max}) of certain receptors and the affinity (K_d) of neurotransmitters for their specific receptors (Bennett, 1978) have opened up new possibilities for research in central nervous tissue. A partial list of brain receptors is given in Table 13.4. It should be emphasized that the number of known brain receptors is continuously increasing. Each of these receptors may represent a target for neurotoxic chemicals. However, an effect on receptors measured *in vitro* is no guarantee of an effect *in vivo*; once a chemical is metabolized, its metabolic products may exert a different effect on receptors from that of the parent compound. The action of metabolite(s) obviously cannot be

Table 13.4 Some drug and neurotransmitter receptor types and subtypes

Subtype	Properties
	Opiate type
μ	Morphine-selective: localized in pain modulating brain regions
$μ_1$	Identified by very high affinity binding of numerous opiates: blocked selectively by naloxonazine; meptazinol a specific agonist; implicated in analgesia but not respiratory depression
δ	Enkephalin-selective; localized in limbic brain regions
k	Mediates sedating, less addicting analgesia; localized to deep layers of cerebral cortex; dynorphin has high affinity; mediates rabbit vas deferens contractions
σ	Naloxone insensitive; mediates psychotomimetic opiate effects; concentrated in hippocampus
ε	β-Endorphin selective; mediates rat vas deferens contractions
Cough-suppressant	Dextromethorphan-selective; reversed stereospecificity; localized to fourth ventricle floor which regulates cough reflexes
	Calcium antagonist type
Dihydropyridine	Binding dependent on Ca^{2+} and blocked by ionic calcium anagonists; regulated allosterically by verapamil; localized to molecular layer dentate gyrus, external plexiform layer olfactory bulb
Verapamil	Inhibited by physiologic Ca^{2+} levels; linked to behavioural activation by diphenylbutylpiperidine neuroleptics, sexual and cardiac effects of the phenothiazine thioridazine, and antidiarrhoeal actions of loperamide and diphenoxalate
Dilitiazem	Can involve same site as verapamil in part; allosterically regulated by dihydropyridines

Adenosine type

A_1 — Labelled by [3H]cyclohexyladenosine, [3H]phenylisopropyladenosine, 2-[3H]chloroadenosine; lowers adenylate cyclase; adenosine analogues potent at nanomolar concentrations; stereospecific for phenylisopropyladenosine; localized to molecular layers of hippocampus and cerebellum, medial geniculate; contained on nerve terminals of cerebellar granule cells and retinal ganglion cell projections to superior colliculus.

A_2 — Stimulates adenylate cyclase; adenosine analogues potent at micromolar concentrations; little stereoselectivity for phenylisopropyl-adenosine; labelled with $5'$-N-[3H]ethylcarboxamide adenosine

α-Adrenergic type

α_1 — Postsynaptic in sympathetic system; prazosin and indoramin-selective; acts through Ca^{2+} channels; little affected by guanine nucleotides

α_2 — Located on sympathetic nerve terminals to regulate norepinephrine release but also postsynaptic, especially in brain; clonidine selective agonist; yohimbine- and piperoxan-selective antagonists; lowers adenylate cyclase

β-Adrenergic type

β_1 — Epinephrine and norepinephrine equally potent agonists; practalol-selective antagonist; more in heart than in lung; regional variations in brain; neuronal localization

β_2 — Epinephrine more potent than norepinephrine; terbutaline- and salbutamol-selective agonists; more in lungs than heart; few regional variations in brain; more on glia than neurons

Muscarinic cholinergic type

M_1 — Concentrated in sympathetic ganglia, corpus striatum, and stomach, pirenzipine-selective antagonist; closes K^+ channels

M_2 — Concentrated in hindbrain, cerebellum and heart; regulated by gallamine and GTP; inhibits adenylate cyclase

---

From Snyder (1984).

Table 13.4 *(continued)*

Subtype	Properties
	GABA type
A	Muscimol-selective; postsynaptic to GABA neurones, inhibited by calcium; antagonized by convulsant bicuculline
B	Baclofen-selective; on GABA and other nerve terminals; stimulated by calcium; bicuculline-resistant
Sedative-convulsant	Labelled by convulsants [³H]dihydropicrotoxinin and [³⁵S]-t-butylbicyclophosphorothionate; regulated by chloride and barbiturates; linked to benzodiazepine and $GABA_A$ receptors
	Dopamine type
D_1	Enhances adenylate cyclase; labelled by [³H]thioxanthenes; absent in pituitary; present in parathyroid
D_2	Lowers adenylate cyclase; labelled by [³H]butyrophenones; present in anterior pituitary; responsible for antipsychotic and extrapyramidal actions
	Serotonin (5HT) type
$5HT_1$	Labelled with [³H]-5HT, which is potent at nanomolar concentrations; classical 5HT antagonists are weak; regulated by guanine nucleotides, possibly linked to adenylate cyclase; mediates contraction of dog basilar artery.
$5HT_2$	Labelled with [³H]spiperone and [³H]ketanserin; micromolar 5HT; less affected by guanine nucleotides; mediates behavioural '5HT syndrome', contraction of oestrous rat uterus, dog and rabbit femoral and rat caudal arteries, and rat and rabbit aorta and jugular vein

detected *in vitro*. An example is trazodone, an antidepressant agent which is transformed in the body into several metabolites, including *m*-chlorophenylpiperazine (Caccia *et al.*, 1981). While trazodone interferes with 5HT2 receptors, the metabolites interact mostly with 5HT1 (Garattini, 1983). Another case is camazepam, a benzodiazepine which interacts very weakly *in vitro* with the benzodiazepine-GABA-chloride receptor complex (IC50 = 950 nM) while its metabolite temazepam shows an IC50 = 24 nM (Garattini *et al.*, 1981).

In some cases, a neurotoxic effect observed *in vitro* may not occur *in vivo* because of problems related to the blood/brain barrier. For example, domperidone is a very active agent that interacts with postsynaptic dopaminergic receptors but does not cross the blood/brain barrier (Laduron and Leysen, 1979).

In addition to the postsynaptic receptors, the brain also contains presynaptic receptors (also known as autoreceptors). These regulate the release of neurochemical mediators from the nerve terminals (Osborne, 1982; Paton, 1979). Although the fundamental role of autoreceptors has not yet been completely elucidated, it may represent another mechanism that may prove useful for detecting neurotoxicity.

Receptors are not stable entities but are continuously modulated so that when there is excessive stimulation, receptor density decreases; when there is reduced stimulation, it increases (Creese and Sibley, 1981). Neurotoxic agents may not affect the receptors *per se* but only their modulation. Furthermore, various neurones do not work in isolation but are connected to each other so that a chemical affecting one type of neurotransmitter is likely indirectly to affect other neurotransmitters too.

There is also recent evidence suggesting that certain nerve terminals contain more than one neurotransmitter (cotransmitters) (Lundberg and Hökfelt, 1983). The neurotransmitters and these interactions represent for the moment a very difficult area of research because of the extreme intricacy of these interrelations. For example, it can be shown that some tricyclic antidepressant agents which, when given in single doses, do not affect the dopaminergic system, elicit marked functional changes of this monoamine after a seven-day treatment (Borsini *et al.*, 1985a,b). These effects can be interpreted as a consequence of changes induced on other chemical neurotransmitters which, in turn, interact with the dopaminergic system.

As an example of how these various biochemical tests can be used in neurotoxicity studies, Table 13.5 summarizes the various effects of lead on neurochemical monoamines (for a review see Winder and Kitchen, 1984). It must be stressed, however, that the significance of these results in the interpretation of the overall toxicity of lead is still doubtful. The concentrations of lead reported to cause effects, especially *in vitro*, are usually higher than those which can be reached *in vivo* (Winder and Kitchen, 1984).

13.4.3 Behavioural effects

Interactions between the various events that occur in the central and peripheral nervous systems are integrated and expressed as behaviour. Behavioural

Table 13.5   Some effects of lead on monoaminergic systems in the CNS

Parameter	Effect	References
Synthesis		
Tyrosine to dopamine	Increase	Wince *et al.*, 1976
Tyrosine hydroxylase	None	Deskin *et al.*, 1980
Uptake		
Dopamine (*in vitro*)	Decrease	Silbergeld, 1977
Dopamine (*in vivo*)	None	Wince *et al.*, 1980
Serotonin (*in vitro*)	None	Silbergeld and Goldberg, 1975
Release		
Dopamine (*in vitro*)	Increase	Bondy *et al.*, 1979
	None	Komulainen and Tuomisto, 1981
Receptors		
Dopamine postsynaptic receptors	Decrease	Wince *et al.*, 1976
Dopamine D_2 (striatum)	Increase	Lucchi *et al.*, 1981
Brain levels		
Noradrenaline	Increase	Dubas and Hrdina, 1978; Jason and Kellogg, 1977
	None	Grant *et al.*, 1976
Dopamine	Decrease	Dubas and Hrdina, 1978; Jason and Kellog, 1977
	None	Golter and Michaelson, 1975
Tyrosine	None	Schumann, 1977
Homovanillic acid	Increase	Silbergeld and Chisholm, 1976
	Decrease	Govoni *et al.*, 1978
Dihydroxyphenyl acetic acid	Decrease	Govoni *et al.*, 1978
Vanilmandelic acid	Increase	Silbergeld and Chisholm, 1976
Serotonin	Decrease	Dubas and Hrdina, 1978
	Increase	Weinreisch *et al.*, 1977
5-hydroxyindolacetic acid	Decrease	Dubas *et al.*, 1978

This is only a partial list of the effects observed by studying lead neurotoxic activity. For a complete analysis, see Winder and Kitchen (1984).

disturbances are, therefore, very important indicators of neurotoxicity. Irwin (1964) developed quantitative methods to monitor many aspects of behaviour in various animal species. A number of tests which can be used for screening effects on behaviour are summarized in Table 13.6; and other tests which could be utilized as second or third order behavioural tests to obtain more detailed information are summarized in Table 13.7.

Although some of these tests require large and expensive laboratory facilities,

Table 13.6   Examples of functional and behavioural tests suitable for screening (Dewar, 1983)

Function	Test	Reference
General	Structured clinical observation (e.g. Irwin screen)	Irwin, 1964
Motor Spontaneous activity	Activity in activity monitor. Open field test. Exploratory behaviour	Tilson and Cabe, 1979; Finger, 1972; Delini Stula *et al.*, 1979
Impairment of motor co-ordination	Inclined plane test Rotarod test. Electrorod test Narrowing bridge test	Graham *et al.*, 1957 Kaplan and Murphy, 1972 Dewar, 1980
Muscular weakness	Forelimb grip Hindlimb exterior	Boissier and Simon, 1960 Cabe and Tilson, 1978; Tilson *et al.*, 1980
Fatigability	Swimming endurance	Bhagat and Wheeler, 1973
Sensory General responsiveness	Startle response, e.g. to puff of air	Tilson and Cabe, 1979

Table 13.6   *(continued)*

Visual	Optokinetic drum	Wallman, 1975
	Evaluation of ocular reflexes: light reflex, menace reflex and corneal reflex	Conquet *et al.*, 1979
	Localization and orientation	Marshall, 1975
	Visual cliff test	Sloane *et al.*, 1978
Olfactory	Orientation in response to odour	Marshall, 1975
Auditory	Startle response	Barlow *et al.*, 1978
	Measurement of threshold sound intensity for Preyer's reflex	Baird and Carter, 1979
Somatosensory/pain/ temperature sensitivity	Tail flick test, hot plate test, Minnesota Thermal disks	Baird and Carter, 1979; Janssen *et al.*, 1963
Orientation in space	Negative geotaxis	Fox, 1965
Physiological behaviour/ Thermoregulation	Measurement of core body temperature	Simonds and Uretsky, 1970
	Measurement of ingestion of food and water	Peters *et al.*, 1979
Learning and memory	One way avoidance task	Clark, 1966

Table 13.7 Examples of second-order and third-order behavioural tests (Dewar, 1983)

Function	Test	Reference
Motor Fine motor control	Operant response force (conditioning of rats to press a lever attached to a force transducer with a designated force for a given period of time)	Falk, 1970
Sensory Sensory deficit	Maze discriminating tests using sensory cues, e.g., T-maze test using visual discrimination	Zenick *et al.*, 1978
Visual, auditory, olfactory	Psychophysical studies—operant responding	Chiba and Ando, 1976
Somatosensory	Vibration sensitivity assessment	Maurissen and Weiss, 1980
Gustatory	Taste discrimination (using quinine)	Kodama *et al.*, 1978
Learning memory	Two-way avoidance Discriminative Y-maze Multiple T water maze	Sobotka *et al.*, 1975 Vorhees, 1974 Vorhees *et al.*, 1978

Table 13.7   *(continued)*

Affective—emotional CNS excitability	Electrical self-stimulation of the brain	Annau, 1978; Ornstein, 1979
Dissociation from environment	Conditioned avoidance response	Corsico, 1979
Physiological/ Thermoregulation	Study of circadian rhythms	Stephan and Nunez, 1977
Specific tests for: Monoamine oxidase inhibitory activity	Potentiation of head twitches by 5-hydroxy-tryptophan and reserpine reversal	Corne *et al.*, 1963; Chessin *et al.*, 1957
Induction of anaesthesia	Potentiation of 2-methoxy-4-allylphenoxy acetic acid diethylamide-induced anaesthesia	Corsico, 1979
Extrapyramidal effects (e.g. side-effects of neuroleptics)	Catalepsy test Test for dopamine receptor hypersensitivity using apomorphine-induced stereotyped behaviour	Bürki, 1979 Worms and Lloyd, 1979
Drug dependence liability	Single dose suppression test (Primates)	Swain, 1979

many others are relatively simple tests. Nevertheless, they call for experienced scientists. An extensive review on the subject has been recently published by Norton (1982) and by Tilson and Harry (1982).

13.5 CONCLUSIONS

It would be naive to believe that any single test could serve to reveal all neurotoxic effects. Even a battery of tests cannot guarantee a complete investigation covering all possible kinds of neurotoxic effects.

At the moment, there are no magic answers in the field of neurotoxicity testing. Each chemical must be studied individually; detection of its possible neurotoxic effects should be regarded not as a routine procedure but as a research project. Chemical and functional analogies may help in establishing the best procedure to be utilized but attention should always be given to unexpected neurotoxic effects.

The importance of *in vitro* tests cannot be overstated; at the present time, *in vitro* tests, although not a complete replacement for *in vivo* experiments, appear to be a complementary tool for understanding mechanisms of action. The specialization of the nervous system is such that it seems impossible to obtain cell lines or organ cultures representative of all these functions for use *in vitro*. Nevertheless, efforts must continue to develop culture conditions for nerve cells that avoid loss of their biochemical characteristics.

In vivo tests also have limitations because all neurotoxic effects are not expressed in detectable symptoms and because compensatory mechanisms operate in the brain. *In vitro* studies following *in vivo* treatment (*ex vivo*) may partially obviate this difficulty. The pressure of some groups to reduce *in vivo* tests because they are not predictive of human neurotoxicity may be understandable, but it is difficult to understand how *in vitro* tests could be more predictive when they obviously suffer from excessive simplification.

Neurotoxic effects in fetuses, newborn and aged organisms represent important aspects of neurotoxicology that deserve special attention. There is also a need to understand better which neurotoxic effects occur in man because of exposure to chemical contaminants. In this respect, epidemiological studies should be encouraged because the results could help in planning more meaningful experimental testing.

REFERENCES

Airoldi, L., Bizzi, A., Salmona, M., and Garattini, S. (1979). Attempts to establish the safety margin for neurotoxicity of monosodium glutamate. In: Filer, L.J. Jr., Garattini, S., Kare, M.R., Reynolds, W.A., and Wurtman, R.J. (Eds), *Glutamic Acid: Advances in Biochemistry and Physiology*, Raven Press, New York, pp. 321–31.
Annau, Z. (1978). Electrical self-stimulation of the brain: A model for the behavioural evaluation of toxic agents. *Environ. Health Perspect.*, **26**, 59–67.

Baird, J.R.C., and Carter, A.J. (1979). Tests for effects of drugs on hearing and balance—screen for assessing the ototoxic potential of aminoglycoside antibiotics. *Pharmacol. Ther.,* **5**, 579–83.

Barlow, S.M., Knight, A.F., and Sullivan, F.M. (1978). Delay in postnatal growth and development of offspring produced by maternal restraint stress during pregnancy in the rat. *Teratology,* **18**, 211–18.

Bennett, J.P. Jr. (1978). Methods in binding studies. In: Yamamura, H.I., Enna, S.J., and Kuhar, M.J. (Eds), *Neurotransmitter Receptor Binding,* Raven Press, New York, pp. 57–90.

Bhagat, B., and Wheeler, M. (1973). Effect of nicotine on the swimming endurance of rats. *Neuropharmacol,* **12**, 1161–5.

Bock, E. (1978). Nervous system specific proteins. *J. Neurochem.,* **30**, 7–14.

Boissier, J., and Simon, P. (1960). L'utilisation du test de la traction (test de Julon-Courvoisier) pour l'etude des psycholeptiques. *Therapie,* **15**, 1171–5.

Bondy, S.C., and Madsen, C.J. (1974). The extent of axoplasmic transport during development, determined by migration of various radioactively labelled materials. *J. Neurochem.,* **23**, 905–10.

Bondy, S.C., Harrington, M.E., Anderson, C.L., and Prasad, K.N. (1979). The effect of low concentrations of an organic lead concentration on the transport and release of putative transmitters. *Toxicol. Lett.,* **3**, 35–41.

Borsini, F., Nowakowska, E., Pulvirenti, L., and Samanin, R. (1985a). Repeated treatment with amitriptyline reduces immobility in the behavioural 'despair' test in rats by activating dopaminergic and beta-adrenergic mechanisms. *J. Pharm. Pharmacol.,* **37**, 137–8.

Borsini, F., Pulvirenti, L., and Samanin R. (1985b). Evidence of dopamine involvement in the effect of repeated treatment with various antidepressants in the behavioural 'despair' test in rats. *Europ. J. Pharmacol.,* **110**, 253–6.

Brightman, M.W. (1977). Morphology of blood–brain interfaces. *Exp. Eye Res. (Suppl.),* **25**, 1–25.

Brosnan, C.G., Bunge, M.B., and Murray, M.R. (1970). The response of lysosomes in cultured neurons to chlorpromazine. *J. Neuropath. Exp. Neurol.,* **29**, 337–53.

Buravlev, V.M. (1978). *In vitro* effect of psychopharmacological drugs on the embryonic brain tissue of the fetuses of schizophrenic mothers. *Zh. Nevropatol. Psikhiatr.,* **78**, 1070–75.

Bürki, H.R. (1979). Extrapyramidal side-effects. *Pharmacol. Ther.,* **5**, 525–34.

Cabe, P.A., and Tilson, H.A. (1978). Hind limb extensor response: a method for assessing motor dysfunction in rats. *Pharmacol. Biochem. Behav.,* **9**, 133–6.

Caccia, S., Ballabio, M., Fanelli, R., Guiso, G., and Zanini, M.G. (1981). Determination of plasma and brain concentratirons of trazodone and its metabolite, 1-m-chlorophenylpiperazine by gas-liquid chromatography. *J. Chromatogr.,* **210**, 311–18.

Caccia, S., Fong, M.H., Garattini, S., and Notarnicola, A. (1985). 1-Aryl-piperazine as active metabolites of drugs with an aryl-piperazine side-chain. *Biochem. Pharmacol.,* **34**, 393–4.

Chessin, M., Kramer, E.R., and Scott, C.C. (1957). Modifications of the pharmacology of reserpine and serotonin by iproniazid. *J. Pharmacol. Exp. Ther.,* **119**, 433–9.

Chiba, S., and Ando, K. (1976). Effects of chronic administration of kanamycin on conditional suppression to auditory stimulus in rats. *Jap. J. Pharmacol.,* **26**, 419–25.

Clark, R. (1966). A rapidly acquired avoidance response in rats. *Psychoanal. Sci.,* **6**, 11–16.

Conquet, P.H., Tardieu, M., and Durand, G. (1979). Evaluation of ocular reflexes during toxicity studies. *Pharmacol. Ther.,* **5**, 585–91.

Corne, S.J., Pickering, R., and Warner, B.T. (1963). A method for assessing the effect of drugs on the central action of 5-hydroxytryptamine. *Brit. J. Pharmacol.,* **20**, 106–12.

Corsico, N. (1979). Proposed for an evaluation schedule of potential CNS activity of various agents. *Pharmacol. Ther.*, **5**, 427–9.

Creese, I., and Sibley, D.R. (1981). Receptor adaptations to centrally acting drugs. *Ann. Rev. Pharmacol. Toxicol.*, **21**, 357–91.

Curtis, D.R. (1979). Problems in the evaluation of glutamate as a central nervous system transmitter. In: Filer, L.J. Jr., Garattini, S., Kare, M.R., Reynolds, W.A., and Wurtman, R.J. (Eds), *Glutamic Acid: Advances in Biochemistry and Physiology*, Raven Press, New York, pp. 163–75.

Damstra, T., and Bondy, S.C. (1982). Neurochemical approaches to the detection of neurotoxicity. In: Mitchell, C.L. (Ed.), *Nervous System Toxicology*, Raven Press, New York, pp. 349–73.

De Jesus, C.P.V., Pleasure, D.E., Asbury, A.K., and Brown, M.J. (1978). Effects of methyl butyl ketone on peripheral nerves and its mechanism of action. Final Report Contract CDG 99-76-16. Cincinnati, National Institute for Occupational Safety and Health.

Delini Stula, A., Radeke, E., Schlicht, G., and Hedwall, P.R. (1979). Detection of CNS-depressant properties of antihypertensives: validity of various test methods in rodents and estimation of therapeutic margin in hypertensive rats. *Pharmacol. Ther.*, **5**, 431–44.

Deskin, R., Bursian, S.J., and Edens, F.W. (1980). An investigation into the effects of manganese and other divalent cations on tyrosine hydroxylase activity. *Neurotoxicology*, **2**, 75–81.

Dewar, A.J. (1980). Neurotoxicity testing—with particular reference to biochemical methods. In: Garrod, J.W. (Ed.), *Testing for Toxicity*, Taylor & Francis, London, pp. 199–217.

Dewar, A.J. (1983). Neurotoxicity. In Balls, M., Riddell, R.J., and Worden, A.N. (Eds), *Animals and Alternatives in Toxicity Testing*, Academic Press, London, pp. 229–84.

Dubas, T.C., and Hrdina, P.D. (1978). Behavioural and neurochemical consequences of neonatal exposure to lead in rats. *J. Environ. Path. Toxicol.*, **2**, 473–84.

Dubas, T.C., Stevenson, A., Singhal, R.L., and Hrdina, P.D. (1978). Regional alterations of brain biogenic amines in young rats following chronic lead exposure. *Toxicology*, **9**, 185–90.

Ericsson, A.-C., and Walum, E. (1984). Cytotoxicity of cyclophosphamide and acrylamide in glioma and neuroblastoma cell lines cocultured with liver cells. *Toxicol. Lett.*, **20**, 251–6.

Falck, B., Hillarp, N.A., Thieme, G., and Torp, A. (1962). Fluorescence of catecholamines and related compounds condensed with formaldehyde. *J. Histochem. Cytochem.*, **10**, 348–54.

Falk, J.L. (1970). The behavioural measurement of fine motor control effects of pharmacological agents. In: Thompson, T., Pickens, R., and Heron, R.A. (Eds), *Readings in Behavioral Pharmacology*, Appleton Century-Crofts, New York, pp. 223–40.

Ferretti, C., Benfenati, F., Cimino, M., Vantini, G., Lipartiti, M., Muccioli, G., Di Carlo, R., and Algeri, S. (1983). Effects of systemic and intracerebro-ventricular domperidone/ treatment on striatal and hypothalamic dopaminergic neurons. *Med. Biol.*, **61**, 331–6.

Finger, F.W. (1972). Measuring behavioral activity. In: Myers, R.D. (Ed.), *Methods in Psychobiology*, Academic Press, New York, pp. 1–25.

Fonnum, F., Karlsen, R.L., Malthe-Sorenssen, D., Sterri, S., and Walaas, I. (1980). High affinity transport systems and their role in transmitter action. In: Cotman, C.W., Poste, G., and Nicolson, G.L. (Eds), *The Cell Surface and Neuronal Function*, North-Holland, Amsterdam, pp. 455–504.

Fox, D.A., Lowndes, H.E., and Bierkamper, G.G. (1982). Electrophysiological techniques in neurotoxicology. In: Mitchell, C.L. (Ed.), *Nervous System Toxicology*, Raven Press, New York, pp. 299–335.

Fox, W.M. (1965). Reflex-ontogeny and behavioural development of the mouse. *Animal Behaviour*, **13**, 234–9.

Fullerton, P.M. (1966). Chronic peripheral neuropathy by lead poisoning in guinea-pigs. *J. Neuropath. exp. Neurol.*, **25**, 214–36.

Fullerton, P.M., and Barnes, J. (1966). Peripheral neuropathy in rats produced by acrylamide. *Brit. J. Industr. Med.*, **23**, 210–22.

Garattini, S. (1979). Evaluation of the neurotoxic effects of glutamic acid. In: Wurtman, R.J., and Wurtman, J.J. (Eds), *Nutrition and the Brain*, volume 4, Raven Press, New York, pp. 79–124.

Garattini, S. (1983). Importance of establishing the presence of drug active metabolites. *Europ. J. Drug Metab. Pharmacokinet.*, **8**, 97–108.

Garattini, S., and Samanin, R. (1977). Selective neurotoxicity of 6-hydroxydopamine. In: Roizin, L., Shiraki, H., and Grcevic, N. (Eds), *Neurotoxicology*, volume 1, Raven Press, New York, pp. 15–23.

Garattini, S., Caccia, S., Mennini, T., Samanin, R., Consolo, S., and Ladinsky, H. (1979). Biochemical pharmacology of the anorectic drug fenfluramine: A review. *Curr. Med. Res. Opin.*, **6**, Suppl. 1, 15–27.

Garattini, S., Caccia, S., Carli, M., and Mennini, T. (1981). Notes on kinetics and metabolism of benzodiazepines. *Adv. Biosci.*, **31**, 351–64.

Golter, M., and Michaelson, I.A. (1975). Growth, behaviour and brain catecholamines in lead exposed neonatal rats: a reappraisal. *Science*, **187**, 359–61.

Goodgold, J., and Eberstein, A. (1977). *Electrodiagnosis of Neuromuscular Diseases*, 2nd Edn., Williams and Wilkins, Baltimore.

Govoni, S., Montefusco, O., Spano, P.F., and Trabucchi, M. (1978). Effect of chronic lead treatment on brain dopamine synthesis and serum prolactin release in the rat. *Toxicol. Lett.*, **2**, 333–7.

Graham, R.C.B., Lu, F.C., and Allmark, M.G. (1957). Combined effect of tranquilizing drugs and alcohol on rats. *Fed. Proc.*, **16**, 302.

Grant, L.D., Kimmel, C.A., Martinez-Vargas, C.M., and West, G.L. (1976). Assessment of developmental toxicity associated with chronic lead exposure. *Environ. Health Perspect.*, **17**, 290.

Heikkila, R., and Cohen, G. (1971). Inhibition of biogenic amine uptake by hydrogen peroxide: A mechanism for toxic effects of 6-hydroxydopamine. *Science*, **172**, 1257–8.

Heikkila, R., and Cohen, G. (1972). Further studies on the generation of hydrogen peroxide by 6-hydroxydopamine. *Mol. Pharmacol.*, **8**, 241–8.

Hendelman, W.J. (1969). The effect of thallium on peripheral nervous tissue in culture: a light and electron microscopic study. *Anatomical Record*, **163**, 198A.

Höhn, K.G., and Wuttke, W.O. (1978). Changes in catecholamine turnover in the anterior part of the mediobasal hypothalamus and the medial preoptic area in response to hyperprolactinemia in ovariectomized rats. *Brain Res.*, **156**, 241–52.

Irwin, S. (1964). Drug screening and evaluation of new compounds in animals. In: Nodine, J.H., and Siegler, P.E. (Eds), *Animal and Clinical Pharmacological Techniques in Drug Evaluation*, Year Book, Chicago, pp. 36–54.

Iversen, L.L. (1970). Inhibition of catecholamine uptake by 6-hydroxydopamine in rat brain. *Europ. J. Pharmacol.*, **10**, 408–410.

Iversen, L.L., and Callingham, B.A. (1971). Adrenergic transmission. In: Bacq, Z.M. (Ed.), *Fundamentals of Biochemical Pharmacology*, Pergamon Press, Oxford, pp. 253–304.

Jacques, Y., Romey, G., Cavey, M.T., Kartalovski, B., and Lazdunski, M. (1980). Interaction of pyrethroids with the Na^+ channel in mammalian neuronal cells in culture. *Biochim. biophys. Acta*, **600**, 882–97.

Janssen, P.A.J., Niemegeers, C.J.E., and Dony, J.G.H. (1963). The inhibitory effect of fentanyl and other morphine-like analgesics on the warm water induced tail withdrawal reflex in rats. *Arzneimittel-Forsch.*, **13**, 502–7.

Jason, K., and Kellogg, C. (1977). Lead effects on behavioural and neurochemical development in rats. *Fed. Proc., 36*, 1008.

Johnson, B.L. (1980). Electrophysiological methods in neurotoxicity testing. In: Spencer, P.S., and Schaumburg, H.H. (Eds), *Experimental and Clinical Neurotoxicology*, Williams and Wilkins, Baltimore, pp. 726–42.

Johnston, G.A.R. (1979). Central nervous system receptors for glutamic acid. In: Filer, L.J. Jr., Garattini, S., Kare, M.R., Reynolds, W.A., and Wurtman, R.J. (Eds), *Glutamic Acid: Advances in Biochemistry and Physiology*, Raven Press, New York, pp. 177–85.

Jones, B.E., and Moore, R.Y. (1977). Ascending projections of the locus coeruleus in the rat. II. Autoradiographic studies. *Brain Res., 127*, 23–53.

Kaplan, M.L., and Murphy, S.D. (1972). Effects of acrylamide on rotorod performance and sciatic nerve β-glucuronidase activity of rats. *Toxicol. Appl. Pharmacol., 22*, 259–68.

Kim, S.U. (1971). Neurotoxic effects of alkyl mercury compounds on myelinating cultures of mouse cerebellum. *Exp. Neurol., 32*, 237–46.

Kodama, J., Fokoshima, M., and Sakata, T. (1978). Impaired taste discrimination against quinine following chronic administration of theophylline in rats. *Physiol. Behav., 20*, 151–9.

Komulainen, H., and Tuomisto, J. (1981). Effect of heavy metals on dopamine, noradrenaline and serotonin uptake and release in rat brain synaptosomes. *Acta Pharmacol. Toxicol., 48*, 199–204.

Laduron, P.M., and Leysen, J.E. (1979). Domperidone, a specific *in vitro* dopamine antagonist, devoid of *in vivo* central dopaminergic activity. *Biochem. Pharmacol., 28*, 2161–5.

Lajtha, A., and Marks, N. (1971). Protein turnover. In: Lajtha, A. (Ed.), *Handbook of Neurochemistry*, volume 5, Plenum Press, New York, pp. 551–629.

Lampert, P., Garro, F, and Pentschew, A. (1970). Tellurium neuropathy. *Acta Neuropathol., 15*, 308–17.

Lamperti, A., and Blaha, G. (1976). The effects of neonatally-administered monosodium glutamate on the reproductive system of adult hamsters. *Biol. Reprod., 14*, 362–9.

Le Quesne, P.M. (1978a). Clinical expression of neurotoxic injury and diagnostic use of electromyograph. *Environ. Health Perspec., 26*, 89–95.

Le Quesne, P.M. (1978b). Neurophysiological investigation of sub-clinical and minimal toxic neuropathies. *Muscle Nerve,1*, 392 5.

Lindvall, O., and Bjorkland, A. (1974). The glyoxylic fluorescence histochemical method: a detailed account of the methodology for the visualization of central catecholamine neurons. *Histochemistry, 39*, 97–127.

Liverani, S.L., and Schaeppi, U. (1979). Electroretinography as an indication of toxic retinopathy in dogs. *Pharmacol. Ther., 5*, 599–602.

Llamas, A., Reinoso-Suarez, F., and Martinez-Moreno, E. (1975). Projections to the gyrus proreus from the brain stem tegmentum (locus coeruleus, raphe nuclei) in the cat demonstrated by retrograde transport of horseradish peroxidase. *Brain Res., 89*, 331–6.

Lotti, M., and Johnson, M.K. (1978). Neurotoxicity of organophosphorus pesticides: predictions can be based on *in vitro* studies with hen and human enzymes. *Arch. Toxicol., 41*, 215–21.

Lucchi, L., Memo, M., Airaghi, M.L., Spano, P.F., and Trabucchi, M. (1981). Chronic lead treatment induces in rat a specific and differential effect on dopamine receptors in different brain areas. *Brain Res., 213*, 397–404.

Lundberg, J.M., and Hökfelt, T. (1983). Coexistence of pesticides and classical neurotransmitters. *TINS, 6*, 325–33.

Marshall, J.F. (1975). Increased orientation to sensory stimuli following medial hypothalamic damage in rats. *Brain Res., 86*, 373–87.

Matsuyama, S. (1970). Studies on experimental obesity in mice treated with MSG. *Jap. J. Vet. Sci.*, **32**, 206.

Maurissen, J.P.J., and Weiss, B. (1980). Vibration sensitivity as an index of somatosensory function. In: Spencer, P.S., and Schaumburg, H.H. (Eds), *Experimental and Clinical Neurotoxicology*, Williams and Wilkins, Baltimore, pp. 767–74.

Mendell, J.R., Saida, K., Ganansia, M.F., Jackson, D.B., Weiss, H., Gardier, R.S., Chrisman, C., Allen, N., Couri, D., O'Neill, J., Marks, B., and Hetland, L. (1974). Toxic polyneuropathy produced by methyl n-butyl ketone. *Science,* **185**, 787–9.

Niemeyer, G. (1979). Electrophysiological testing of the function of the vertebrate retina. *Pharmacol. Ther.,* **5**, 593–7.

Norton, S. (1982). Methods in behavioural toxicology. In: Hayes, A.W. (Ed.), *Principles and Methods of Toxicology,* Raven Press, New York, pp. 353–73.

Olney, J.W. (1969). Brain lesions, obesity and other disturbances in mice treated with monosodium glutamate. *Science,* **164**, 719–721.

Olney, J.W., Sharpe, L.G., and DeGubareff, T. (1975). Excitotoxic amino acids. Presented at the Fifth Annual Meeting of the Society of Neurosciences, New York, **1**, 371.

Omata, S., Sakimura, K., Tsubaki, H., and Sugano, H. (1978). *In vivo* effect of methylmercury on protein synthesis in brain and liver of the rat. *Toxicol. Appl. Pharmacol.,* **44**, 367–78.

Ornstein, K. (1979). Drug evaluation by use of rewarding brain stimulation. *Pharmacol. Ther.,* **5**, 417–22.

Osborne, N.N. (Ed.) (1982). *Biology of Serotonergic Transmission.* Wiley, Chichester.

Partridge, W.M. (1979). Regulation of amino acid availability to brain: Selective control mechanisms for glutamate. In: Filer, L.J. Jr., Garattini, S., Kare, M.R., Reynolds, W.A., and Wurtman, R.J. (Eds), *Glutamic Acid: Advances in Biochemistry and Physiology*, Raven Press, New York, pp. 125–37.

Paton, D.M. (Ed.) (1979). *The Release of Catecholamines from Adrenergic Neurons,* Pergamon Press, Oxford.

Perez, V.J., and Olney, J.W. (1972). Accumulation of glutamic acid in the arcuate nucleus of the hypothalamus of the infant mouse following subcutaneous administration of monosodium glutamate. *J. Neurochem.,* **19**, 1777–83.

Perez, V.J., Olney, J.W., and Robin, S.J. (1973). Glutamate accumulation in infant mouse hypothalamus: influence of temperature. *Brain Res.,* **59**, 181–9.

Perkins, M.A., and Westfall, T.C. (1978). The effect of prolactin on dopamine release from rat striatum and medial basal hypothalamus. *Neuroscience,* **3**, 59–63.

Peters, G., Besseghir, K.P., Kasermann, H.P., and Peters-Haefeli, L. (1979). The effects of drugs on ingestive behaviour. *Pharmacol. Ther.,* **5**, 485–504.

Pickel, V.M., Segal, M., and Bloom, F.E. (1974). A radioautographic study of the efferent pathways of the nucleus locus coeruleus. *J. Comp. Neurol.,* **55**, 15–42.

Pizzi, W.J., Barnhart, J.E., and Fanslow, D.J. (1977). Monosodium glutamate administration to the newborn reduces reproductive ability in female and male mice. *Science,* **196**, 452–4.

Saida, T. (1984). A study of methylmercury intoxication in cultured nervous tissue. *J. Kyoto Prefectural University Medicine,* in press.

Saunders, N.R. (1977). Ontogeny of the blood-brain barrier. *Exp. Eye Res.,* **25**, Suppl. 523–50.

Savolainen, H., and Jarvisalo, J. (1977). Effects of acute CS_2 intoxication on protein metabolism in rat brain. *Chem. Biol. Interact.,* **17**, 51–9.

Schechter, P.J., Trainen, Y., and Grove, J. (1979). Gabaculine and isogabaculine: *In vivo* biochemistry and pharmacology in mice. *Life Sci.,* **24**, 1173–82.

Schotman, P., Gipon, L., Jennekens, F.G.I., and Gispen, W.H. (1978). Polyneuropathies and CNS protein metabolism. III. Changes in protein synthesis induced by acrylamide intoxication. *J. Neuropath. Exp. Neurol.*, **37**, 820–37.

Schrier, B.K. (1982). Nervous system cultures as toxicologic test systems. In: Mitchell, C.L. (Ed.), *Nervous System Toxicology*, Raven Press, New York, pp. 337–48.

Schumann, A.M. (1977). The effects of inorganic lead on the central catecholaminergic system of the rodent with emphasis on postnatally exposed rats and mice. *Diss. Abstr.*, **38**, 5880.

Seppaläinen, A.M., and Hernberg, S. (1972). Sensitive technique for detecting subclinical lead neuropathy. *Brit. J. Industr. Med.*, **29**, 443–50.

Shank, R.P., and Aprison, M.H. (1979). Biochemical aspects of the neurotransmitter function of glutamate. In: Filer, L.J. Jr., Garattini, S., Kare, M.R., Reynolds, W.A., and Wurtman, R.J. (Eds), *Glutamic Acid: Advances in Biochemistry and Physiology*, Raven Press, New York, pp. 139–150.

Shore, P.A., and Giachetti, A. (1978). Reserpine: basic and clinical pharmacology. In: Iversen, L.L., Iversen, S.D., and Snyder, S.H. (Eds), *Handbook of Psychopharmacology*, volume 10, Plenum Press, New York, pp. 197–219.

Silbergeld, E.K. (1977). Interactions of lead and calcium on the synaptosome uptake of dopamine and choline. *Life Sci.*, **20**, 309–18.

Silbergeld, E.K., and Chisholm, J.J. Jr. (1976). Lead poisoning: altered urinary catecholamine metabolites as indicators of intoxication in mice and children. *Science*, **192**, 153–5.

Silbergeld, E.K., and Goldberg, A.M. (1975). Pharmacological and neurochemical investigations of lead induced hyperactivity. *Neuropharmacology*, **14**, 431–44.

Simonds, M.A., and Uretsky, N.J. (1970). Central effects of 6-hydroxydopamine on the body temperatures of the rat. *Brit. J. Pharmacol.*, **40**, 630–36.

Simson, E.L., Gold, R.M., Standish, L.J., and Pellett, P.L. (1977). Axon-sparing brain lesioning technique: the use of monosodium-L-glutamate and other amino acids. *Science*, **198**, 515–17.

Sloane, S.A., Shea, S.L., Procter, M.M., and Dewsbury, D.A. (1978). Visual cliff performance in 10 species of muroid rodents. *Animal Learning Behav.*, **6**, 244–50.

Snyder, S.H. (1984). Drug and neurotransmitter receptors in the brain. *Science*, **224**, 22–31.

Sobotka, T.J., Brodie, R.E., and Cook, M.P. (1975). Psychophysiologic effects of early lead exposure. *Toxicology*, **5**, 175–91.

Sokoloff, L., Reivich, M., Kennedy, C., Des Rosiers, M.H., Patlak, C.S., Pettigrew, K.D., Sakurada, O., and Shinohara, M. (1977). The ^{14}C-deoxyglucose method for the measurement of local cerebral glucose utilization: theory, procedure and normal values in the conscious and anaesthetized albino rat. *J. Neurochem.*, **28**, 897–916.

Spencer, P.S., Peterson, E.R., Madrid, R., and Raine, C.S. (1973). Effects of thallium salts on neuronal mitochondria in organotypic cord–ganglia–muscle combination cultures. *J. Cell Biol.*, **58**, 79–95.

Starkey, P.R., and Brimijoin, S. (1979). Stop-flow analysis of axonal transport of DOPA decarboxylase. *J. Neurochem.*, **32**, 437–42.

Stephan, P.K., and Nunez, A. (1977). Elimination of circadian rhythms in driving, activity, sleep and temperature by isolation of the suprachiasmatic nuclei. *Behav. Biol.*, **20**, 1–8.

Swain, H.H. (1979). The use of primates in screening dependence liability. *Pharmacol. Ther.*, **5**, 519–22.

Takeuchi, Y., and Hisanaga, N. (1977). The neurotoxicity of toluene: EEG changes in rats exposed to various concentrations. *Brit. J. Industr. Med.*, **34**, 314–20.

Tilson, H.A., and Cabe, P.A. (1979). Studies on the neurobehavioural effects of polybrominated biphenyls in rats. *Ann. N.Y. Acad. Sci.*, **320**, 325–34.

Tilson, H.A., Cabe, P.A., and Burne, T.A. (1980). Behavioural procedures for the assessment of neurotoxicity. In: Spencer, P.S., and Schaumburg, H.H. (Eds), *Experimental and Clinical Neurotoxicology*, Williams and Wilkins, Baltimore, pp. 743–57.

Tilson, H.A., and Harry, G.J. (1982). Behavioural principles for use in behavioural toxicology and pharmacology. In: Mitchell, C.L. (Ed.), *Nervous System Toxicology*, Raven Press, New York, pp. 1–27.

Van den Bercken, J., Akkermans, L.M.A., and Van der Zalm, J.M. (1973). DDT-like action of allethrin in the sensory nervous system of xenopus lae vis. *Europ. J. Pharmacol.*, **21**, 95–106.

Vorhees, C.V. (1974). Some behavioural effects of maternal hypervitaminosis A in rats. *Teratology*, **10**, 269–73.

Vorhees, C.V., Brunner, R.L., McDaniel, C.R., and Butcher, R.E. (1978). The relationship of gestational age to vitamin A induced postnatal duplication. *Teratology*, **17**, 271–5.

Wallman, J. (1975). A simple technique using an optomotor response for visual psychophysical measurements in animals. *Vision Res.*, **15**, 3–8.

Walum, E., and Peterson, A. (1983). Acute toxicity testing in cultures of mouse neuroblastoma cells. *Acta Pharmacol. Toxicol.*, **52** (Suppl. II), 100–114.

Weindl, A. (1973). Neuroendocrine aspects of circumventricular organs. In: Ganong, W.F., and Martini, L. (Eds), *Frontiers in Neuroendocrinology*, Oxford University Press, Oxford, pp. 3–32.

Weinreich, K., Stelte, W., and Bitsch, I. (1977). Effect of lead acetate on the spontaneous activity of young rats. *Nutr. Metab.*, **21**, Supp. I, 201–3.

Wiesel, T.N., Hubel, D.H., and Lam, D.K. (1974). Autoradiographic demonstration of ocular dominance columns in the visual cortex revealed by a reduced silver stain. *Brain Res.*, **79**, 273–9.

Wince, L.C., Donovan, C.A., and Azzaro, A.J. (1976). Behavioural and biochemical analysis of the lead-exposed hyperactive rat. *Pharmacologist*, **18**, 198.

Wince, L.C., Donovan, C.A., and Azzaro, A.J. (1980). Alterations in the biochemical properties of central dopamine synapses following chronic postnatal $PbCO_3$ exposure. *J. Pharmacol. Exp. Ther.*, **214**, 642–50.

Winder, C., and Kitchen, I. (1984). Lead neurotoxicity: a review of the biochemical, neurochemical and drug induced behavioural evidence. *Progr. Neurobiol.*, **22**, 59–87.

Wolfson, L.I., and Brown, L. (1976). Glucose utilization and dopamine agonists. *Neurosci. Abstr.*, **2**, 510.

Worms, P., and Lloyd, K.G. (1979). Predictability and specificity of behavioural screening tests for neuroleptics. *Pharmacol. Ther.*, **5**, 445–50.

Yonezawa, T., Bornstein, M.B., and Peterson, E.R. (1980). Organotypic cultures of nerve tissue as a model system for neurotoxicity investigation and screening. In: Spencer, P.S. and Schaumburg, H.H. (Eds), *Experimental and Clinical Neurotoxicology*, Williams and Wilkins, Baltimore, pp. 788–802.

Zenick, H., Padich, R., Tokarek, T., and Aragon, P. (1978). Influences of prenatal and postnatal lead exposure on discrimination learning in rats. *Pharmacol. Biochem. Behav.*, **8**, 347–56.

Short-term Toxicity Tests for Non-genotoxic Effects
Edited by P. Bourdeau *et al.*
© 1990 SCOPE. Published by John Wiley & Sons Ltd

CHAPTER 14

Methods for Assessing the Effects of Chemicals on the Endocrine System

J. H. CLARK AND F. X. R. VAN LEEUWEN

14.1 INTRODUCTION

The endocrine system is an important integrating system of the body. The various endocrine glands influence the following major physiological functions: (1) maintenance of homeostatis (involving enzymes, substrates and co-factors) which provides for an optimum environment for the basic biochemical reactions of the body; (2) regulation of growth maturation; (3) reactions to exogenous stimuli such as stress, starvation and infection; (4) regulation of reproductive processes.*

Finely-regulated hormonal mechanisms make the endocrine system particularly sensitive to toxic effects of exogenous compounds. These effects can interfere with the action, biosynthesis and release of hormones, and result in alterations in hormonal target cells. In this review, methods are discussed that are useful for the short-term testing of chemicals that affect the endocrine system.

14.1.1 Important human and other mammalian health problems

Interaction of chemical compounds with endocrine structures leading to dysfunction of the endocrine glands may result in a broad variety of metabolic or neoplastic alterations (De Bruin, 1976; IARC, 1979). For example, the therapeutic use of lithium salts for the treatment of manic-depressive disorders has provided much information about the toxic action of relatively high doses of lithium on the endocrine system of man and animals (Cooper *et al.*, 1979; Fauerholdt and Vendsborg, 1981; Bagchi *et al.*, 1982). On the other hand, relatively little information is available about the effects of low doses of lithium from routine toxicity tests.

Barsano (1981) reviewed the occurrence of thyroid dysfunction as a consequence of exposure to polyhalogenated biphenyls. Rats exposed to polychlorinated

---

*A chapter dealing specifically with reproductive processes is included in this volume. This chapter deals with reproduction only in so far as this is influenced by endocrine organs other than the gonads (e.g. pituitary, thyroid, adrenal gland and the endocrine pancreas).

biphenyls (PCBs) and polybrominated biphenyls (PBBs) exhibited decreased serum thyroxine (T4) levels and goitrogenesis. From epidemiological evaluations, it appeared that PBBs might induce primary hypothyroidism although it has also been suggested that this effect was a PBB-induced exacerbation of pre-existing, but subclinical, thyroid disease. Exposure to antithyroid agents (e.g. thiourea or ethylenethiourea) impaired the biosynthesis of thyroid-hormones with a consequential decrease in thyroid hormone release (Graham and Hansen, 1972; Graham *et al.*, 1973). This, in turn, caused an enhanced secretion of pituitary thyrotropin (TSH) to promote proliferation of tumour cells in the target organ. In this way, chemical compounds may act, via the endocrine system, as tumour promotors.

These examples serve to show that the study of endocrine systems in routine toxicity tests is important, not only from a mechanistic point of view, but also to ensure reliable evaluation of the safety of chemicals.

14.1.2 General comments on successes and failures using routine *in vivo* toxicity tests

In the past, the endocrine system was not a common subject for study in toxicological investigations. Few effects have been described in either short-term or long-term experiments except for those influencing the thyroid. Thus, increased thyroid weight and induced hyperplastic alterations consisting of nodular or microfollicular goitre in rat have been observed following the administration of tetrasul (Verschuuren *et al.*, 1973a,b), and enlargement of the thyroid and activation of thyroid tissue after exposure to sodium bromide (Van Logten *et al.*, 1974, 1976), strontium chloride (Kroes *et al.*, 1977) and zinc phosphide (Muktha Bai *et al.*, 1980).

Recent developments in immunochemistry have resulted in the availability of a number of species-specific antibodies which have greatly expanded the possibilities to determine circulating hormone levels using radioimmunoassay (RIA) or enzyme-linked immunosorbent assay (ELISA) techniques. These allow the detection of specific hormone-producing cells in tissue sections and enable one to carry out organ specific function tests.

The following procedures are suggested to detect effects on the endocrine systems in routine *in vivo* toxicity experiments: (1) determination of the weight of the endocrine organs and histology (haematoxylin/eosin) as screening parameters; (2) determination of circulating hormones or tropic hormones in combination with morphological or immunocytochemical methods; and (3) specific function tests and biochemical methods to determine dysfunction of the endocrine organ under study.

The use of such an approach in toxicity experiments has provided insight into the mechnisms of action and the toxicity of chemical compounds. In the case of sodium bromide, a decreased concentration of thyroxin and corticosterone in the serum of rats was found by radioimmunoassay. Using immunocytochemical techniques (peroxidase–anti-peroxidase antibody method or indirect peroxidase-labelled antibody method), a decrease was observed in the amount of thyroxin in the thyroid while the immunoreactivity of thyroid stimulating hormone and adrenocorticotropic hormone-producing cells in the pituitary gland was increased. Concomitantly, the serum TSH concentration was increased and a decrease in vacuolization of the zona fasciculata of the adrenals was observed (van Leeuwen *et al.*, 1983; Loeber *et al.*, 1983). From these observed changes, it was possible to conclude that bromide directly disturbs thyroid and adrenal function while changes in the pituitary are due to feedback regulation.

This combined biochemical and morphological approach has also been applied in toxicity studies in organotin compounds (Funahashi *et al.*, 1980; Manabe and Wada, 1981; Krajnc *et al.*, 1984). After a single oral dose of triphenyltin fluoride (TPTF) to rabbits, Manabe and Wada (1981) described a decrease in fasting glucose, inhibition of insulin release in response to glucose, glucagon and arginine, and a normal pancreatic islet morphology. They concluded that the diabetogenic activity of TPTF is due to the inhibition of insulin release. However, hypoinsulinaemia observed in rats treated with Bis(tri-*n*-butyltin) oxide (TBTO), was not accompanied by changes in immunochemical reactivity of insulin and glucagon in the pancreas (Krajnc *et al.*, 1984). In the latter case, it was suggested that the decreased insulin levels may reflect a decreased metabolic rate, possibly as a consequence of the decreased thyroxin concentration that was observed. This effect was accompanied by a marked increase in immunoreactivity for TSH in the pituitary, with a consequently reduced serum TSH concentration. No effect was seen on the ACTH (adrenocorticotropic hormone) producing cells in the anterior pituitary. Furthermore, increased stainability of LH (luteinizing hormone) cells and the absence of effects on FSH (follicle stimulating hormone) cells and the absence of effects on FSH (follicle stimulating hormone) cells was accompanied by decreased serum LH and normal FSH levels. These striking correlations between radioimmunochemical and cyto-chemical findings indicate that a combination of radioimmunoassay and immuno-cytochemistry can be a sensitive and reliable method to detect chemically induced dysfunction of the endocrine system.

14.1.3   Consideration of particular problems

The rat is the species most frequently used in routine toxicity tests. The rat has also served as an excellent model for the study of endocrine mechanisms. Thus, it would appear reasonable to study the endocrine system as part of toxicity experiments as they are presently performed. This offers the advantage of studying effects of chemicals on the system at the same time that other facets of endocrine toxicity are studied in the same species. However, stress, housing conditions, diet, age and sampling procedures can all influence the results obtained and lead to conflicting results. Therefore, special attention should be given to the experimental conditions. It has been known for a long time that animals housed in groups are particularly sensitive to non-specific stimuli such as environmental change (transport stress), noise, weighing and injections (Barrett and Stockham, 1963). Handling the animals daily over a period of some weeks in order to get them accustomed to the experimental manipulations can improve the reliability of the results obtained.

The choice of a suitable blood sampling method is of great importance if reliable measurements of hormones are to be obtained. Decapitation without anaesthesia has been shown to result in less stress compared with cardiac or retro-orbital sinus puncture under ether anaesthesia, abdominal aorta puncture under chloroform anaesthesia, or decapitation after treatment with Nembutal ® (Dohler *et al.*, 1977). Nevertheless, daily handling of the animals (during which the decapitation procedure is simulated) remains a prerequisite.

In order to properly evaluate endocrine effects, it is necessary to establish baseline levels of circulating hormones. Systematic determinations of the circadian rhythm in the selected species and strain have to be performed. By selection of the appropriate time for sampling, the variance of the endocrine parameters within the test groups can be reduced, with improved resolution of the endocrine tests.

Little is known about the influence of perinatal exposure or exposure *in utero* to toxic compounds on the endocrine system. There is evidence to suggest that the developing endocrine system is more susceptible than the mature one.

Changes in dietary composition can affect the functioning of the endocrine system and hence influence the effects of toxic compounds. The purity, type and amount of nutrients and minerals in diets should be carefully controlled to enable toxic effects on the endocrine system to be properly interpreted, and to ensure comparability between different investigations. For example, if the amount of iodide in the diet is too high, tests to determine thyroid dysfunction will lose sensitivity due to the presence of excess substrate for thyroid hormone synthesis. Furthermore, depending on the protein source of the diet, goitrogens can be present (Liener, 1979). The total amount of protein is also of importance (Singh *et al.*, 1971). Carbohydrate and lipid composition of the diet should be established, since both influence pancreatic (Maji *et al.*, 1980) and adrenal function (Lawson *et al.*, 1981). Adequate calcium, magnesium and phosphate content of the diet is important because of the influence of these compounds on calcitonine-parathyroid hormone mechanisms, particularly in relation to the occurrence of a sex-linked nephro- calcinosis in female Wistar rats (Harwood, 1982). The same is true for other minerals, particularly potassium and sodium for which high dietary concentrations might mask and low dietary concentrations might enhance the effects of toxic compounds on mineral corticoid secretions.

Although most toxicological experiments involve exposure by the oral route (intubation or ingestion), impairment of pituitary and thyroid function has been described after short-term inhalatory exposure (Clemons and Garcia, 1980; Atwal and Pemsingh, 1984). It is, therefore, likely that systemic effects of chemical compounds on the endocrine system can be determined in short-term toxicity experiments regardless of the route of exposure.

14.2 *IN VIVO* STUDIES

14.2.1 Clinical observations

In general, the effects of chemicals on the non-reproductive endocrine organs are not easily observed clinically. In contrast to gonadal dysfunction, which is easily detected in reproductive studies, growth depression or changes in protein or carbohydrate metabolism ascribable to impaired pituitary, thyroid or pancreatic function can also result from other, non-endocrinal effects.

14.2.2 Morphology

Weight changes and histopathological findings are frequently indications of impairment of the endocrine system. Routine histological staining procedures for tissue sections (e.g. haematoxylin and eosin staining) do not reveal alterations in the number of the specific hormone-producing cells, or the amount of hormone in the endocrine organs following exposure to toxic agents. Immunocytochemical (and especially immunoperoxidase) techniques can be used to localize specific hormone-producing cells. In general, the use of these methods has the great advantage that many antigens can be demonstrated in paraffin sections of formalin fixed tissue. Sometimes, pre-treatment with proteolytic enzymes such as trypsin is necessary to unmask antigenic sites (Mepham *et al.*, 1979). In particular, fixation with formaldehyde solution containing mercuric chloride (sublimate) offers good preservation of antigens; the sublimate must be removed before the staining procedure. Apart from application on paraffin sections, however, recent advances in immunocytochemistry allow the localization of antigens in plastic-embedded material both in light-microscopic and immunoelectron-microscopic techniques (Dell'orto *et al.*, 1982; Casanova *et al.*, 1983; Figueroa *et al.*, 1984). A critical review of the applications of immunocytochemistry to the endocrine system has been given at El Etreby (1981).

Different immunoperoxidase techniques are used to achieve localization of anti gents in tissue sections. These include the peroxidase-labelled antibody method (which can be divided into direct and indirect methods according to Nakane and Pierce, 1966), the unlabelled antibody method of peroxidase–anti-peroxidase (PAP) (Sternberger, 1979) and the avidin–biotin–peroxidase complex (ABC) method (Hsu *et al.*, 1981). In each of these techniques, peroxidase is localized in areas of tissue antigen through an antigen–antibody reaction. The sites of peroxidase localization are made visible through addition of a substrate that reacts with the peroxidase label to result in an insoluble staining product. Substrates commonly used are 3,3'-diaminobenzidine or 3-amino-9-ethylcarbazole dissolved in N,N'-dimethyl- formamide in combination with hydrogen peroxide. These methods achieve intense staining with minimal non-specific background staining; they have sufficient sensitivity to stain the cells with high dilutions of antiserum. The addition of compounds such as imidazole can enhance the cytochemical reaction for peroxidase

(Straus, 1982). For a comparison of the sensitivity and efficiency of the indirect peroxidase labelled antibody method with the peroxidase–antiperoxidase technique, the reader is referred to Bosman *et al.* (1983).

The techniques mentioned above were applied in the experiments described in Section 14.1.2. For the investigation of toxic effects on the endocrine system, information about pituitary function is of main importance. For the determination of the different tropic hormones, species-specific antisera are needed. Many of these antisera were obtained from the Rat Pituitary Hormone Distribution Programme, National Institute of Arthritis, Metabolism and Digestive Disease (NIAMDD), Bethesda, Maryland, USA.

A recent and very interesting development in the fields of immunochemistry involves the use of monoclonal antibodies. Their defined specificity for tissue compounds enables them to be used in double staining procedures for the simultaneous localization of antigens on membrane structures or intracellular components (Boorsma, 1984).

14.2.3   Biochemistry of tissue and biological fluids

Radioimmunoassay appears to be the most appropriate technique for the determination of hormones in body fluids and tissue homogenates. In this review, methods are not discussed in detail, but the reader is referred to recent reviews or handbooks (Abraham, 1977; Lorraine and Bell, 1981; Hunter and Corrie, 1982). Radioimmunoassay can also be applied as a post-column detection method after chromatographic separation of various hormones (Loeber, 1984).

The availability of many commercial clinical radioimmunassay kits for steroids and thyroid hormones has undoubtedly stimulated the attention of toxicologists to these types of hormones. However, the use of these kits in routine animal toxicity tests has some disadvantages. Most kits require a relatively large sample size so that the method must be modified to a microscale for use in tests involving small animals. Furthermore, differences in the metabolism of steroids between humans and rats may lead to unexpected cross-reactions with metabolites that cause interference.

In general, serum or plasma can be used in RIA methods; in practice, serum is preferred because of coagulation that occurs during thawing of frozen plasma samples. In principle, radioimmunoassays can also be performed with urine although one should realize that steroids are present in urine as conjugated glucuronides or sulphates.

Hormones may be present in two physical forms in blood; as free compounds or bound to serum proteins. Because of its high concentration, albumin is a major absorbent for circulating hormones although specific binding proteins also exist. In the rat, transcortin is the binding protein for corticosterone, whereas (in contrast to the human) the rat does not possess the specific thyroxin-binding globulin (TBG). Therefore, the determination of free-T4 used in clinical chemistry is of no additional value in rat toxicity experiments because the effect of toxic compounds on T4 levels will parallel changes in free-T4.

Nevertheless, the concept of bound versus free hormones is of importance for the evaluation of changes in circulating hormone levels. A decrease in total concentration as measured with RIA methods does not indicate, *per se*, a physiologically important effect because the concentration of the biologically active free form might be unchanged while the total amount might be reduced due to a decrease in binding protein.

No kits are commercially available for the determination of tropic hormones in animal toxicity investigations because it is necessary to use specific antisera for the species used. For method development, antisera for tropic hormones are provided by NIAMDD in the Rat Pituitary Hormone Distribution Programme. Iodination is generally carried out using the Chloramine-T technique according to Hunter and Greenwood (1962), whereas counting data can be evaluated using the computer program developed by Rodbard and Lewald (1970).

New methods have been developed recently as an alternative to the use of radio-isotopically labelled materials. However, the sensitivity of luminescent immunoassays as compared with RIAs has not yet been fully evaluated. Schall and Tenoso (1981) reviewed the possibilities of various labels as substitutes for radio-isotopes; they concluded that there was no single, all-round best label to replace the radioisotopes. But any new label might have its own advantages over radioimmunoassays. Improvements in luminescence-measuring equipment are likely; a promising development in this respect might be the introduction of fibre-optics (Whitehead *et al.*, 1979).

Biochemical analysis of endocrine tissue from animals exposed *in vivo* is an important tool for elucidating the mechanisms of action of toxic compounds. A recent development, for instance, is the application of lipid-free homogenates for study by two-dimensional chromatography or high-performance liquid chromatography in order to determine the various thyroid hormones and their precursors (Gordon *et al.*, 1982). The determination of thyroid-peroxidase activity can also be important, since changes in iodide-dependent or guaiacol-dependent activity might reflect alterations in the incorporation of iodine in tyrosine residues or in the coupling of iodinated tyrosine residues in thyroglobulin, respectively.

14.2.4   Function tests

Function tests are a valuable tool in assessing the endocrine toxicity of chemical compounds. Due to the complexity of the endocrine system, there is no single overall function test, but the various endocrine organs have their own specific tests based upon the uptake of radioisotopes or their reaction on 'externally' added hormonal stimuli. The need for undertaking function tests of the endocrine system is indicated by changes in organ weights or morphology, or by changes in circulating hormone levels observed in screening studies.

Release tests are very suitable for the study of endocrine organ function. For the anterior pituitary, the function of various tropic-hormone producing cells can be examined by stimulation with hypothalamic-releasing factors. Following intravenous injection of 1 µg/kg^{-1} body weight of luteinizing hormone-releasing hormone (LHRH), also called luliberin, the release of luteinizing hormone (LH) and follicle-stimulating-hormone (FSH) can be determined in serum using RIA. In a similar manner, thyrotopin-releasing hormone (TRH or thyroliberin) induces the secretion of thyroid-stimulating hormone (TSH) and prolactin into the serum, and corticotropic-releasing homone (CRH or corticoliberin) affects the adrenocorticotropic hormone (ACTH)-producing cells.

Following the administration of ACTH, the concentration of corticosterone can be determined in the serum as a measure of adrenal cortex function.

For the study of pancreatic function, administration of glucose by the measurement of immuno-reactive insulin (IRI) is most appropriate. It should be noted that oral administration of glucose produces higher insulin levels than parenteral administration, leading to equal hyperglycaemia (McIntyre *et al.*, 1964).

At the National Institute of Public Health and Environmental Hygiene (NIPHEH) in Bilthoven, the Netherlands, various release tests are performed consecutively in the same animals. This necessitates the collection of blood samples without killing the animal and under conditions of minimal stress. This can be achieved by inserting a silicon rubber cannula into the jugular vein under Nembutal ® anaesthesia. Two to three days after surgery, the animals are fasted overnight and blood samples taken (without anaesthesia) before and 3, 5, 10, 15 and 20 minutes after intravenous injection of glucose (4 mol/kg^{-1} body weight) for IRI determination. Pituitary function is tested in the same animals 48 hours later with a 48–72 hour interval between the administration of TRH and LHRH (1 µg/kg^{-1} body weight). Blood samples are taken before, and 8, 20 and 60 minutes after injection. The various hormone concentrations in the serum of individual animals are plotted and the area above the zero-time value is calculated and statistically evaluated. This method offers the advantage of requiring the use of a small number of animals while providing reliable results.

Another type of function test is the uptake of radiolabel. For the assessment of thyroid function, for instance, a well-known technique is the determination of the uptake of parenterally administered 125 or 131-iodine (2–2.5 µC/kg^{-1} body weight) by the thyroid. Radioactivity can be determined in excised thyroid glands, but it is also possible to anaesthetize the animals and put them between the detectors of a gamma counter. In this way, individual rats can be screened for the uptake as well as release function, by determining the radioactivity 6, 24 and 48 or 72 hours after administration of the radioisotope.

Function studies can also be performed with non-invasive techniques. The determination of 17-hydroxy-corticosteroids in 24 hour urine samples is an effective way to determine adrenocortical activity. An increase in 24-hour levels, whether or not after ACTH administration, regularly reflects hyperadrenocorticism. For a differential diagnosis, determining the suppression of corticosteroid production by metyrapone might be useful.

Although there are some ethical drawbacks, function tests can also be applied in toxicity experiments in humans. This facilitates the comparison with animal models as a predictive model for human risk assessment.

14.2.5　Surgically modified animals

As an alternative to studies of endocrine function by hormone determinations and function tests, surgically-modified animals (in which particular organs have been removed) can be used to establish the effects of impairment of the endocrine system, or to rule out the involvement of particular endocrine organs in the toxic action of chemicals. This approach is not only valuable in endocrine toxicity studies, but also in experiments to determine hormone mediated immune alterations (Vos and Dean, this volume). By using adrenalectomized or hypophysectomized rats, for example, it can be shown that alterations in glucocorticoid or growth hormone concentrations in the circulation are not the cause of thymic involution observed in animals exposed to TCDD (Van Logten *et al.*, 1980).

14.3　*IN VITRO* TESTING

In theory, every known aspect of cell regulation can be tested *in vitro* and the effects of toxic substances on these control mechanisms can be examined. However, *in vitro* techniques have not been used extensively in practice; consequently, little is known concerning the toxic effects of chemicals in such systems. For this reason, much of the following discussion relates to test systems that may prove useful in the future. The methods proposed do not cover all systems or all possible endocrine interactions; rather, examples have been provided for selected systems which may be broadly applicable to others.

14.3.1　Thyroid

The synthesis and secretion of thyroxin (T_4) and triiodothyronine (T_3) involves several steps that can be influenced by exposure to toxins. Dietary iodine is taken up as iodide by the thyroid in response to the binding of thyrotrophin (TSH) to cell membranes. Once inside the thyroid cell, iodide is oxidized and combined with tyrosine residues of thyroglobulin to form monoiodotyrosyl or diodotyrosyl residues. T_4 and T_3 are formed by the coupling of iodotyrosyl residues within the thyroglobulin molecule and secretion of T_4 and T_3 occurs following proteolytic cleavage of these hormones from thyroglobulin. Methods for the analysis of these various steps in the biosynthetic pathway are considered in Sections 14.2.1.1 to 14.3.1.3.

14.3.1.1   Uptake of iodide

The inhibition of the uptake ^{125}I can be readily measured in thyroid tissue or cell culture (Weiss *et al.*, 1984). Several substances, such as perchlorate, nitrate and thiocyanate, are known to act as competitive inhibitors of the TSH-regulated, Na/K-ATPase mediated transport. Such inhibitors can be used as reference standards in toxicological studies. Thyroid glands or cell cultures can be used to examine the effects of toxins on iodide transport (Weiss *et al.*, 1984).

14.3.1.2   TSH receptor binding

The binding of TSH to plasma membrane fractions which contain the receptor for TSH can also be assessed (Tate *et al.*, 1975; Pekonen and Weintraub, 1979). Potential inhibitors of TSH binding can be examined by competitive inhibition analysis to determine the effects on the number of receptors and relative binding affinities. Such inhibition would be expected to correlate with decreased synthesis and secretion of T_4 and T_3. The binding of TSH to membrane receptors is associated with the stimulation of adenylate cyclase and increased production of cyclic AMP (Lefort *et al.*, 1984; Carayon *et al.*, 1978). Therefore, any interference of TSH binding would likely be involved in inhibiting adenylate cyclase activity. However, TSH binding and adenylate cyclase activity should be examined in conjunction in order that the validity of any assumptions made about physiological effects which might result from toxic inhibition of TSH receptor interactions may be determined. An example of discrepancies that might occur is found in the work of Marshall *et al.* (1977) who showed that D-propanalol increased the binding of TSH to thyroid membranes but this increase was not associated with an increase stimulation of adenylate cyclase.

14.3.1.3   Oxidation and coupling reaction

The oxidation and coupling reactions that lead to formation of T_3 and T_4 are inhibited by substances such as propylthiouracil and methylmercaptoimidazole. These compounds inhibit thyroid peroxidase, a membrane-bound haemoprotein which catalyses both oxidation and coupling reactions in thyroid tissue (Taurog, 1970). Toxic substances could be tested in thyroid membrane preparations for their ability to inhibit thyroid peroxidase, and thiourelylene drugs could be used as model inhibitors to establish relative potencies (Engler *et al.*, 1982). Such inhibition could be examined further by measuring the amount of monoiodothyronine and di-iodothyronine in thyroid glands grown in culture.

14.3.2   Adrenal gland

The adrenal cortex is responsible for the synthesis and secretion of glucocorticoid steroid hormones which regulate many important functions of the body. The pituitary hormone adrenocorticotropin (ACTH) binds to membrane receptors on adreanl cortical cells which activate the adenylate cyclase systems and ultimately stimulate the synthesis of glucocorticoid hormones. The biosynthetic pathway for these hormones involves many enzymatic steps and utilizes cholesterol as the primary precursor. Cholesterol is accumulated in the adrenal cortex by the endocytosis of lipoproteins from the blood; this process is under the control of ACTH. The mineralocorticoid hormone, aldosterone, is also synthesized by the adrenal cortex. However, its synthesis is primarily controlled by plasma sodium levels and angiotensin II. The various control functions (such as receptors, enzyme activation and synthesis, pituitary secretion of ACTH, angiotensin II production and action of adrenal steroids on target cells) present a complex array of possible points at which toxins could interfere with proper adrenal function. Some of the possible *in vitro* methods that may be useful to determine effects on adrenal function are reviewed in Sections 14.3.2.1 to 14.3.2.3.

14.3.2.1   *ACTH receptor interactions*

Radiolabelled ACTH can be used to establish saturation curves for the assessment of binding parameters of adrenal cells or plasma membrane preparations (Simonian *et al.*, 1982). The effects of chemicals on either the dissociation constant or binding capacity (number of receptors) in these systems may provide an indication of toxicity. Should specific alterations in these receptor characteristics be found, it would be important to establish whether they were associated with alterations in adenylate cyclase activity or alterations in the biosynthesis of adrenal steroids. Such a system has been described for bovine adrenal cells in serum-free media which respond to ACTH by synthesizing the appropriate corticoids (Simonian *et al.*, 1982).

14.3.2.2   *Lipoprotein uptake by adrenal cells*

Although the adrenal gland synthesizes cholesterol from acetate, it also acquires cholesterol by endocytosis of low density lipoprotein (LDL) from the blood (Brown *et al.*, 1979). It is conceivable that lipophilic toxins could not only be delivered to cells by this route, but also interfere with the uptake process. ^{125}I-LDL could be examined and the effects of toxic substances on binding parameters assessed. The influence of toxicants transferred by means of LDL-endocytosis on the activity of HMG CoA reductase (the rate limiting enzyme in cholesterol synthesis), acyl-CoA : cholesterol acyltransferase (the enzyme which reesterifies excess cholesterol for storage as cholesterylesters) and synthesis of LDL receptors could be examined in adrenal cells or in cultured fibroblasts (see Brown *et al.*, 1981).

14.3.2.3   *Biosynthesis of adrenal steroids and enzyme inhibition*

The biosynthesis of adrenal steroids involves a complex pathway consisting of many enzymatic steps. The overall effect of a toxicant could be examined by adding ^{14}C-cholesterol to adrenal cells or to glands in culture and measuring the production of ^{14}C-corticosterone and/or ^{14}C-aldosterone. The individual enzymatic steps could also be examined. One of the most important of these would be the conversion of cholesterol to pregnenolone which is performed by the desmolase enzyme complex; this is the rate-limiting step in steroid biosynthesis. Other important enzymes in the pathway, such as 3B-hydroxysteroid dehydrogenase, 17 $\propto$-hydroxylase, 21-hydroxylase and 11B-hydroxylase, could also be examined by precursor-product analysis.

14.3.3   Adrenal hormone action at the target cell

14.3.3.1   Glucocorticoids

As indicated previously, the glucocorticoid hormones secreted by the adrenal cortex influence many important physiological functions. The concentration and activity of several liver enzymes are increased by glucocorticoid treatment (Rousseau and Baxter, 1979). These increases appear to result from the binding of glucocorticoids to their respective receptor which stimulates the transcription of specific mRNAs that code for the synthesis of these enzymes. The binding of glucocorticoid receptor complexes to nuclear sites is closely correlated with the level of enzymatic stimulation. Thus occupancy of the receptor by hormone is closely coupled with response.

Although there are clear-cut examples of the stimulator (anabolic) effects of glucocorticoids, these hormones also have an inhibitory or catabolic effect in many systems. These include: the suppression of DNA synthesis, the promotion of protein breakdown in muscle, the suppression of immunological and inflammatory responses, and the inhibition of cell proliferation in lymphoid, fibroblastic, epithelial and bone cells. Although the mechanism of action of glucocorticoids in these inhibitory responses is not known, it appears to involve hormone–receptor interactions. Therefore, regardless of the stimulatory or inhibitory actions, the binding of glucocorticoids to cellular receptors is important for their action. Since a great deal is known about hormone–receptor interactions in these systems, and since such interactions are likely to be involved in toxic interference of hormonal regulation, a study of these receptor systems may provide valuable insight about the effects of toxic substances.

Glucocorticoid receptors are present in many tissues and several cell lines are available (Gasson and Bourgeois, 1983). Receptors are present in the cytosol and nuclei of homogenized cells or tissues and the binding parameters (numbers of sites and dissociation constant) can be determined by saturation analysis (for a discussion of the principles and methods involved, see Chapter 2, Clark and Peck, 1979). Toxic agents can be added in these systems. Classical competitive inhibition curves are easily performed and provide a rapid method for the determination of relative binding affinity. If substances are found that inhibit the binding of [^{3}H]-

glucocorticoids to the cytosol receptor, it is possible that such a substance may interfere with glucocorticoid action. That is, the binding of a chemical to the glucocorticoid receptor may interfere with nuclear accumulation of the hormone receptor complex. This possibility can be tested by measuring the nuclear accumulation of receptor following exposure of cells or tissues to both toxin and [^{3}H]-glucocorticoid. Although a blockade or reduction in the binding of [^{3}H]-glucocorticoid receptor complexes in the nucleus would be suggestive of an inhibitory action, it is possible that such substances might form stable receptor–toxin complexes in the nucleus and act as glucocorticoid agonists. However, it would require analysis of the response parameters (such as enzyme synthesis) in order to establish whether the chemical is acting in an agonistic or an antagonistic manner.

14.3.3.2   Mineralocorticoids

Mineralocorticoids, such as aldosterone, regulate electrolyte balance in the kidney, salivary glands, sweat glands and the gastrointestinal tract. Aldosterone augments the transport of sodium across epithelia by stimulating the synthesis of proteins that are involved in increasing the permeability of the apical membrane to sodium and the energy metabolism of the cell.

Aldosterone receptors are present in target organs for mineralocorticoids, such as the kidney and toad bladder (Marver *et al.*, 1978). These receptors form activated nuclear bound complexes in a fashion similar to those of other steroids. The mechanism by which aldosterone controls sodium transport probably involves the synthesis of proteins involved in the function of the sodium channel and energy production (ATP). Aldosterone stimulates an increase in the number of sodium-specific apical membrane channels and increases the activity of at least four mitochondrial enzymes. Therefore, the major effect of aldosterone is to increase the activity of enzymes involved in the generation of ATP. The increased ATP acts as an energy source for the sodium pump and also may increase the number of sodium pumps. In addition to these effects, aldosterone also stimulates phospholipase activity, fatty acid synthesis and acyltransferase activity. All of these actions are probably involved in altering the membrane functions in the renal cell.

The assessment of toxic effects of mineralocorticoid actions could involve any one of the above steps; however, most of these would involve difficult methodology that would be unsuitable for use in routine testing. The most easily accessible parameter for testing would be receptor binding interactions analogous to those discussed for the glucocorticoid system.

14.3.4   Hypothalamic–pituitary system

The hypothalamus produces releasing hormones that stimulate the secretion of pituitary hormones which control many other endocrine gland functions. Although toxic effects could interfere with many aspects of these complex pathways (some of these have been discussed in previous sections) *in vitro* analysis would best be done at the pituitary level. For this reason, interactions with pituitary cells or glands in culture are the focus of potential methods discussed here.

The plasma membrane of anterior pituitary cells contains specific receptors for the various releasing hormones produced by hypothalamic neurones. These hormones include: corticotropin releasing hormone (CRF), which stimulates secretion of ACTH; thyrotropin releasing hormone (TRF), which stimulates secretion of TSH; and growth hormone releasing hormone (GRH), which stimulates the secretion of somatotropin (STH). Not included in this list are the gonadotropin releasing hormone and prolactin inhibitory factor since these are discussed in relation to reproduction by Nadolney *et al.* (Chapter 16, this volume).

The binding of each of the releasing hormones is important for the production of pituitary hormones, and thus could be an important point at which toxic substances could interfere with pituitary function. This interference may be tested by measuring the ability of toxins to inhibit or enhance the binding of radiolabelled releasing hormones to pituitary glands *in vitro*, pituitary cells in culture or to pituitary membrane preparations. Any observed effects on the binding parameters of hormone receptor interactions could be coupled to the release of specific pituitary hormones from cells or glands in culture. Radioimmunoassays are available for each of the pituitary hormones so that effects on stimulated release into the culture medium could be checked readily.

The effects of opiate drugs on TSH secretion by superfused anterior pituitaries can serve as an example of this type of analysis (Judd and Hedge, 1983). Beta-endorphin, and endogenous opioid, and other opiate drugs, stimulate TSH secretion from the anterior pituitary *in vitro*. Thus, model compounds are available to serve as reference standards. Nothing is known about the mechanisms involved; however, it is possible that stimulation may be due to enhanced TRF binding. Toxic substances with similar activity would be potential inducers of hyperthyroidism. It should be noted, however, that opioid peptides decrease plasma TSH, *in vivo*, rather than enhance its secretion. This action is presumed to be at the level of the hypothalamus where opioids cause a decrease in TRF. Therefore, it would be important to verify *in vitro* observations and predictions using *in vivo* tests.

In addition to the effects of releasing hormones on the secretion of pituitary hormones, chemicals could also interfere with the normal steroid homrone feedback mechanisms. For example, glucocorticoids suppress the ability of CRF to stimulate ACTH secretion. This feedback inhibition is necessary for the maintenance of normal stimulation and secretion of adrenal steroids. Cultured anterior pituitary cells respond to CRF by increasing the production of cyclic AMP which results in the stimulation of secretion of ACTH (Bilezikjian and Vale, 1983). These responses are inhibited by the addition of glucocorticoid hormones to the medium. Such a system could be established to identify toxic substances which interfere with feedback mechanisms.

14.4   STRATEGY AND FUTURE DEVLEOPMENTS

Due to the complex nature of the endocrine system, it is obvious that no single test exists that can provide all the data that are necessary to assess the potency of compounds that may disturb endocrine functions. *In vivo* function tests of the various endocrine organs are indicated when the potential for chemicals to affect the endocrine system is established by:

(1)   changes in weight of the endocrine organs;
(2)   morphological alterations, detected with conventional as well as immuno-cytochemical staining;
(3)   changes in circulating hormone concentrations.

In vitro tests are potentially useful in order to ascertain:

(1)   mechanisms of action (e.g. receptor binding studies, determination of enzymatic activity, release tests), although it should also be emphasized that *in vitro* metabolic activation of the compound should be taken into account;
(2)   the relative potency of chemical compounds (or their metabolites) that interfere with endocrine function.

Most of the *in vitro* test systems need validation; in particular, the correlation between *in vivo* and *in vitro* tests remains to be clarified.

In the near future, techniques already in use in clinical medicine should be explored for their suitability for use in animal studies. In general, the use of non-invasive, *in vitro* techniques should be encouraged since these offer the possibility to obtain sample material under conditions of minimal stress and may reduce the number of animals required in toxicity studies.

REFERENCES

Abraham, G.E. (1977). *Handbook of Radioimmunoassay*, Dekker, New York.
Atwal, O.S., and Pemsingh, R.S. (1984). Occurrence of mallory body-like inclusion in para-thyroid chief cells of ozone-treated dogs. *J. Pathol.*, **142**, 169–74.
Bagchi, N., Brown, T.R., and Mack, R.E. (1982). Effect of chronic lithium treatment on hypothalamic-pituitary regulation of thyroid function. *Horm. Metablol. Res.*, **14**, 92–3.
Barrett, A.M., and Stockham, M.A. (1963). The effect of housing conditions and simple experimental procedures upon the corticosterone level in the plasma of rats. *J. Endocrinol.*, **26**, 97–105.
Barsano, C.P. (1981). Environmental factors altering thyroid function and their assessment. *Environ. Health Perspect.*, **38**, 71–82.
Bilezikjian, L.M., and Vale, W.W. (1983). Glucocorticoids inhibit corticotropin-releasing factor induced production of adenosine 3,5'-monophosphate in cultured anterior pituitary cells. *Endocrinology*, **113**, 657–62.

Boorsma, D.M. (1984). Direct immunoenzyme double staining applicable for monoclonal antibodies. *Histochemistry, 80*, 103–6.

Bosman, F.T., Cramer-Knijnenburg, G., and Van Bergen Henegouw, J. (1983). Efficiency and sensitivity of indirect immunoperoxidase methods. *Histochemistry, 77*, 185–94.

Brown, M.S., Kovanen, P.T., and Goldstein, J.L. (1979). Receptor mediated uptake of lipoprotein-cholesterol and its utilization for steroid biosynthesis. *Recent Prog. Horm. Res., 35*, 215–49.

Brown, M.S., Kovanen, P.T., and Goldstein, J.L. (1981). Regulation of plasma cholesterol by lipoprotein receptors. *Science, 212*, 628–35.

Carayon, P., Guibout, M., and Lissitzky, S. (1978). Thyrotropin receptor adenylate cyclase system in plasma membranes from normal and diseased human thyroid glands. *J. Endocrinol. Invest., 1*, 321–8.

Casanova, S., Donini, U., Zini, N., Morelli, R., and Zucchelli, P. (1983). Immunohistochemical staining on hydroxyethyl-methacrylate-embedded tissues. *J. Histochem. Cytochem., 31*, 1000–04.

Clark, J.H., and Peck, E.J. Jr. (1979). Female sex steroids: receptors and function. *Monographs in Endocrinology*, Springer-Verlag, New York.

Clemons, G.K., and Garcia, J.F. (1980). Changes in thyroid function after short-term ozone exposure in rats. *J. Environ. Pathol., Toxicol., 4*, 359–69.

Cooper, T.B., Gershon, S., Kline, N.S., and Shou, M. (1979). Lithium: controversies and unresolved issues. Proc. Int. Lithium Conf., New York, 1978. Excerpta Medica, Amsterdam.

De Bruin, A. (1976). *Biochemical Toxicology of Environmental Agents*, Elsevier/North-Holland and Biomedical Press.

Dell'orto, P., Viale, G., Columbi, R., Braidotti, P., and Copggi, G. (1982). Immunohistochemical localization of human immunoglobulins and lysozyme in epoxy-embedded lymph nodes. *J. Histochem. Cytochem., 307*, 630–36.

Dohler, K.D., Von zur Muhlen, A., Gartner, K., and Dohler, U. (1977). Effect of various blood sampling techniques on serum levels of pituitary and thyroid homrones in the rat. *J. Endocrinol., 74*, 341–2.

El Etreby, M.F. (1981). Practical applications of immunocytochemistry to the pharmacology and toxicology of the endocrine system. *Histochem. J., 13*, 821–37.

Engler, H., Taurog, A., and Dorris, M.L. (1982). Preferential inhibition of thyroxine and 3,5,3'-triiodothyronine formation by propylthiouracil and methylmercaptoimidazole in thyroid peroxidase catalyzed iodination of thyroglobulin. *Endocrinology, 110*, 190–97.

Fauerholdt, L., and Vendsborg, P. (1981). Thyroid gland morphology after lithium treatment. *Acta Pathol. Microbiol. Scand. Sect., A 89*, 339–41.

Figueroa, C.D., Caorsi, I., Subiabre, J., and Vio, C.P. (1984). Immunoreactive kallikrein localization in the rat kidney: an immuno-electron-microscopic study. *J. Histochem. Cytochem., 32*, 117–21.

Funahashi, N., Iwasaki, I., and Ide, G. (1980). Effects of bis(tri-*n*-butyltin) oxide on endocrine and lymphoid organs of male rats. *Acta Pathol. Jpn., 30*, 955–66.

Gasson, J.C., and Bourgeois, S. (1983). Determinants of glucocorticoid resistance in lymnphoid cell lines. In: Chabner, B.A. (Ed.), *UCLA Symposia on Molecular and Cellular Biology: Rational Basis for Chemotherapy*, Alan Liss Inc., New York, pp. 153–76.

Gordon, J.T., Crutchfield, F.L., Jenning, A.S., and Dratman, M.B. (1982). Preparation of lipid-free tissue extracts for chromatographic determination of thyroid hormones and metabolites. *Arch. Biochem. Biophys., 216*, 407–15.

Graham, S.L., and Hansen, W.H. (1972). Effects of short-term administration of ethylenethiourea upon thyroid function of the rat. *Bull. Environ. Contam. Toxicol., 7*, 19–25.

Graham, S.L., Hansen, W.H., Davis, K.J., and Perry, C.H. (1973). Effects of one year administration of ethylenethiourea upon the thyroid of the rat. *J. Agric. Food Chem.*, **21**, 324–9.

Harwood, E.J. (1982). The influence of dietary magnesium on reduction of nephrocalcionosis in rats fed purified diet. *Laboratory Animal*, **16**, 314–18.

Hsu, S.M., Raine, L., and Fanger, H. (1981). The use of avidin-biotin-peroxidase complex (ABC) in immunoperoxidase techniques: a comparison between ABC and unlabelled antibody (PAP) procedures. *J. Histochem. Cytochem.*, **29**, 577–80.

Hunter, W.M., and Corrie, J.E.T. (1982). *Immunoassays for Clinical Chemistry*, Livingstone, Edinburgh.

Hunter, W.M. and Greenwood, F.C. (1962). Preparation of iodine-131 labelled human growth hormone of high specific activity. *Nature*, **94**, 495–6.

International Agency for Research on Cancer (1979). IARC Monographs on the Evaluation of the Carcinogenic Risk of Chemicals to Humans. *Sex Hormones (II)*, volume 21, IARC, Lyon.

Judd, A.M., and Hedte, G.A. (1983). Direct pituitary stimulation of thyrotropin secretion by opioid peptides. *Endocrinology*, **113**, 706–10.

Krajnc, E.I., Wester, P.W., Loeber, J.G., Van Leeuwen, F.X.R., Vos, J.G., Vaessen, H.A.M.G., and Van der Heijden, C.A. (1984). Toxicity of bis(tri-n-butyltin)oxide in the rat. I. Short-term effects on general parameters and on the endocrine and lymphoid systems. *Toxicol. Appl. Pharmacol.*, **75**, 363–86.

Kroes, R., Den Tonkelaar, E.M., Minderhoud, A., Speijers, G.J.A., Vonk-Visser, D.M.A., Berkvens, J.M., and Van Esch, G.J. (1977). Short-term toxicity of strontium chloride in rats. *Toxicology*, **7**, 11–21.

Lawson, N., Jenning, R.J., Pollard, A.D., Shirten, R.G., Ralph, S.J., Marsden, C.A., Fears, R., and Brindley, P.N. (1981). Effect of chronic modification of dietary fat and carbohydrate in rats. *Biochem. J.*, **200**, 265–73.

Lefort, G.P., Amr, S., Carayon, P., and Nisula, B.C. (1984). Relevance of the low and high affinity thyrotropin binding sites of human thyroid membranes to the stimulation of adenylate cyclase. *Endocrinology*, **114**, 1005–11.

Liener, I. (1979). Significance for humans of biologically active factors in soybeans and other food legumes. *J. Am. Oil Chem. Soc.*, **56**, 121–9.

Loeber, J.G. (1984). Radioimmunoassay as a post-column detection method. In: Hancock, W.S. (Ed.), *Handbook for the HPLC Separation of Amino Acids, Peptides and Proteins*, volume I, CRC Press Inc., Boca Raton, pp. 277–332.

Loeber, J.G., Franken, M.A.M., and van Leeuwen, F.X.R. (1983). Effect of sodium bromide on endocrine parameters in the rat as studied by immunochemistry and radioimmunoassay. *Good Chem. Toxicol.*, **21**, 391–404.

Lorraine, J.A., and Bell, E.T. (1981). *Hormone Assays and Their Clinical Application*, 4th edn, Livingstone, Edinburgh.

Maji, T., Yoshida, A., and Ashida, K. (1980). Effect of alternate high carbohydrate and high fat diets on insulin function. *Nutrit. Rep. Int.*, **21**, 437–45.

Manabe, S., and Wada, O. (1981). Triphenyltin fluoride (TPTF) as a diabetogenic agent. TPTF induces diabetic lipemia by inhibiting insulin secretion from morphologically intact rabbit B-cell. *Diabetes*, **30**, 1013–21.

Marshall, N.J., Von Borcke, S., Florin-Christensen, A., and Ekins, R.P. (1977). Propranolol increases binding of thyrotropin to thyroid membranes. *Nature* (London), **268**, 58–60.

Marver, D., Stewart, J., Funder, J.W., Feldman, D., and Edelman, I.S. (1978). Renal aldosterone receptors: studies with [^{3}H]aldosterone and the anti-mineralocorticoid [^{3}H]spirolactone (SC-26304). *Proc. Nat. Acad. Sci. (USA)*, **71**, 1431–5.

McIntyre, N., Holdsworth, C.D., and Turner, D.S. (1964). New interpretation of oral glucose tolerance. *Lancet*, **2**, 20–21.

Mepham, B.L., Frater, W., and Mitchell, B.S. (1979). The use of proteolytic enzymes to improve immunoglobulin staining by the PAP technique. *Histochem. J.*, **11**, 345–57.

Muktha Bai, K., Krishnakamari, M.K., Ramesh, H.P., Shivanandappa, T., and Majumder, S.K. (1980). Short-term toxicity of zinc phosphide in albino rats. *Indian J. Exp. Biol.*, **18**, 854–7.

Nakane, P.K., and Pierce, J.B. (1966). Enzyme-labelled antibodies: Preparation and application for localization of antigens. *J. Histochem. Cytochem.*, **14**, 929–31.

Pekonen, F., and Weintraub, B.C. (1979). Thyrotropin receptors on bovine thyroid membranes. Two types with different affinities and specificities. *Endocrinology*, **105**, 352–9.

Rodbard, D., and Lewald, J.E. (1970). Computer analysis of radioligand assay and radioimmunoassay data. *Acta Endocrinol. Suppl.*, **147**, 79–103.

Rousseau, G.G., and Baxter, J.D. (1979). Glucocorticoid receptors. In: Baxter, J.D., and Rousseau, G.G. (Eds), *Glucocorticoid Hormone Action,* Springer-Verlag, New York, .pp. 49–77.

Schall, R.F., and Tenoso, H.J. (1981). Alternatives to radioimmunoassay: Labels and methods. *Clin. Chem.*, **27**, 1157–64.

Simonian, M.H., White, M.L., and Gill, G.N. (1982). Growth and function of cultured bovine adrenocorticol cells in a serum-free defined medium. *Endocrinology*, **111**, 919–27.

Sing, D.V., Anderson, R.R., and Turner C.W. (1971). Effect of decreased dietary protein on the rate of thyroid hormone secretion and food consumption in the rats. *J. Endocrinol.*, **50**, 445–50.

Sternberger, L.A. (1979). *Immunocytochemistry*, John Wiley & Sons, New York, pp. 104–69.

Straus, W. (1982). Imidazole increases the sensitivity of the cytochemical reaction for peroxidase with diaminobenzidine at a neutral pH. *J. Histochem. Cytochem.*, **30**, 491–3.

Tate, R.L., Schwarz, H.I., Holmers, J.M., Kohn, L.D., and Winand, R.J. (1975). Thyrotropin receptors in thyroid plasma membranes. *J. Biol. Chem.*, **250**, 6509–15.

Taurog, A. (1970). Thyroid peroxidase and thyroxine biosynthesis. *Rec. Prog. Horm. Res.*, **26**, 189–247.

Van Leeuwen, F.X.R., Den Tonkelaar, E.M., and Van Logten, M.J. (1983). Toxicity of sodium bromide in rats: effects on endocrine system and reproduction. *Food Chem. Toxicol.*, **21**, 383–9.

Van Logten, M.J., Wolthuis, M., Rauws, A.G., Kroes, R., Den Tonkelaar, E.M., Berkvens, H., and Van Esch, G.J. (1974). Semichronic toxicity study of sodium bromide in rats. *Toxicology*, **2**, 257–67.

Van Logten, M.J., Rauws, A.G., Kroes, R., Den Tonkelaar, E.M., and Van Esch, G.J. (1976). Semichronic toxicity studies of sodium bromide in rats on a normal diet and a low chloride diet. *Meded. Fac. Landbouww. Rijksuniv. Gent.*, **412**, 1499–1507.

Van Logten, M.J., Gupta, B.N., McConnell, E.E., and Moore, J.A. (1980). Role of the endocrine system in the action of 2,3,7,8-tetrachloro-dibenzo-*p*-dioxin (TCDD) on the thymus. *Toxicology*, **15**, 135–44.

Verschuuren, H.G., Kroes, R., and Van Esch, G.J. (1973a). Toxicity studies on tetrasul. I. Acute, long-term and reproduction studies. *Toxicology*, **1**, 63–78.

Verschuuren, H.G., Kroes, R., and Den Tonkelaar, E.M. (1973b). Toxicity studies on tetrasul. III. Short-term comparative studies in rats with tetrasul and structurally related acaricides. *Toxicology*, **1**, 113–23.

Weiss, S.J., Philp, N.J., and Grollman, E.F. (1984). Iodide transport in a continuous line of cultured cells from rat thyroid. *Endocrinology*, **114**, 1090–98.

Whitehead, T.P., Kricka, L.J., Carter, T.J.N., and Thorpe, G.H.G. (1979). Analytical luminescence: its potential in the clinical laboratory. *Clin. Chem.*, **25**, 1531–46.

Short-term Toxicity Tests for Non-genotoxic Effects
Edited by P. Bourdeau *et al.*
© 1990 SCOPE. Published by John Wiley & Sons Ltd

CHAPTER 15

Methods for Assessing the Effects of Chemicals on the Immune System

J. G. VOS AND J. H. DEAN

15.1 INTRODUCTION

In this review, methods to assess chemically-induced lesions of acquired cellular and humoral immunity as well as natural resistance will be discussed. Not included are tests for the assessment of the allergic potential of chemicals.

15.1.1 Relevant human and other mammalian health considerations

Exposure of rodents to certain chemicals at doses that do not cause overt toxicity can produce immune alterations sufficient to result in altered host resistance to infectious agents (e.g. bacteria, viruses and parasites) and neoplastic cells (see reviews by Golstein *et al.*, 1976; Vos, 1977; Vos *et al.*, 1980; Faith *et al.*, 1980; Dean *et al.*, 1982, 1986a). Exposure to chemicals of environmental concern has likewise been shown to adversely affect the immune system of man. For example, accidental exposure of Michigan dairy farmers and factory workers to polybrominated biphenyls (Bekesi *et al.*, 1978) and exposure of Chinese to polychlorinated biphenyl contaminated with polychlorinated dibenzofurans (Chang *et al.*, 1982) resulted in demonstrable immune alterations. In 1981, an outbreak of pneumonitis occurred in Spain which was linked to the ingestion of chemically-altered cooking oil (Centers for Disease Control, 1981b). It has been suggested that this 'toxic oil syndrome' was a chemically-induced graft versus host disease caused by the presence of isothiocyanate-derived, imidazolidinethione compounds in adulterated rapeseed oil (Kammuller *et al.*, 1984). Additionally, an increased incidence of pulmonary infections in humans has been associated with exposure to noxious gases and airborne particulates (Lunn, *et al.*, 1967; French *et al.*, 1973), similar to effects seen in rodents exposed by inhalation to these same airborne contaminants (see reviews by Ehrlich, 1966; Gardner, 1984; Dean and Adams, 1985).

During the past decade, substantial evidence has accumulated indicating that there is an association between the therapeutic use of immunosuppressive drugs or congenital immune deficiency diseases and an increased incidence of infectious and neoplastic diseases in humans (see reviews by Gatti and Good, 1971; Koers *et al.*, 1975; Allen, 1976; Penn, 1978, 1985). For example, an increased incidence of lymphomas and leukaemias has been observed in patients with congenital immunodeficiency disorders (Gatti and Good, 1971). Allograft recipients chronically receiving immunosuppressive agents (mainly corticosteroids and anti-metabolites (such as azathioprine) have a remarkable frequency of secondary cancer (26 per cent at 1 year and 47 per cent at 10 years); the types of tumours found included non-Hodgkin's lymphoma, Kaposi's sarcoma, carcinoma of the cervix, and skin and lip cancer (Penn, 1985). Likewise, the prevalence of opportunistic infections and Kaposi's sarcoma among individuals with acquired immune deficiency syndrome (AIDS) (Centre for Disease Control, 1981a) also suggests a central role for T-cell mediated immunity in host resistance to tumours and infectious agents.

In animal models, a variety of immunosuppressive treatments including x-irradiation, neonatal thymectomy, or lymphocytoxic drugs have been shown to result in enhanced tumour incidence, growth rate and/or metastases. Furthermore, support for an immune-based component in the regulation of infectious disease or tumour growth is provided by *in vitro* and *in vivo* observations indicating that specific cells of the host (e.g. lymphocytes and macrophages) can recognize and destroy tumour cells and infectious agents (see Section 15.2).

Toxicological manifestations in the immune system following xenobiotic exposure in experimental animals may appear as: changes in lymphoid organ weights and/or histology; quantitative or qualitative changes in cellularity of lymphoid tissue, bone marrow or numbers of peripheral leukocytes; impairment of immune cell function; and increased susceptibility to infectious agents or transplantable tumours.

The use of the immune system as a sensitive parameter for detecting subclinical toxic injury is justified for several reasons: functionally immunocompetent cells are required for host resistance to opportunistic infectious agents or neoplasia; immunocompetent cells require continued proliferation and differentiation for self-renewal and are thus susceptible to agents which affect cell proliferation or differentiation; and the immune system is a tightly regulated organization of lymphoid cells which are interdependent in function.

Immunocompetent cells communicate through soluble mediators or cell–cell interactions and any agent altering this delicate regulatory balance, affecting a particular cell type or altering intercellular communications, can lead to an immune alteration. An imbalance of the immune system resulting from cellular injury might be expressed as either immune enhancement (e.g. possibly leading to autoimmunity or hypersensitivity) or immune suppression (e.g. immune dysfunction or altered host resistance). Some investigators are of the opinion that any immune alteration observed in rodents following xenobiotic exposure is of potential consequence for man. An alternative opinion is that only those immune alterations in rodents which are associated with hypersensitivity or altered host resistance to infectious agents or neoplastic cells are of major concern. In either case, the interpretation of immune alterations observed in toxicity studies in terms of risk for man deserves special and continued consideration. The incorporation of reliable methods for assessing immune parameters into routine toxicity testing will provide useful and necessary information for a rational approach to the safety assessment of chemicals.

15.1.2   General comments on successes and failures using routine *in vivo* toxicity testing

Procedures currently used to detect immune alterations in routine *in vivo* toxicity studies include: weight and histology of thymus, spleen, mesenteric or popliteal lymph nodes; peripheral lymphocyte and monocyte counts; and serum IgG and IgM levels (Vos, 1977). Using this abbreviated approach, a total of seventeen pesticides were screened at three dose levels for possible immunotoxicity during subacute toxicity studies in weaned male rats receiving the test compounds through the diet (Vos *et al.*, 1983b). More recently, the pesticide tributyltin oxide was studied using this protocol (Krajnc *et al.*, 1984). From these experiments, it appeared that seven chemicals (benomyl, chlorfenson, *pp'*-DDT, diuron, dinitro-*o*-cresol, endosulphan and lead acetate) did not cause, or caused only marginal, effects on the immune system. Six compounds (azinphosmethyl, chlor IPC, quintozene, 2,4,5-trichlorophenoxyacetic acid, zineb and hexachlorobenzene) affected both immunological and general toxicological parameters. Finally, five chemicals (atrazine, captan, lead arsenate, triphenyltin hydroxide and tributyltin oxide) significantly altered one or more immune parameters which appeared to be the most sensitive criterion of their toxicity.

Immune function tests comprising cell-mediated immunity, humoral immunity and non-specific resistance (Vos *et al.*, 1983b; 1984a, b) were performed in rats exposed pre- and post-natally and after weaning to atrazine, captan, lead arsenate, triphenyltin hydroxide and hexachlorobenzene (HCB). Functional immune effects were virtually absent in rats exposed to captan and lead arsenate. Of the different parameters of cell-mediated immunity (CMI) studied, the main effect exhibited by triphenyltin hydroxide was a suppression of delayed-type hypersensitivity (DTH). Tributyltin oxide caused a pronounced suppression of different parameters of CMI; of thymus-dependent antibody responses; and of natural resistance (e.g. macrophage phagocytosis and tumoricidal activity, and natural killer cell activity). In contrast, HCB markedly enhanced the antibody response to tetanus toxoid. Combined pre- and post-natal exposure to HCB, at a dose that did not alter liver weight or morphology, also enhanced the DTH response to antigen. From the results of this screening study, it was concluded that eleven of eighteen chemicals tested affected the immune system. Results of immune function assays indicated that in the rat model, alterations in lymphoid organ weights, histology, or cellularity of lymphoid organs did not necessarily equate with functional immune alterations. Likewise in mice, House *et al.* (1985) recently reported thymus atrophy in mice following exposure to ethylene glycol monomethyl ether and its metabolite methoxyacetic acid without a functional immune defect.

It is too early to draw definite conclusions on the absolute reliability of this battery of screening procedures to predict immune dysfunction. For example, pronounced thymic atrophy produced in the rat by diethylstilboestrol exposure did not cause suppression of thymus-dependent immunity (Vos, unpublished data) while, in the mouse, such treatment resulted in severe immunosuppression (reviewed by Dean *et al.*, 1982). Species differences are the most likely explanation of this discrepancy.

Differences in the immunotoxic effects of chemicals may also be linked to different modes of action. For example, both 2,3,7,8-tetrachlorodibenzo-*p*-dioxin (TCDD) and organotin compounds produce thymus atrophy and immunotoxicity in the rat. However, pre- and post-natal exposure (i.e. during immune ontogenesis in the rat) may be a prerequisite for pronounced immunosuppression by TCDD (reviewed by Vos *et al.*, 1980; Dean and Lauer, 1984), whereas organotin compounds also appear to depress thymus-dependent immunity in young adult rats (Seinen, 1981; Vos *et al.*, 1984a, b). Thus, exposure during immune ontogenesis is not prerequisite for the organotins to produce immune dysfunction. In contrast to the direct cytotoxic effects of the organotins for thymic lymphocytes, recent studies (Greenlee *et al.*, 1984; Nagarkatti *et al.*, 1984) suggest that thymic epithelial cells, which promote thymocyte proliferation and differentiation, are a possible target for TCDD-induced immunotoxicity. Impaired production of thymic hormones or inappropriate cell–cell interaction might explain the TCDD-induced thymic atrophy and immune dysfunction.

15.1.3   Consideration of experimental parameters

In designing protocols for immunotoxicity assessment of chemicals, special attention should be given to the choice of species and strain, age of animals, duration and level of exposure, as well as the route of exposure.

For practical reasons, it is desirable to use the same species and strain of animal for immune function studies that is being used in the routine toxicity study. This allows immune studies to be evaluated against the background of other standard toxicological parameters, thus eliminating the need for dose–response comparisons between different species or strains. The rationale for selecting the mouse for immunotoxicity studies is based on the fact that the immune system of the mouse is better characterized, and functional assays are better defined. However, the rat is the rodent most frequently used in routine toxicity assessment. Most of the immunological methods developed in the mouse can, with minor modifications, be adapted for use in the rat (see Section 15.2).

It is well established that the most profound effects of compounds that interfere with the immune response occur when the animal is exposed during ontogenesis of the lymphoid system (as with TCDD for example (discussed by Vos, 1977)). Thus, *in utero* and neonatal exposure appear to be the most sensitive method especially for chemicals that affect the thymus by impairing the proliferation and differentiation of the thymocytes. The second best choice is to use weaning animals.

The exposure interval required for a chemical to produce immune dysfunction differs and depends on a number of variables such as the type of immunological injury, chemical threshold, and the toxicokinetics of the compound. Few systematic studies have been done in this respect; in general, a subacute exposure regimen of 14–30 days is employed prior to assessment of immune parameters.

Dose selection is likewise critical. High doses producing overt toxicity should be avoided since severe stress and malnutrition are known to impair immune responses. For proper dose selection, information on the effect of the chemical on general toxicological parameters (e.g. LD50, LD10 and type of acute or subchronic toxicity associated with exposure) is important. To establish dose–effect relationships, two or three exposure levels are recommended. The highest dose selected for exposure should be less than the LD10, and ideally have no associated mortality.

The route of exposure should be the same as the natural route of exposure in man whenever possible. For the majority of environmental chemicals, the oral route of exposure (i.e. feeding or gavage) is preferred. In the case of airborne agents, inhalation exposure is commonly utilized.

15.2 *IN VIVO* STUDIES

15.2.1 Clinical observation

It is unlikely that immunotoxicity will be manifested by changes that can be easily observed clincally with the exception of an increased incidence of infectious disease or neoplasia. In studies involving animals that are not specified pathogen-free, immune suppression might result in the appearance of spontaneous infections. For example, Hansen *et al.* (1971) reported the development of fungus-like skin lesions in fish after PCB exposure.

If severe growth depression is observed in animals exposed to the test compound during the perinatal period, an immunologically-based wasting syndrome might be suspected. This wasting syndrome was first described by Miller (1962) in mice that were thymectomized at birth. In these mice, thymus-dependent immunological responses were severely impaired whereas adult thymectomy had only slight effects and did not produce wasting. Examples of compounds that can produce an immune-based wasting syndrome are cortisone (Ioachim, 1971), busulphan (Pinto-Machado, 1970) and TCDD (Vos and Moore, 1974).

15.2.2 Morphology

In many studies, it has been shown that routine histopathology of lymphoid organs is useful in assessing the immunotoxicity of a chemical (in particular, when these data are combined with the effects observed on the weight of thymus, spleen and peripheral lymph nodes). Because of the structural division of the spleen and lymph nodes into thymus-dependent and thymus-independent areas, a qualitative assessment can be made regarding the relative effects of the chemical for T or B cell compartments. It is also sometimes necessary to examine bronchus- or gut-associated lymphoid tissue (BALT and GALT) depending on the route of chemical exposure. Atrophy of the thymus and thymus-dependent areas of the spleen and lymph nodes were observed after di-*n*-octyltindichloride exposure (Seinen and Willems, 1976). In contrast, exposure to certain chemicals may lead to immune stimulation and lymphoid tissue hypertrophy. For example, pre- and post-natal treatment of rats with hexachlorobenzene caused proliferation of the high-endothelial venules in thymus-dependent areas of lymph nodes and in thymus-dependent areas of the Peyer's patches of the small intestine. These changes correlated with an enhanced immune response upon immune functional assessment (Vos *et al.*, 1983a).

Since the bone marrow is an integral part of the immune system (containing multipotent stem cells capable of differentiating along haemopoietic lines to B and T lymphocytes and macrophages), morphological analysis of this tissue is essential in immunotoxicity assessment. Morphological analysis can be done on tissue sections, marrow smears or on cytospin preparations of cells collected from the bone marrow. The latter technique has the advantage that the cell number and viability can be determined. In studies with TCDD, bone marrow cellularity proved to be a sensitive indicator of toxicity (Luster *et al.*, 1980). Similarly, enumeration and characterization of free alveolar macrophages obtained by bronchoalveolar lavage appears to be a good quantitative method to determine the effect of inhalation exposure to a compound (Bingham *et al.*, 1972). Macrophage quantitation and functional assessment has yielded insights into the function of immune and inflammatory processes in the human lung (Hunninghake *et al.*, 1979; Dean *et al.*, 1986b; for a review see Dean and Adams, 1985).

In routine toxicity studies, histopathologic examination depends mostly on haemotoxylin and eosin staining. Immunofluorescence methods, enzyme immune histochemistry and electron microscopy are techniques that are of great value to better understand the nature of chemically-induced lesions of the immune system. For example, enzyme histochemistry appears to be a useful method for the identification and enumeration of macrophages by staining for non-specific esterase activity (Koski *et al.*, 1976). However, the requirement of specially prepared tissue, expensive instrumentation, and experienced personnel has prevented the widespread use of fluorescence, enzyme histochemistry or ultrastructural methods.

Recent progress in immunohistochemistry, namely, the development of immunoperoxidase techniques, has made it possible to adapt this highly sensitive and specific technique not only to diagnostic pathology (Mukai and Rosai, 1980) but also to toxicology. The major application in toxicology has been the identification of hormones (see Clark and Van Leeuwen, chapter 14, this volume). Different immunoperoxidase techniques are used to localize antigens in tissue sections. These include the peroxidase-labelled antibody method, the unlabelled antibody method of peroxidase–anti-peroxidase (PAP) and the avidin–biotin–peroxidase complex (ABC) method (reviewed by Falini and Taylor, 1983). In all techniques, peroxidase is localized through an antigen–antibody reaction in areas where specific antigen is present. The sites of peroxidase localization are visualized by addition of a substrate solution which reacts with the peroxidase label to form an insoluble coloured product.

Most cytoplasmic antigens (e.g. immunoglobulins) are readily demonstrated in fixed paraffin sections. Cell surface antigens (e.g. surface markers used for the demonstration of macrophages, T-helper cells and T-suppressor lymphocytes), which are only present in small amounts, are better preserved in frozen sections. With a proper fixative, paraffin embedding can now also be employed (Gendelman *et al.*, 1983). Thin, methacrylate-embedded tissue sections (Casanova *et al.*, 1983; Franklin, 1984) have potential application for immunohistochemistry techniques. The enhanced histological detail obtained with micro-thin, plastic-embedded sections is also useful in examining bone marrow, thymus and other lymphoid tissue. By staining thin methacrylate-embedded sections with monoclonal antibodies to cell surface determinants, lymphoid subpopulations in tissue sections can be identified (Hancock *et al.*, 1982).

A difficulty for the pathologist in the evaluation of often minor chemically-induced lesions is making objective classifications. By randomizing and coding the slides, bias in reading can be avoided and qualitative analysis is possible. Classification is being improved by morphometric analysis since quantitative measurements on cells and tissues can be made by this method. In this context, it is of interest to mention that recent developments in monoclonal antibody technology, computer image processing and cytometric instrumentation has led to the new field of clinical flow cytometry. This field has already found specific applications in diagnostic immunopathology, including the study of congenital and acquired immune deficiency diseases (reviewed by Lovett *et al.*, 1984). The application of this technique to immunotoxicology may be of value (e.g. enumeration of bone marrow stem cell populations which are currently only identified by complex culture methods). Flow cytometric analysis (FACS) of T and B lymphocytes in the spleen of rats exposed to tributyltin oxide revealed a reduction of T-cells which correlated with the results of immune functional studies (Vos *et al.*, 1984a) and histopathological observations (Krajnc *et al.*, 1984). Similar observations have been made in mice exposed to tumour-promoting phorbol diesters (Murray *et al.*, 1985b). In contrast, these techniques will not always replace functional analysis since Dean *et al.* (1986b) reported functional defects in mice exposed to dimethyl-benzanthracene although the percentage of T- and B-cells and subpopulations of T-cells were unaltered.

15.2.3   Serum analysis

Information on the immunotoxicity of a compound can also be obtained by analysis of serum from animals that are not used for functional studies *in vivo*. Serum analysis can be used for the quantification of the different immunoglobulin classes (e.g. IgM and IgG). Alterations in serum immunoglobulin levels were observed following tributyltin oxide exposure in rats (Krajnc *et al.*, 1984). The classical analytical method for quantitating Ig levels is the single radial immunodiffusion assay. An alternative method is the 'sandwich' enzyme-linked immunosorbent assay (ELISA) of Engvall and Perlmann (1971). This procedure is more sensitive, easier to automate, and requires smaller amounts of antiserum than does the radial immunodiffusion assay (Vos *et al.*, 1982).

In addition to specific humoral immunity mediated by immunoglobulins, the body is also protected by non-specific antimicrobial factors. Non-specific humoral factors include interferon (IFN) production, which functions in defence against viruses; complement (C') proteins which mediate their effects through at least two important mechanisms (namely by direct killing of micro-organisms and by facilitated opsoninization); and, bactericidal enzymes such as lysozyme. Non-specific factors, for the most part, have received little attention in immunotoxicity studies, although they are of potential importance. For example, Gainer (1972) demonstrated that arsenicals inhibited the synthesis and action of IFN in mice which accounted for the increased susceptibility of these mice to viral infections. Practical and sensitive microassays for determining serum IFN and C' activity have been described (Klerx *et al.*, 1983; Campbell *et al.*, 1978).

15.2.4   Use of surgically-manipulated animals

Immunotoxicity may be secondary to other effects such as malnutrition or altered endocrine balance. An interaction of the chemical with the endocrine system should always be considered since various endogenous hormones (e.g. glucocorticosteroids) modify immune functions (White and Goldstein, 1972). For this reason, it is necessary to weigh and histologically examine the adrenals. An alternative method of identifying an endocrine effect is through the use of surgically-manipulated animals. For example, adrenalectomized rats were used to demonstrate that effects on the immune system produced by oxisuran (van Dijk *et al.*, 1975) and cholera toxin Morse *et al.*, 1975) were mediated by adrenal hormones. In contrast, thymic atrophy induced in the rat by di-*n*-octyltindichloride (Seinen and Willems, 1976) and TCDD (van Logten *et al.*, 1980) was not prevented by adrenalectomy, thus ruling out the possible role of glucocorticoids. Similarly, hypophysectomized rats were used to demonstrate that pituitary hormones were not involved in TCDD-induced thymic atrophy (van Logten *et al.*, 1980).

15.2.5 Immune function tests

Tests selected for the evaluation of immune dysfunction induced by xenobiotic exposure should meet at least two criteria: (1) the tests should result in data that can be extrapolated to the human experience; and (2) the tests should be adaptable to practical considerations such as expense, simplicity and reproducibility. A 'single' immunological test that would identify chemicals or drugs with potential risk is most desirable. However, because of the enormous complexity of the immune system, no single assay can accomplish this task. Thus, a tiered panel of selected functional assays (Dean *et al.*, 1982; Vos *et al.*, 1983b, 1984a) that have been validated in experimental rodent models and that are relevant to human clinical studies is recommended.

During the past ten years, numerous functional tests have been developed and refined to examine cell-mediated immunity, humoral immunity and natural resistance. The assembly of these tests is slightly different among the various groups working in immunotoxicology, partly because of the selection of different animal species. This is particularly true for bacterial, viral and tumour challenge models, since many of these host resistance models are not yet developed in the rat. Selection of functional assays also depends on whether inbred or random-bred animals are employed. For example, at the National Institute of Public Health and Environmental Protection (RIVM) in Bilthoven, the Netherlands, random-bred Wistar rats are utilized in toxicity testing, and immunotoxicity screening is included as part of subacute toxicity study protocols (see also Section 15.1.2). When the results of screening studies indicate that a chemical is immunotoxic, function tests are performed as part of a confirmatory tier in the same random-bred strain. The RIVM panel of immune function tests is shown in Table 15.1. Technical details of these models are provided elsewhere (Vos *et al.*, 1984a).

On the other hand, initial screening (Tier 1) for immunotoxicity at the Chemical Industry Institute of Toxicology (CIIT) and in the National Toxicology Program's (NTP) Special Studies Panel for Immunotoxicology (Dean *et al.*, 1982; Moore *et al.*, 1982) includes functional and host resistance assessment (Table 15.2). In CIIT and NTP studies, a hybrid mouse designated B6C3F1, resulting from a cross between male inbred C3H and female C57B1/6 mice, is routinely used since this mouse was selected by the NTP for the cancer bioassay of chemicals and allows the use of semisyngeneic tumour challenge models.

In the following sections, various immune function tests designed to assess acquired and natural immune resistance will be described. Detailed information on these assays and the effects of environmental chemicals on immune function are given in several reviews (Vos, 1977; Luster *et al.*, 1982; Dean *et al.*, 1982, 1986a). It should be noted that the *in vitro* assays described here are performed following *in vivo* exposure of the animal to the test compound (i.e. *ex vivo – in vitro*).

Table 15.1   Function tests for detecting immunotoxic alterations in the rat currently being used at RIVM, Bilthoven, the Netherlands

Parameters	Procedures
Cell-mediated immunity	Sensitization to T-cell dependent antigens (e.g. ovalbumin and tuberculin) and skin test challenge
	Mitogen response and one-way mixed leukocyte cultures
Humoral immunity	Serum titration of IgM and IgG response to T-dependent antigens (e.g. ovalbumin, tetanus toxoid and *Trichinella spiralis*, including IgE) and T-independent IgM response to LPS.
Macrophage function	*In vitro* phagocytosis and killing of *Listeria monocytogenes* by adherent spleen and peritoneal cells
	Cytolysis of YAC-1 lymphoma cells by adherent spleen and peritoneal cells
Natural killer cell function	Cytolysis of YAC-1 lymphoma cells by non-adherent spleen and peritoneal cells
Host resistance	*Trichinella spiralis* challenge (muscle larvae counts and worm expulsion)
	Listeria monocytogens challenge (splenic clearance)
	Endotoxin hypersensitivity

15.2.5.1   *Cell-mediated immunity*

Assays to examine cell-mediated immunity (CMI) include both *in vivo* (delayed hypersensitivity) and *in vitro* techniques (lymphocyte transformation, one-way mixed lymphocyte culture response and cytotoxicity). Currently, allograft rejection and graft versus host reaction are not used since both techniques are very labour intensive. In addition, the former technique is quite insensitive for detection of cell-mediated immune dysfunction, while the latter procedure depends on the use of a large number of recipient animals.

   A delayed-type hypersensitivity (DTH) reaction is initiated by sensitized T cells which respond specifically to an antigen through release of lymphokines (Godfrey and Gell, 1978). Although *in vitro* assays appear more sensitive, the *in vivo* test remains a widely accepted means of assessing CMI and correlates well with decreased CMI in humans and host resistance to infectious agents (MacLean, 1979). Animals are sensitized to a T-dependent antigen (e.g. keyhole limpet haemocyanin, ovalbumin, tuberculin, bovine gammaglobulin, or DNCB) and then challenged

Table 15.2　Procedures for detecting immunotoxic alterations in the mouse currently being used at CIIT, Research Triangle Park, North Carolina

Parameters	Procedures
Immunopathology	Routine haematology*
	Lymphoid organ weights (spleen, thymus) and histology.* Spleen and bone marrow cellularity*
Cell-mediated immunity	Mitogen responses and one-way mixed leukocyte cultures*
Surface markers	Quantification of lymphocyte subpopulations using monoclonal antibodies
Antibody-mediated immunity	Antibody plaque-forming cells (PFC) response*
Macrophage function	Resident peritoneal macrophage number, phagocytosis, cytostasis and enzyme levels in activated and non-activated cells
Host resistance	Tumour challenge model: 　PYB6 sarcoma* 　B16F10 melanoma Bacterial challenge model: 　*Listeria monocytogenes**

* Currently included in the National Toxicology Program's Special Studies Tier for Immunotoxicity Assessment.

intradermally with antigen (elicitation). Radiometric assays for quantifying the response provide greater sensitivity than measuring the swelling reaction but have the disadvantage of relying on the *in vivo* use of radioactive agent. It is recommended that animals be sensitized during or immediately following chemical exposure to approximate conditions which occur in humans.

Lymphoproliferative responses are a widely used correlate of CMI and can be defective in the absence of lymphocytopenia (Oppenheim and Rosenstreich, 1976). In the microculture assay, T or B cell mitogens (e.g. plant lectins, bacterial products), or allogeneic leukocytes (e.g. tissue transplantation antigens) in unidirectional mixed leukocyte cultures (MLC) are used to selectively stimulate lymphocyte blastogenesis as measured by [^{3}H]TdR incorporation into DNA. Specific depressed responses in humans or animals with normal numbers of lymphocytes are usually interpreted as a defect in cell activation.

The generation of cytotoxic T lymphocytes (CTL) is another manifestation of CMI which represents an important acquired effector mechanism in resistance to viral infections and surveillance against neoplastically transformed cells. Induction to CTL can be accomplished *in vivo* by immunization with allogeneic lymphocytes or tumour cells, or *in vitro* in a one-way mixed lymphocyte culture, or mixed lymphocyte tumour cell interaction. The cytolytic activity of the CTL is usually assessed in a 4-hour ^{51}Cr-release assay. In contrast to the ease with which mouse lymphocytes can be sensitized, it is rather difficult to generate CTL activity in MLC of rat origin (Weiss and Fitch, 1977). Measurement of CTL activity has proven to be a valuable tool in immunotoxicity testing and has been reported to be suppressed by exposure to polycyclic aromatic hydrocarbon carcinogens (e.g. DMBA, MCA, DBA) (Dean *et al.*, 1986b; Wojdani *et al.*, 1983) and extremely low doses of TCDD (Nagarkatti *et al.*, 1984; Clark *et al.*, 1981). The CTL assay is still considered a second tier assay used for mechanistic studies and is not routinely performed in Tier 1.

15.2.5.2   *Humoral immunity*

Functional assessment of humoral activity is commonly accomplished by quantifying the antibody plaque-forming cell (PFC) response, or specific serum antibody titers.

The modification by Cunningham (1965) of the Jerne and Nordin (1963) plaque assay is extensively used. In this test, lymphoid cells from an animal immunized four days previously with T-dependent antigen (e.g. sheep red blood cells (SRBC)) are incubated in a slide chamber with the target erythrocytes and lytic complement. Plaques (haemolysis) in the SRBC lawn are observed around each antibody-producing cell due to complement lysis of SRBC that are coated with specific antibody produced by sensitized B cells. The PFC assay can be applied to other antigens including T-independent antigens (e.g. TNP-LPS or TNP-Ficoll) by coating them on the surface of the SRBC. The PFC assay has been shown to be sensitive for detecting chemically-induced alterations in humoral immunity. In the assay most commonly employed, only antibodies of the IgM-type are detected, because of the high haemolytic activity of this isotype.

Currently, sensitive immunoassays such as the enzyme-linked immunosorbent assay (ELISA) (Vos *et al.*, 1982) are used for the quantification of specific serum antibodies. In the ELISA, antigen is coupled to a solid phase sorbent which is then incubated with serial dilutions of the test serum. The amount of specific antibody bound to the solid phase sorbent is titrated by enzyme-labelled anti-immunoglobulins (e.g. anti-IgM and anti-IgG). Thus, classes of specific antibodies can be quantified. Because of its extreme sensitivity, the ELISA could be useful for the measurement of specific IgE (Giallongo *et al.*, 1982) and become an alternative method to the *in vivo* measurement of specific IgE by the passive cutaneous anaphylaxis reaction.

15.2.5.3   *Macrophage function*

It is now well established that macrophages provide not only non-specific phagocytic and cytotoxic functions but also are directed and regulated by lymphokines. In addition, they provide interactions as well as products which have feedback and regulatory roles (i.e. prostaglandins and monokines) in immune responses. Thus, an understanding of macrophage function is becoming central to our understanding of immune responses and any assessment of a chemical's immunotoxicity would not be complete without examining some macrophage function parameters. Dysfunction of the mononuclear phagocytic system (MPS) can lead to indirect tissue damage through altered host resistance to infectious agents or neoplastically transformed cells, or through direct tissue injury by the mononuclear phagocytes themselves or their cellular products (e.g. autoimmune diseases). Environmental agents, especially fibres, particulates and gases are well known to alter macrophage function (Gardner, 1984). Chemicals and drugs have also been found to alter the MPS (Ehrlich, 1966; see reviews by Loose *et al.*, 1981; Dean and Adams, 1985). The effects of environmental agents upon macrophage function have been difficult to characterize precisely. This difficulty may be attributable, in part, to the fact that the functions of macrophages are closely related to their stage of maturation and to the fact that development of macrophages follows a complex and dynamic cascade of differentiation starting with bone marrow precursors (Adams and Marino, 1984). The effects of chemical exposure are also often pleiotropic so that a rational basis for understanding, studying and characterizing dysfunction of the MPS has been difficult to establish.

Studies from several laboratories have recently demonstrated that murine macrophages develop in stages (Hibbs *et al.*, 1977; Meltzer, 1981) and that the stages of development can be clearly identified by quantifying certain objective biological and enzymatic makers, the expression of which characterizes each of the stages (Johnson *et al.*, 1983). This system of analysis has been used to characterize modulation of macrophage development including those produced by agents of environmental concern (Adams and Dean, 1982). Thus, an understanding of macrophage function is pivotal to our understanding of immune responses and assessment of chemically-induced immunotoxicity.

Techniques measuring the uptake of ^{125}I-triolein (Di Luzio and Riggi, 1964) or the clearance of colloidal carbon (Stuart *et al.*, 1973) are often used for *in vivo* measurement of the phagocytic capacity of mononuclear phagocytes. For *in vivo* assessment of phagocytosis and macrophage bactericidal capacity, infection with *Listeria monocytogenes* is widely employed (see Host resistance, Section 15.2.5.6).

A *Listeria monocytogenes* model can also be used for the *in vitro* assessment of macrophage bactericidal function (van Furth and van Zwet, 1973). It has the advantage that the processes of phagocytosis and intracellular killing can be assessed independently. By using only the adherent-cell population, phagocytosis by mononuclear cells can be analysed independently of granulocyte phagocytosis. However, a main difficulty of this test lies in removing adherent, non-phagocytosed bacteria from the macrophages. The test is also quite labour-intensive for routine use.

Besides their capacity for intracellular digestion, macrophages can destroy cells by a process of exocytosis and are thought to play a role in surveillance against malignancies (Keller, 1978; Adams and Snyderman, 1979). Tumour cytolytic activity of macrophages is commonly assessed in a microcytotoxicity assay by measuring the release of ^{51}Cr from tumour target cells added to cultures of adherent peritoneal effector cells. More recently, the measurement of macrophage ecto- and lysosomal enzymes appears to offer another promising approach (Dean and Adams, 1985).

15.2.5.4   *Natural killer cell function*

Spontaneous cytotoxicity is an important cytolytic effector mechanism in natural resistance to tumours and viral diseases. Natural killer (NK) cells are active in tumour surveillance (Warner and Dennert, 1982) and can limit viral infections (Bukowski *et al.*, 1983). NK tumoricidal activity is assessed in a 4-hour microcytotoxicity assay by culturing splenocytes or peripheral blood lymphocytes with a ^{51}Cr-labelled cell line sensitive to NK lysis (e.g. YAC-1 or K562 lymphoma cells).

15.2.5.5   *Granulocyte function*

Granulocyte function can be assessed by measuring physiological activities such as phagocytosis, chemotactic activity, bactericidal activity or nitro blue tetrazolium (NBT) dye reduction. Perhaps the best single assay is the NBT dye reduction procedure which has been extensively employed in the diagnosis of persons with chronic granulomatous disease. Failure of granulocytes to reduce NBT was found to correlate with an impaired enzymatic ability to kill phagocytosed bacteria. The number of granulocytes reducing dye can be easily quantified histochemically. This procedure can be utilized if altered bacterial resistance is observed in the presence of normal humoral, CMI and macrophage function.

15.2.5.6   *Host resistance*

Models assessing host resistance are needed in order to improve the human risk assessment data base for the evaluation of relevant chemically-induced immunotoxicity and provide *in vivo* correlates for the numerous *in vitro* immune function assays. This interest in providing better correlation and interpretation between an alteration in one or several measurable immunological parameters and host resistance stems from the established associations between patients with well-defined immunodeficiencies and the concomitant increase of infectious diseases or neoplasia (see Section 15.1.1).

Infectious agent challenge models. The application of host resistance assays following exposure of rodents to chemicals has indicated that certain chemicals can alter host resistance to bacteria, viruses and parasites (see reviews of Vos, 1977; Bradley and Morahan, 1982; Dean *et al.*, 1982; Faith *et al.*, 1980). Workers have employed such infectious agents as *Klebsiella pneumoniae, Listeria monocytogenes, Streptococcus pyogenes, Salmonella bern, Salmonella typhimurium*, pseudorabies virus, duck hepatitis virus, encephalomyocarditis virus, *Trichinella spiralis* and *Plasmodium berghei*. Resistance in most models appears to require T-cell immunity and functional, mononuclear phagocytes. Resistance to *Streptococcus pyogenes* and *Plasmodium berghei* are exceptions and require phagocytic cells whose function is facilitated by opsonizing antibodies.

Resistance to *Listeria monocytogenes* involves a combination of non-specific phagocytosis by macrophages which limits the growth or kills the organism during the first few days (1–3 days) after infection, and CMI which develops from day 2 post-infection (Tripathy and Mackaness, 1969; Cheers *et al.*, 1978). Non-specific phagocytosis and killing can be measured on days 1 and 2 after an intravenous inoculation of *Listeria*, at a time when acquired CMI is not yet developed. Spleens of the infected animals are homogenized, and serial dilutions of each humogenate are plated in bacteriological media to determine the viable *Listeria* count. Challenge of mice and rats with *L. monocytogenes* has proven to be a reproducible model for detecting altered macrophage or T-cell function after chemical exposure (Dean *et al.*, 1980, 1981; Vos *et al.*, 1984a).

Resistance to the nematode *Trichinella spiralis* is thymus-dependent as shown by a strongly retarded expulsion of adult worms from the intestine, increased numbers of muscle larvae and absence of IgM, IgG and IgE antibodies in athymic nude mice (Ruitenberg *et al.*, 1977), and nude rats (Vos *et al.*, 1983c). Both CMI (Larsh *et al.*, 1974) and humoral immunity (particularly the IgE isotype, Dessein *et al.*, 1981) appear to play an important role in the resistance to *Trichinella*. This model has been shown to be useful in detecting chemically-induced immune dysfunction (Dean *et al.*, 1980; Faith *et al.*, 1979; Vos *et al.*, 1984a).

Transplantable tumour challenge models. Of recent interest has been the demonstration that resistance to transplantable syngeneic tumour cells is also a sensitive parameter for detecting altered host resistance following chemical exposure (Dean *et al.*, 1980, 1982; see Murray *et al.*, 1985a for a review). Tumour models commonly used include the sarcoma MKSA and Madison 109 lung tumour of BALB/c mice and the sarcoma PYB6, B16F10 melanoma and Moloney virus-induced sarcoma of C57BL/6 mice. Almost any tumour model in which resistance is dependent on T-cell immunity, natural killer cells or macrophages could be employed. The selection of a specific tumour model for transplantation experiments will depend primarily on the species and strain of animal tested since the tumour must be syngeneic or semisyngeneic to the host. Tumour models that have been well characterized in terms of antitumour effector cell mechanisms are preferred.

The ability of an animal to reject a challenge of syngeneic tumour cells inoculated at a dose previously titrated to produce a low tumour incidence in control animals (i.e. TD 10–30 per cent) has been proposed as a sensitive *in vivo* assessment of general immunocompetence. Tumour challenge models using MKSA (BALB/c background) and PYB6 (C57BL/6 background) tumour cells have been validated for detecting immune alterations following *in vivo* administration of the immuno-suppressive chemotherapeutic agent, cyclophosphamide (Dean *et al.*, 1979). Like-wise, exposure to a variety of immunotoxic chemicals has been found to alter host susceptibility in terms of capacity to reject a low concentration challenge (TD 10–30 per cent with these tumour cells which generally correlates with deficits in T-lym-phocyte function.

Chemically-induced immune suppression is expressed in these models as an increased incidence of tumours, a decreased latency to tumour appearance, an increased tumour growth rate, and/or decreased mean survival time. Conversely, agents which stimulate immune function may facilitate resistance to tumour de-velopment through enhancement of transplantation rejection mechanisms. Immune enhancement can be detected in these models using a higher challenge level of tumour cells (e.g. TD 70–90 per cent).

Several metastatic models adaptable for host tumour resistance evaluation are available. The B16F10 melanoma model provides a convenient and reproducible means for detecting modulation of host resistance parameters involved in the growth of solid, transplantable tumours and metastases. Intravenous challenge with the B16F10 subline results in haematogenous dissemination of tumour cells; their sub-sequent growth in the lungs (i.e. experimental metastasis) can be determined by either of two methods. Since the B16 melanoma forms pigmented metastatic foci, visual quantitation of organ-associated metastases is relatively simple. Alter-natively, radioisotopic labelling of tumour cells *in vivo* provides a reliable means of determining relative organ tumour burden between control and treated mice. In this method (Murray *et al.*, 1985b), animals receive an intraperitoneal injection of ^{125}I–iododeoxyuridine, a radiolabelled DNA precursor which is incorporated into the nuclei of proliferating cells, following an initial tumour growth period (21 days). The mice are sacrificed 18 hours after the isotope injection and organs are removed and counted for incorporated radioactivity.

Bacterial endotoxin detoxification. The detoxification of Gram-negative bacterial endotoxin is believed to be accomplished primarily by liver parenchymal cells and macrophages (Cook *et al.*, 1975). Increased mortality following endotoxin challenge has been observed following the administration of known mononuclear phagocyte system (MPS) stimulants as well as a variety of environmental chemicals which depress MPS function (Faith *et al.*, 1979; Vos, 1977). It should be noted that endotoxin hypersensitivity has not been found to relate to any known macrophage function or activational state.

15.3 *IN VITRO* STUDIES

In recent years, *in vitro* lymphoid cell models for defining toxicological effects have received increasing attention because of the interest of alternatives to animal testing. The main reasons for this interest involve the burden and expense of the large number of toxicological studies currently required, and the ethical motive to limit *in vivo* animal experimentation.

The *in vitro* approach has been particularly successful in the screening of a multitude of compounds for genotoxic potential. For immunotoxicity screening, *in vitro* assays have only been used to a limited extent. Results of *in vitro* studies should be critically evaluated regarding their *in vivo* significance, because of the enormous complexity of the immune system.

Currently, the most widely utilized *in vitro* system for studying immunotoxic effects of chemicals is the *in vitro* immunization, antibody plaque-forming cell assay of Mishell and Dutton (1967). Archer *et al.* (1978) screened various food additives and metabolites for potential immunosuppressive properties by relating the cytotoxic dose with the quantity of the compound inhibiting the antibody plaque-forming cell responses. The same assay was used by Kutz *et al.* (1980) in studying food additives and environmental compounds including organometals and polychlorinated biphenyls. Disconcerting was the fact that some chemicals found to be immunosuppressive *in vivo*, were not immunosuppressive in the Mishell–Dutton assay. In order to widen the applicability of the *in vitro* models to include immunosuppressive chemicals which are not direct acting (i.e. those requiring metabolic activation), Tucker *et al.* (1982) successfully interfaced a system for metabolic activation using the microsomal fraction, S9, with three *in vitro* assays (Mishell–Dutton, lymphocyte transformation and bone marrow cell culture), using the immunosuppressive drug cyclophosphamide which requires metabolic activation. Dean *et al.* (1986b) recently found that the *in vitro* generation of CTL could be inhibited by direct addition of polycyclic aromatic hydrocarbon carcinogens to the cultures. *In vitro* assays have also been used by several investigators to assess macrophage function. For example, Graham *et al.* (1975) and Greenspan and Morrow (1984) showed that the phagocytic activity of alveolar macrophages was reduced by *in vitro* treatment with cadmium. These results correlated with findings of *in vivo* treatment.

In vitro assays are of great value in determining the mechanism of action of established immunotoxic compounds and investigating their immunotoxic potential for man. Seinen *et al.* (1977) showed that di-*n*-butyltindichloride, a compound with cytotoxic properties for rat thymocytes but not mouse or guinea-pig thymocytes, was also cytotoxic for human thymocytes. A good example of the efficiency of *in vitro* assays in defining the mode of action of chemicals comes from the work of Greenlee *et al* (1984) who treated thymic epithelial cells with TCDD and found impaired thyocyte maturation suggesting that the thymic epithelium is one of the target sites for TCDD.

In vitro assays can be designed to study the different phases of an immune response by separately adding (e.g. cellular depletion/reconstitution experiments) the various cell types involved. It is in the area of mechanisms of immunotoxicity that *in vitro* models provide much insight.

15.4 STRATEGY

The application of immunologic methods for toxicity assessment has developed rapidly and has been widely accepted. Programmes to determine the immunotoxic potential of chemicals and drugs are being developed in many governmental, university and industrial laboratories throughout the world. Since a single immune function assay cannot be used to comprehensively evaluate deleterious effects on the immune system following exposure to chemicals or drugs, tiers of sensitive *in vivo* and *in vitro* assays are used to assess immunotoxicity in rodents and are currently being further refined and validated in several laboratories. The tier approach to immunotoxicity assessment consists of a screening panel of assays selected from Tier I which enables the quick identification of compounds which may produce immune alterations. Agents shown to be positive in Tier I assays can be further evaluated with assays selected from a more comprehensive panel (Tier II). Tier II assays allow confirmation and in-depth evaluation of the underlying mechanism(s) of immunotoxicity.

Further development in this area should include an international interlaboratory validation of test methods using compounds with known immunotoxic effects and should ultimately provide a more standardized protocol for immunotoxicity testing. Such a tier of validated methods should rely not only on function tests, but incorporate immunopathology, monoclonal antibody, immunohistochemistry and flow cytometry methods as well. Future research needs include the development of protocols to assess mucosal and local immunity (Bienenstock and Befus, 1980), better models for studying chemically-induced autoimmunity and more mechanistic studies focused at the cellular and molecular level. Current immunotoxciology procedures emphasize systemic immunity. Even in programmes that evaluate the immunotoxicity of airborne contaminants, emphasis is given to the lower respiratory tract where the immune response is of the systemic type, while mucosal immune responses of the upper respiratory tract are much less investigated. The same holds true for the local immunity in the intestines, despite the fact that mucosal surfaces are the main sites of entry of foreign compounds, including chemicals that might have immunotoxic potential.

The next ten years presents a new era and challenge to immunotoxicology because of the required safety assessment of new recombinant biologicals (e.g. growth hormones, interferons, interleukins and new vaccines); biological response modifiers (i.e. drugs such as muramyl dipeptide) designed to enhance immunoresponsiveness against tumours and infections; and, monoclonal antibodies designed as drug delivery vehicles or for detoxification.

REFERENCES

Adams, D.O., and Dean, J.H. (1982). Analysis of macrophage activation and biological response modifier effects by use of objective markers to characterize the stages of activation. In: Herberman, R.B. (Ed.), *NK Cells and Other Natural Effector Cells,* Academic Press, New York, pp. 511–18.

Adams, D.O., and Marino, P.A. (1984). Activation of mononuclear phagocytes for destruction of tumor cells as a model for study of macrophage development. In: Gordon, A.S., Loboe, J., and Silber, R. (Eds), *Contemporary Haematology/Oncology,* volume III, Plenum Publishing Corp., New York, pp. 69–136.

Adams, D.O., and Snyderman, R. (1979). Do macrophages destroy nascent tumors? *J. Natl. Cancer Inst.,* **62**, 1341–5.

Allen, J.C. (1976). Infection complicating neoplastic disease and cytotoxic therapy. In: Allen, J.C. (Ed.), *Infection and the Comprised Host,* Williams and Wilkins, Baltimore, pp. 151–71.

Archer, D.L., Smith, B.G., and Bukovic-Wess, J.A. (1978). Use of an *in vitro* antibody-producing system for recognizing potentially immunosuppressive compounds. *Int. Arch. Allergy Appl. Immunol.,* **56**, 90–93.

Bekesi, J.G., Holland, J.F., Anderson, H.A., Fischbein, A.S., Rom, W., Wolff, M.S., and Selikoff, I.J. (1978). Lymphocyte function of Michigan dairy farmers exposed to polybrominated biphenyls. *Science,* **199**, 1207–9.

Bienenstock, J., and Befus, A.D. (1980). Mucosal immunity. *Immunology,* **41**, 249–70.

Bingham, E., Barkley, W., Zerwas, M., Stemmer, K., and Taylor, P. (1972). Responses of alveolar macrophages to metals. I. Inhalation of lead and nickel. *Arch. Env. Health,* **25**, 406–14.

Bradley, S.G., and Morahan, P.S. (1982). Approaches to assessing host resistance. *Environ. Health Perspect.,* **43**, 61–9.

Bukowski, J.F., Woda, B.A., Habu, S., Okumura, K., and Welsh, R.M. (1983). Natural killer cell depletion enhances virus synthesis and virus-induced hepatitis *in vivo. J. Immunol.,* **131**, 1531–8.

Campbell, J.B., Grunberger, T., Kochman, M.A., and White, S.L. (1978). A microplaque reduction assay for human and mouse interferon. *Can. J. Microbiol.,* **21**, 1247–53.

Casanova, S., Domini, U., Zini, N., Morelli, R., and Zucchelli, P. (1983). Immunohistochemical staining on hydroxyethyl-methacrylate-embedded tissues. *J. Histochem. Cytochem.,* **31**, 1000–4.

Centers for Disease Control (1981a). Kaposi's sarcoma and pneumocystis pneumonia among homosexual men—New York City, California. *Morbid. Mortal. Weekly Rep.,* **30**, 305–8.

Centers for Disease Control (1981b). Follow-up on toxic pneumonia—Spain. *Morbid. Mortal. Weekly Rep.,* **30**, 436–8.

Chang, K.J., Hsieh, K.H., Tang, S.Y., Tung, T.C., and Lee, T.P. (1982). Immunologic evaluation of patients with polychlorinated biphenyl poisoning: Evaluation of delayed-type skin hypersensitive response and its relation to clinical studies. *J. Tox. Environ. Health,* **9**, 217–23.

Cheers, C., McKenzie, I.F.C., Pavlov, H., Waid, C., and York, J. (1978). Resistance and susceptibility of mice to bacterial infection: Course of listeriosis in resistant or susceptible mice. *Infect. Immun.,* **19**, 763–70.

Clark, D.A., Gauldie, J., Szewczuk, M.R., and Sweeney, G. (1981). Enhanced suppressor cell activity as a mechanism of immunosuppression by 2,3,7,8-tetrachlorodibenzo(p)dioxin. *Proc. Soc. Expt. Biol. Med.,* **168**, 290–99.

Cook, J.A., Di Luzio, N.R., and Hoffmann, E.O. (1975). Factors modifying susceptibility to bacterial endotoxin: the effect of lead and cadmium. *CRC Crit. Rev. Tox.,* **3**, 201–29.

Cunningham, A.J. (1965). A method of increased sensitivity for detecting single antibody-forming cells. *Nature,* **207**, 1106–7.

Dean, J.H., and Lauer, L.D. (1984). Immunological effects following exposure to 2,3,7,8-tetrachlorodibenzo-p-dioxin: a review. In: Lowrance, W.W. (Ed.), *Public Health Risk of the Dioxins,* William Kaufman, Inc., Los Altos, CA, pp. 275–94.

Dean, J.H., and Adams, D.O. (1985). The effect of environmental agents on cells of the mononuclear phagocyte system. In: Hadden, J.W., and Szentivany, A. (Eds), *The Reticuloendothelial System: A Comprehensive Treatise,* volume 8, *Pharmacology,* Plenum Press, New York, pp. 389–409.

Dean, J.H., Padarathsingh, M.L., Jerrells, T.R., Keys, L., and Northing, J.W. (1979). Assessment of immunobiological effects induced by chemicals, drugs or food additives. II. Studies with cyclophosphamide. *Drug Chem. Toxicol.,* **2**, 133–53.

Dean, J.H., Luster, M.I., Boorman, G.A., Luebke, R.W., and Lauer, L.D. (1980). The effect of adult exposure to diethylstilbestrol in the mouse: alterations in tumor susceptibility and host resistance parameters. *J. Reticuloendoth. Soc.,* **28**, 571–83.

Dean, J.H., Luster, M.I., and Boorman, G.A. (1982). Immunotoxicology. In Sirois, P., and Rola-Pleszczynski, M. (Eds), *Immunopharmacology,* Elsevier Biomedial Press, Amsterdam, pp. 349–97.

Dean, J.H., Lauer, L.D., House, R.V., Murray, M.J., Stillman, W.S., Irons, R.D., Steinhagen, W.H., Phelps, M.C., and Adams, D.O. (1984). Studies of immune function and host resistance in B6C3F1 mice exposed to formaldehyde. *Toxicol. Appl. Pharmacol.,* **72**, 519–29.

Dean, J.H., Murray, M.J., and Ward, E.C. (1986a). Toxic responses of the immune system. In: Klaassen, C.D., Amdur, M.O., and Doull, J. (Eds), *Casarett and Doull's Toxicology: The Basic Science of Poisons,* 3rd Edn, MacMillan Publishing Co., New York, pp. 245–85.

Dean, J.H., Ward, E.C., Murray, M.J., Lauer, L.D., House, R.V., Stillman, W., Hamilton, T.A., and Adams, D.O. (1986b). Immunosuppression following 7,12-dimethylbenz(a)anthracene exposure in B6C3F1 mice. II. Altered cell-mediated immunity and tumor resistance. *Int. J. Immunopharmacol.,* **8**, 189–98.

Dessein, A.J., Parker, W.L., James, S.L., and David, J.R. (1981). IgE antibody and resistance to infection. I. Selective suppression of the IgE antibody response in rats diminishes the resistance and the eosinophil response to *Trichinella spiralis* infection. *J. Exp. Med.,* **153**, 423–36.

Di Luzio, N.R., and Riggi, S.J. (1964). The development of a lipid emulsion for the measurement of reticuloendothelial function. *J. Reticuloendoth. Soc.,* **1**, 136–49.

Ehrlich, R. (1966). Effects of nitrogen dioxide on resistance to respiratory infections. *Bacteriol. Rev.,* **30**, 604–14.

Engvall, E., and Perlmann, P. (1971). Enzyme-linked immunosorbent assay (ELISA). Quantitative assay of immunoglobulin G. *Immunochemistry,* **8**, 871–4.

Faith, R.E., Luster, M.I., and Kimmel, C.A. (1979). Effect of chronic developmental lead exposure on cell-mediated immune functions. *Clin. Exp. Immunol.,* **35**, 413–20.

Faith, R.E., Luster, M.I., and Vos, J.G. (1980). Effects on immunocompetence by chemicals of environmental concern. In: Hodgson, E., Bend, J.R., and Philpot, R.M. (Eds), *Reviews in Biochemical Toxicology,* volume 2, Elsevier–North-Holland, New York, pp. 173–211.

Falini, B., and Taylor, C.R. (1983). New developments in immunoperoxidase techniques and their application. *Arch. Pathol. Lab. Med.,* **107**, 105–17.

Franklin, R.M. (1984). Immunohistochemistry on semi-thin sections of hydroxypropyl methacrylate embedded tissues. *J. Immunol. Methods,* **68**, 61–72.

French, J.G., Lowrimore, G., Nelson, W.C., Finklea, J.F., English, T., and Hertz, M. (1973). The effect of sulfur dioxide and suspended sulfates on acute respiratory disease. *Arch. Env. Health,* **27**, 129–33.

Gainer, J.H. (1972). Effects of arsenicals on interferon formation and action. *Am. J. Vet. Res.,* **33**, 2579–86.

Gardner, D.E. (1984). Alterations in macrophage functions by environmental chemicals. *Environ. Health Perspect.,* **55**, 343–58.

Gatti, R.A., and Good, R.A. (1971). Occurrence of malignancy in immunodeficiency disease: a literature review. *Cancer,* **28**, 89–98.

Gendelman, H.E., Moench, T.R., Narayan, O., and Griffin, D.E. (1983). Selection of a fixative for identifying T-cell subsets, B-cells and macrophages in paraffin-embedded mouse spleen. *J. Immunol. Methods,* **65**, 137–45.

Giallongo, A., Kochoumain, L., and King, T.P. (1982). Enzyme and radioimmunassays for specific murine IgE and IgG with different solid-phase immunosorbents. *J. Immunol. Methods,* **52**(3), 379–93.

Godfrey, H.P., and Gell, P.G.H. (1978). Cellular and molecular events in the delayed-onset hypersensitivities. *Rev. Physiol. Biochem. Pharmacol.,* **84**, 1–92.

Goldstein, E., Jordan, G.W., MacKenzie, M.R., and Osebold, J.W. (1976). Methods for evaluating the toxicological effects of gaseous and particulate contaminants on pulmonary microbial defense systems. *Ann. Rev. Pharm. Tox.,* **16**, 447–63.

Graham, J.A., Gardner, D.E., Waters, M.D., and Coffin, D.L. (1975). Effect of trace metals on phagocytosis by alveolar macrophages. *Infect. Immun.,* **11**, 1278–83.

Greenlee, W.F., Dold, K.M., and Irons, R.D. (1984). 2,3,7,8-Tetrachlorodibenzo-p-dioxin (TCDD) inhibits the induction by thymic epithelial cells of T-lymphocyte mitogen responsiveness. *The Toxicologist,* **4**, 188.

Greenspan, B.J., and Morrow, P.E. (1984). The effects of *in vitro* and aerosol exposures to cadmium on phagocytosis by rat pulmonary macrophages. *Fund. Appl. Toxicol.,* **4**, 48–57.

Hancock, W.W., Becker, G.J., and Atkins, R.C. (1982). A comparison of fixatives and immunohistochemical technics for use with monoclonal antibodies to cell surface antigens. *Am. J. Clin. Pathol.,* **78**, 825–31.

Hansen, D.J., Parish, P.R., Lowe, J.I., Wilson, Jr., A.J., and Wilson, P.D. (1971). Chronic toxicity, uptake, and retention of Aroclor 1254 in two estuarine fishes. *Bull. Environ. Contam. Toxicol.,* **6**, 113–19.

Hibbs, J.B. Jr., Taintor, R.R., Chapman, H.A. Jr., and Weinberg, J.B. (1977). Macrophage tumor killing: influence of the local environment. *Science,* **197**, 279–82.

House, R.V., Lauer, L.D., Murray, M.J., Ward, E.C., and Dean, J.H. (1985). Immunological studies in B6C3F1 mice following exposure to ethylene glycol monomethyl ether and its principal metabolite methoxyacetic acid. *Toxicol. Appl. Pharmacol.,* **77**, 358–62.

Hunninghake, G.W., Gadek, J.E., Kawanami, O., Ferrans, V.J., and Crystal, R.G. (1979). Inflammatory and immune processes in the human lung in health and disease: Evaluation by bronchoalveolar lavage. *Am. J. Pathol.,* **97**, 149–206.

Ioachim, H.L. (1971). The cortisone-induced wasting disease of newborn rats: Histopathological and autoradiographic studies. *J. Pathol.,* **104**, 201–5.

Jerne, N.K., and Nordin, A.A. (1963). Plaque formation in agar by single antibody-producing cells. *Science,* **140**, 405–7.

Johnson, W.J., Marino, P.A., Schreiber, R.D., and Adams, D.O. (1983). Sequential activation of murine mononuclear phagocytes for tumor cytolysis: Differential expression of markers by macrophages in the several stages of development. *J. Immunol.,* **131**, 1038–43.

Kammüller, M.E., Penninks, A.H., and Seinen, W. (1984). Spanish toxic oil syndrome is a chemically induced GVHD-like epidemic. *Lancet,* **i**, 1174–5.

Keller, R. (1978). Macrophage-mediated natural cytotoxicity against various target cells *in vitro*. I: Macrophages from diverse anatomical sites and different strains of rats and mice. *Br. J. Cancer,* **37**, 732–41.

Klerx, J.P.A.M., Beukelman, C.J., van Dijk, H., and Willers, J.M.N. (1983). Microassay for colorimetric estimation of complement activity in guinea pig, human and mouse serum. *J. Immunol. Methods*, **63**, 215–20.

Koski, I.R., Poplack, D.G., and Blaese, R.M. (1976). A non-specific esterase strain for the identification of monocytes and macrophages. In: Blood, B., and David, J.R. (Eds), *In Vitro Methods in Cell-Mediated and Tumor Immunity*, Academic Press, New York, pp. 359–62.

Krajnc, E.I., Wester, P.W., Loeber, J.G., van Leeuwen, F.X.R., Vos, J.G., Vaessen, H.A.M.G., and van der Heijden, C.A. (1984). Toxicity of bis (tri-*n*-butyltin)oxide in the rat. I: Short-term effects on general parameters and on the endocrine and lymphoid systems. *Toxicol. Appl. Pharmacol.*, **75**, 363–86.

Kroes, R., Weiss, J.W., and Weisburger, J.H. (1975). Immune suppression and chemical carcinogenesis. *Recent Results Cancer Res.*, **52**, 65–75.

Kutz, S.A., Hinsdill, R.D., and Weltman, D.J. (1980). Evaluation of chemicals for immunomodulatory effects using an *in vitro* antibody-producing assay. *Environ. Research*, **22**, 368–76.

Larsh, J.E. Jr., Race, G.J., Martin, J.H., and Weatherly, N.F. (1974). Studies on delayed (cellular) hypersensitivity in mice infected with *Trichinella spiralis*. VIII: Serologic and histopathologic responses of recipients injected with spleen cells from donors suppressed with ATS. *J. Parasitol.*, **60**, 99–109.

Loose, L.D., Silkworth, J.B., Charbonneau, T., and Blumenstock, F. (1981). Environmental chemical-induced macrophage dysfunction. *Environ. Health Perspect.*, **39**, 79–91.

Lovett, E.J., Schnitzer, B., Keren, D.F., Flint, A., Hudson, J.L., and McClatchey, K.D. (1984). Application of flow cytometry to diagnostic pathology. *Lab. Invest.*, **50**, 115–40.

Lunn, J.E., Knowelden, J., and Handyside, A.J. (1967). Patterns of respiratory illness in Sheffield infant schoolchildren. *Br. J. Prev. Soc. Med.*, **21**, 7–16.

Luster, M., Boorman, G.A., Dean, J.H., Harris, M.W., Luebke, R.W., Padarathsingh, M.L., and Moore, J.A. (1980). Examination of bone marrow, immunologic parameters and host susceptibility following pre- and post-natal exposure to 2,3,7,8-tetrachlorodibenzo-*p*-dioxin (TCDD). *Int. J. Immunopharmacol.*, **2**, 301–10.

Luster, M.I., Dean, J.H., and Moore, J.A. (1982). Evaluation of immune functions in toxicology. In: Hayes, A.W. (Ed.), *Principles and Methods of Toxicology*, Raven Press, New York, pp. 561–86.

MacLean, L.D. (1979). Host resistance in surgical patients. *J. Trauma*, **19**, 297–304.

Meltzer, M.S. (1981). Tumor cytotoxicity by lymphokine-activated macrophages: Development of macrophage tumoricidal activity requires a sequence of reactions. *Lymphokines*, **3**, 319–43.

Miller, J.F.A.P. (1962). Effect of neonatal thymectomy on the immunological responsiveness of the mouse. *Proc. Royal Soc. B.*, **156**, 415–28.

Mishell, R.I., and Dutton, R.W. (1967). Immunization of dissociated spleen cell cultures from normal mice. *J. Exp. Med.*, **126**, 423–42.

Moore, J.A., Huff, J.E., and Dean, J.H. (1982). The National Toxicology Program and immunological toxicology. *Pharm. Reviews*, **34**, 13–16.

Morse, S.I., Stearns, C.D., and Goldsmith, S.R. (1975). Lymphocyte depletion induced by cholera toxin; relationship to adrenal cortical function. *J. Immunol.*, **114**, 665–670.

Mukai, K., and Rosai, J. (1980). Application of immunoperoxidase techniques in surgical pathology. In: Fenoglio, C.M., and Wolff, M. (Eds), *Progress in Surgical Pathology*, volume 1, Masson Publishing USA, New York, pp. 15–49.

Murray, M.J., Kerkvliet, N.I., Ward, E.C., and Dean, J.H. (1985a). Models for the evaluation of tumor resistance following chemical or drug exposure. In: Dean, J.H., Munson, A.E., Luster, M.I., and Amos, H.E. (Eds), *Immunotoxicology and Immunopharmacology*, Target Organ Toxicology Series, Raven Press, New York, pp. 113–22.

Murray, M.J., Lauer, L.D., Luster, M.I., Luebke, R.W., Adams, D.O., and Dean, J.H. (1985b). Correlation of murine susceptibility to tumor, parasite and bacterial challenge with altered cell-mediated immunity following systemic exposure to the tumor promotor phorbol myristate acetate. *Int. J. Immunopharmacol.,* **7**, 491–500.

Nagarkatti, P.S., Sweeney, G.D., Gauldie, J., and Clark, D.A. (1984). Sensitivity to suppression of cytotoxic T cell generation by 2,3,7,8-tetrachlorodibenzo-*p*-dioxin (TCDD) is depenent on the *Ah* genotype of the murine host. *Toxicol. Appl. Pharmacol.,* **72**, 169–76.

Oppenheim, J.J., and Rosenstreich, D.L. (1976). *Mitogens in Immunobiology,* Academic Press, New York.

Penn, I. (1978). Development of cancer in transplant patients. *Adv. Surg.,* **12**, 155–91.

Penn, I. (1985). Neoplastic consequences of immunosuppression. In: Dean, J.H., Luster, M.I., Munson, A.E., and Amos, H. (Eds), *Immunotoxicology and Immunopharmacology,* Raven Press, New York, pp. 79–89.

Pinto-Machado, J. (1970). Influence of prenatal administration of busulfan on the postnatal development of mice. Production of a syndrome hypoplasia of the thymus. *Teratology,* **3**, 363–70.

Ruitenberg, E.J., Elgersma, A., Kruizinga, W., and Leenstra, F. (1977). *Trichinella spiralis* infection in congenitally athymic (nude) mice. Parasitological, serological and haematological studies with observations on intestinal pathology. *Immunology,* **33**, 581–7.

Seinen, W. (1981). Immunotoxicity of alkyltin compounds. In: Sharma, R.P. (Ed.), *Immunologic Considerations in Toxicology,* volume 1, CRC Press, Boca Raton, pp. 103–19.

Seinen, W., and Willems, M.I. (1976). Toxicity of organotin compounds. I. Atrophy of thymus and thymus-dependent lymphoid tissue in rats fed di-*n*-octyltindichloride. *Toxicol. Appl. Pharmacol.,* **35**, 63–75.

Seinen, W., Vos, J.G., van Spanje, I., Snoek, M., Brands, R., and Hooykaas, H. (1977). Toxicity of organotin compounds. II. Comparative *in vivo* and *in vitro* studies with various organotin and organolead compounds in different animal species with special emphasis on lymphocyte cytotoxicity. *Toxicol. Appl. Pharmacol.,* **42**, 197–212.

Stuart, A.E., Habeshaw, J.A., and Davidson, A.E. (1973). Phagocytes *in vitro.* In: Weir, D.M. (Ed.), *Handbook of Experimental Immunology,* 2nd Edn, Blackwell Scientific, Oxford, Chapter 24.

Tripathy, S.P., and Mackaness, G.B. (1969). The effect of cytotoxic agents on the primary immune response to *Listeria monocytogenes. J. Exp. Med.,* **130**, 1–16.

Tucker, A.N., Sanders, V.M., Hallett, P., Kauffmann, B.M., and Munson, A.E. (1982). *In Vitro* immunotoxicological assays for detection of compounds requiring metabolic activation. *Environ. Health Perspect.,* **43**, 123–7.

van Dijk, H., Bakker, I.A., Testerink, J., Bloksma, N., and Willers, J.M. (1975). Oxisuran and immune reactions: mediation of oxisuran action by the adrenal glands. *J. Immunol.,* **115**, 1587–91.

van Furth, R., and van Zwet, T.L. (1973). *In vitro* determination of phagocytosis and intracellular killing by polymorphonuclear and mononuclear phagocytes. In: Weir, D.M. (Ed.), *Handbook of Experimental Immunology,* 2nd Edn, Blackwell Scientific, Oxford, Chapter 36.

van Logten, M.J., Gupta, B.N., McConnell, E.E., and Moore, J.A. (1980). Role of the endocrine system in the action of 2,3,7,8-tetrachloro-dibenzo-*p*-dioxin (TCDD) on the thymus. *Toxicology,* **15**, 135–44.

Vos, J.G. (1977). Immune suppression as related to toxicology. *CRC Crit. Rev. Toxicol.,* **5**, 67–101.

Vos, J.G., and Moore, J.A. (1974). Suppression of cellular immunity in rats and mice by maternal treatment with 2,3,7,8-tetrachlorodibenzo-*p*-dioxin. *Int. Arch. Allergy Appl. Immunol.,* **47**, 777–94.

Vos, J.G., Brouwer, G.M.J., van Leeuwen, F.X.R., and Wagenaar, S. (1983a). Toxicity of hexachlorobenzene in the rat following combined pre- and post-natal exposure: Comparison of effects on immune system, liver and lung. In: Gibson, G.G., Hubbard, R., and Parke, D.V. (Eds), *Immunotoxicology,* Academic Press, London, pp. 219–35.

Vos, J.G., Faith, R.E., and Luster, M.I. (1980). Immune alterations. In Kimbrough, R.D. (Ed.), *Halogenated Biphenyls, Terphenyls, Naphthalenes, Dibenzodioxins and Related Products,* Elsevier–North-Holland Biomedical Press, Amsterdam, pp. 241–66.

Vos, J.G., Krajnc, E.I., and Beekhof, P. (1982). Use of the enzyme-linked immunosorbent assay (ELISA) in immunotoxicity testing. *Environ. Health Perspect.,* **43**, 115–21.

Vos, J.G., Krajnc, E.I., Beekhof, P.K., and van Logten, M.J. (1983b). Methods for testing immune effects of toxic chemicals: evaluation of the immunotoxicity of various pesticides in the rat. In: Miyamoto, J., and Kearney, P.C. (Eds), *Pesticide Chemistry: Human Welfare and the Environment,* volume 3. Pergamon Press, Oxford, pp. 497–504.

Vos, J.G., Ruitenberg, E.J., van Basten, N., Buys, J., Elgersma, A., and Kruizinga, W. (1983c). The athymic nude rat. IV. Immunocytochemical study to detect T-cells, and immunological and histopathological reactions against *Trichinella spiralis. Parasite Immunol.,* **5**, 195–215.

Vos, J.G., de Klerk, A., Krajnc, E.I., Kruizinga, W., van Ommen, B., and Rozing, J. (1984a). Toxicity of bis)tri-*n*-butyltin)oxide in the rat. II. Suppression of thymus-dependent immune responses and of parameters of nonspecific resistance after short-term exposure. *Toxicol. Appl. Pharmacol.,* **75**, 387–408.

Vos, J.G., van Logten, M.J., Kreeftenberg, J.G., and Kruizinga, W. (1984b). Effect of triphenyltin hydroxide on the immune system of the rat. *Toxicology,* **29**, 325–36.

Warner, J.F., and Dennert, G. (1982). Effects of a cloned cell line with NK activity on bone marrow transplants, tumour development and metastasis *in vivo. Nature,* **300**, 31–4.

Weiss, A., and Fitch, F.W. (1977). Macrophages suppress CTL generation in rat mixed leukocyte cultures. *J. Immunol.,* **119**, 510–16.

White, A., and Goldstein, A.L. (1972). Hormonal regulation of host immunity. In: Borek, F. (Ed.), *Immunogenicity. Frontiers of Biology,* volume 25, North-Holland Publishing Co., Amsterdam, pp. 334–64.

Wojdani, A., Nieto, M., Alfred, L.J., and Drew, C.R. (1983). Carcinogenic PAH compounds suppressed cell-mediated immune functions, and alter T-cell subsets in splenic lymphocyte populations. *Proc. Amer. Assoc. Cancer Res.,* **24**, 242.

Short-term Toxicity Tests for Non-genotoxic Effects
Edited by P. Bourdeau *et al.*
© 1990 SCOPE. Published by John Wiley & Sons Ltd

CHAPTER 16

Potential Short-term Tests to Detect Chemicals Capable of Causing Reproductive and Developmental Dysfunction

CARLTON H. NADOLNEY, NEIL CHERNOFF, ROBERT L. DIXON, KUNDAN S. KHERA, RALF KROWKE, BORIS V. LEONOV, DIETHER NEUBERT AND SONIA TABACOVA

16.1 INTRODUCTION

The reproductive cycle encompasses a wide variety of complex interactions at the molecular, cellular and structural levels within a specific chronological sequence. The cycle starts with gametogenesis and includes all the differentiational and developmental processes occurring during the prenatal and postnatal periods. A broad spectrum of biological processes is represented, and includes cellular replication, tissue development and differentiation, neuroendocrine regulation, peptide and steroid hormone synthesis and action, secretory processes, and smooth muscle function, among others. Each of these processes is vulnerable to a multiplicity of toxic interferences. It is, therefore, extremely unlikely that a small number of 'simple' tests will ensure the identification of all possible adverse reproductive and developmental effects.

In recent years, a great number of short-term tests for assessing reproductive toxicity has become available and can be performed in *in vivo* and *in vitro* systems. These have been recently reviewed in Vouk and Sheehan (1983). These tests have been developed as adjuncts to the existing array of primary test batteries and are designed to: (a) rank compounds for scheduling further testing; (b) generate more specific data on the basic biological processes which are involved in the reproductive cycle; and (c) further characterize the mode(s) of action of agents known to affect essential biological processes of the reproductive cycle.

In vivo tests evaluate reproductive performance and perinatal toxicity. *In vitro* methods assess responses to test chemicals and other toxic agents (for example, ionizing and non-ionizing radiation), employing systems involving the growth and development of cells, tissues and organs of invertebrate and vertebrate origins, and whole-embryo cultures of each. As our knowledge of basic mechanisms increases, it may also be possible to programme computer simulation models for quantitative analyses of the qualitative processes associated with particular developmental dysfunctions.

We seek to understand how foreign chemicals perturb essential biological processes and cause physiological dysfunction. Information is sought at all levels of hierarchical biological organization, but especially at the molecular level involving interaction between the exogenous chemical and its 'receptor' for toxicity. As our understanding of mechanisms of toxicity increases, laboratory testing to define toxicological hazards, and clinical examination for the identification of the earliest effect(s) of chemical exposure become more objective. In many cases, methods become more efficient, more time- and cost-effective, better conserve laboratory test animals, and involve fewer investigations. However, most short-term tests have not been validated for regulatory use.

16.2   EFFECTS ON THE MALE REPRODUCTIVE SYSTEM

In general, damage to gonads and their functions can result from: (a) direct actions of chemicals on germs cells; (b) actions affecting the accessory sex organs; and (c) actions on overall hormonal systems at either the gonadal or the hypothalamic-pituitary level. Temporally, these actions can occur either prenatally or during different time periods of postnatal life. The processes by which a chemical exerts its effects, whether through direct action, through interference with receptor interactions, or through altered steroid-metabolizing enzymes, is ultimately important for extrapolation to other chemicals or species. Evidence suggests that environmental chemicals have exerted their effects on reproduction via each of these mechanisms, often affecting more than one (World Health Organization, 1984).

16.2.1   Male accessory sex organs

The male accessory sex organs (namely, prostate, seminal vesicles and bulbourethral gland) produce secretions which serve as a buffer, vehicle or source of nutrients for sperm. In man, about 30 per cent of the semen volume comes from the prostate, while 60 per cent is produced by the seminal vesicles (Vouk and Sheehan, 1983).

Prostatic secretions are rich in acid phosphatase, lysozymes, citric acid, citric acid aminotransferase, dehydrogenases, zinc and magnesium, among other substances, while seminal vesicle secretions are rich in fructose and prostaglandins (Vouk and Sheehan, 1983). These biochemical constituents are androgen-dependent and can be measured to assess androgenic activity of toxicants, using testosterone as a reference standard.

Seminal vesicle fructose has been used as a sensitive indicator for testosterone and other androgens. It decreases following castration and can be restored by androgen administration. Fructose can be measured spectrophotometrically by several different techniques (Thomas *et al.*, 1968). Prostate citric acid (Humphrey and Mann, 1949) and zinc (Gunn and Gould, 1956) concentrations can also be used to assess androgenic activity. These chemical indicator tests for androgens are more sensitive than gravimetric responses used in bioassay procedures (Thomas and Bell, 1982). Androgen-binding protein (ABP) can also be quantified.

Short-term *in vivo* bioassays based on the response of male sex accessory organs to androgens have been traditionally used to assess androgenic substances (Zarrow *et al.*, 1964). Newer techniques make use of radioimmunoassays (RIAs), enzyme immunosorbent assays (ELISAs), and high pressure liquid chromatography (HPLC).

16.2.2   Effects on androgen production and androgen receptors

Androgens are the principal sex hormones produced by the testis. The most important of these is testosterone secreted by the Leydig cells. The conversion of testosterone to oestrogen is thought to take place in the Sertoli cells. Although the precise hormonal regulation of spermatogenesis is not completely understood, current information suggests that testosterone is involved in such key processes as the generation of spermatogonia and the first meiotic division of diplotene cells at puberty. The androgen-protein (ABP) produced by Sertoli cells transports androgens to differentiating germ cells. The Sertoli cells have recently been the subject of much research (Mather *et al.*, 1982).

A potential testicular toxin could be studied by exposing primary cultures and continuous cell lines of rat or mouse Leydig cells to various concentrations of the toxin in the presence of luteinizing hormone (LH) and then comparing the amount of testosterone produced to that produced by LH alone. The amount of testosterone produced by the Leydig cells can be measured in the culture medium by radioimmunoassay (Furuyama *et al.*, 1970; Kinouchi *et al.*, 1973). The sensitivity of the RIA techniques continues to be refined to detect very low levels.

Androgen production and transport are regulated by the anterior pituitary gonadotropins. Follicle-stimulating hormone (FSH) stimulates Sertoli cells to produce androgen-binding protein (ABP). LH stimulates the synthesis of androgens in the interstitial cells.

Chemicals can interfere with androgen production by either directly affecting steroid synthesis in interstitial cells or by interfering with the regulation of steroid synthesis by the pituitary gonadotropins. Effects of chemicals on the production of testosterone and ABP have been studied *in vivo* and are now being investigated in *in vitro* cultures of Leydig and Sertoli cells. The responsiveness of Sertoli cells (preferably from post-pubertal males) in culture can be used to assess ABP following stimulation by FSH and incubation with the test chemical.

Cytoplasmic and nuclear androgen receptors in the target tissues are being actively studied and toxicologic applications are being increasingly sought. Gonadotropin receptors also have been demonstrated in the testes of some species.

Affinity constants of these receptors can be estimated and the effects of various exogenous chemicals on hormone–receptor interactions determined.

16.2.3 Effects on sperm

Substances can pass from blood into semen via the fluid from the excurrent ducts and the male accessory glands and could be spermicidal or alter sperm function. Such effects can be tested *in vitro* by exposing sperm (incubated in a protein-rich buffer at 37°C for 4 to 8 hours) for various periods (up to 8 hours) of time. The decline in percentage of motile sperm over time is a suitable criterion to study dose–response relationships. Other criteria, such as integrity of the acrosome and plasma membrane, oxygen consumption, adenosine 5'-triphosphate content, or degree of agglutination could be used. Methods are available for extended semen analysis, including survival and motility patterns, metabolic patterns, intracellular constituents, as well as sperm penetration of cervical mucus (Eliasson, 1978). It is felt, however, that this latter test is not a reliable indicator for predicting spermicidal action of agents *in vivo* (ORNL, 1982).

16.2.4 Biotransformation of toxicants in testicular tissues

Exogenous chemicals introduced into an organism may undergo chemical transformations resulting in metabolites which may be more toxic than the parent compound. The toxic effects of certain polycyclic hydrocarbons in tissues have been demonstrated to be due to metabolites (an epoxide) which interact with DNA, RNA and other macromolecules. The rate of epoxide formation and detoxifying enzyme activities in tissues or cells are important determinants of tissue-specific toxicity and of the sensitivity of cells to the toxicant's actions.

Appreciable activities of aryl hydrocarbon hydroxylase (AHH), epoxide hydrase (EH), glutathione transferase (GSH-SY), and cytochrome P-450 have been found in isolated, perfused testicular tissues (Mukhtar *et al.*, 1978). The distribution of these enzymes in the interstitial and germ cell compartments indicates that AHH activity and cytochrome P-450 content of microsomes from the interstitial cells are nearly twice that in the seminiferous tubules. In contrast, the specific activity of the detoxication enzymes EH and GSH-ST in seminiferous tubules is twice that in the interstitial cells. Although AHH activity in interstitial cells has been found to be only 5 per cent that of hepatic microsomes, its close proximity to the germ cells may increase its importance with regard to the effects of enzyme-activated toxic chemicals on germ cells. However, haemodynamics and the blood–testis barrier must be considered when drug- or toxicant-metabolizing activity is determined *in vitro*.

Factors affecting induction of AHH and cytochrome P-450 may play a significant role in germ cell toxicity. Both testicular and prostatic AHH activity and cytochrome P-450 are significantly induced by 2,3,7,8-tetrachlorodibenzo-*p*-dioxin(TCDD). TCDD doubled the AHH activity in the rat testis and increased

AHH activity in the prostate 150 times (Dixon and Lee, 1980a). Thus, exposure to environmental chemicals can induce significant activation of enzymes in the testis as well as in the prostate, thereby suggesting modulation of potential germ cell toxicity. The isolation of a toxicant from specific testicular tissues and the measurement of drug-metabolizing enzyme activities in these tissues following exposure to chemicals can be used as an indicator of such effects. The velocity sedimentation technique (Lee and Dixon, 1972) can be used to separate physically complex spermatogenic cell populations into homogeneous subpopulations capable of normal function. This technique also can be used to determine the cellular affinity of specific spermatogenic cells for chemicals, including trace metals (Lee and Dixon, 1973).

16.2.5   DNA damage, synthesis, and repair in spermatogenic cells

DNA repair by spermatogenic cells is a sensitive indicator of chemically-induced DNA damage. Evidence for this form of repair has come from the detection of unscheduled DNA synthesis (UDS), sometimes called 'repair synthesis'. The uptake of ^{3}H-thymidine into cells that are not in S-phase is generally taken as an indicator of UDS (Dixon and Hall, 1982).

Cellular fractionation of tissue demonstrates that the uptake of thymidine label is normally confined to spermatogonial cells, which indicates that these cells are uniquely involved in normal DNA synthesis (Dixon and Lee, 1980b). Following administration of DNA-damaging chemicals (such as methyl-methanesulphonate), thymidine incorporation has been demonstrated not only in spermatogonia but also in the leptotene, zygotene, pachytene, and diplotene cells (Lee and Dixon, 1978). Because the postmeiotic cell types do not normally incorporate thymidine, they are sensitive dosimeters of DNA damage when the repair mechanism is triggered.

16.3   EFFECTS ON THE FEMALE REPRODUCTIVE SYSTEM

The ovary is responsible for two roles in reproduction: nurture and release of gametes and hormone production. Xenobiotic compounds can alter both these aspects of ovarian function. The assessment of oocyte and follicle toxicity of chemicals is of great significance because the effect is irreversible: there is no mechanism for repopulation of oocytes in the ovary.

16.3.1   Assessment of oocyte and follicle toxicity

A short-term *in vivo* murine assay has been recommended as a sensitive indicator for xenobiotic effect on oogenesis (ORNL, 1982). The test is performed on inbred mouse strains which have been shown to be the most sensitive test strains for oocyte and follicle toxicity assays (Mattison, 1979). Prenatal as well as postnatal treatments are employed. After treatment, mice are sacrificed at varying time intervals and their ovaries removed, fixed, serially sectioned and stained. Oocytes and follicles are counted, and stages of follicular development are quantified and compared (Pedersen and Peters, 1968). The percentage of atretic follicles and the relative percentages of primordial, growing and graafian follicles are calculated. The assay appears to be a much more sensitive indicator of oocyte and follicle damage than alterations in fertility. Evidence suggests that as many as 90 per cent of all oocytes have to be destroyed before alterations in fertility of the female can be observed.

Assessment of oocyte and follicle toxicity of chemicals can also be performed *in vitro* in ovarian organ cultures by morphological assessment of follicular and oocytic growth and maturation, incidence of follicular artresia, and biochemical analysis of follicular fluid composition.

Effects of chemicals on oogonia can be evaluated *in vivo* by cytological quantitation. The test compound is administered to the experimental animal on the day of maximal oogonial proliferation. The day of sacrifice is based on the time when most of the oogonia are in dictyale stage. Gametotoxicity is assessed using indices of oogonial mitosis and germ cell degeneration. Germ cell responses to toxicants have been shown not only by a decrease in the total number of oocytes, but also by a change in the relative number of oocytes at different stages of meiosis. Similar methods utilizing *in vitro* organ cultures of fetal ovaries from humans and other mammals have also been used (Neal and Baker, 1974; Kurilo *et al.*, 1983).

16.3.2 Effects on ovarian steroid synthesis

The predominant steroids produced by the ovary are oestrogen (primarily 16β-oestradiol), progesterone, and androgens. Follicular oestrogen is produced by direct cell secretion or granulosa cell aromatization of thecal androgen (Armstrong and Dorrington, 1977). Androgens are produced by thecal and interstitial cells. Progesterone is produced by the corpus luteum formed from both granulosa and thecal compartments after ovulation. Under the influence of the hypophyseal gonadotropins, endocrine activity of the ovary is diphasic: (i) secretion of oestrogen during the first, follicular phase; (ii) excretion of both oestrogen and progesterone produced by the corpus luteum in the second, luteal phase. A drop in both steroids occurs at the time of menses in a non-conceptive cycle. Androgens are secreted throughout a non-conceptive cycle, with a slight rise in midcycle. An alteration in steroidogenic processes can have major effects on the reproductive function.

In vitro models are valuable for assessment of the effect of toxicants on steroid synthesis because of the direct action of toxicants on the culture components. The following aspects are of importance in developing a model system: (a) the cell-type specific steroids to be measured; (b) the cycle-related variations in sex steroid production; and (c) the key biochemical rate-limiting steps in steroid biosynthesis.

Adequate methodology is currently available for isolation of ovarian cell types (Haney and Schomberg, 1978; McNatty *et al.*, 1979), tissue or organ culture, and direct RIA of media for individual steroids (Butcher *et al.*, 1974; Korenman, 1969).

Because of the ease of culture, purity of cell type, and active basal steroidogenesis, isolated granulosa cell cultures represent attractive models for evaluation of a toxicant's potential effect on steroidogenesis.

Biochemical rate-limiting steps in gonadal steroid secretion include: (a) substrate (cholesterol) availability; (b) follicle-stimulating hormone (FSH) induction of granulosa cell aromatase activity converting thecal androgens to oestrogens; and (c) luteinizing hormone (LH) induction of enzyme steps converting cholesterol to pregnenolone.

It should be noted that the removal of the cells from their approximation to the thecal layer, contact with follicular fluid, or disruption of intricate cell-to-cell contact, may alter their steroidogenic potential and morphologic apearance *in vitro*. For these reasons, the use of intact follicle cells, without separation of the thecal and granulosa compartments, may have to be considered as a test system, if problems are encountered with isolated cell systems.

To detect long-acting oestrogenic compounds with slow clearance *in vivo* such as clomiphene and nafoxidine, oestrogen receptor assays can be done *in vivo* (Clark *et al.*, 1978; 1979). These assays involve injecting various dose levels of the compound into immature rats and measuring the nuclear accumulation and cytoplasmic depletion of oestrogen receptors in the uterine tissues (Clark *et al.*, 1979). The test is sensitive, easy to perform and requires relatively few animals.

Short-term *in vivo* tests used routinely for assessment of oestrogenic activity involve determination of the time of vaginal opening and uterine epithelial cell hypertrophy in the rat after treatment with the test compound shortly after birth (Gellert *et al.*, 1972; Clark and McCormack, 1980). The tests are simple, reproducible and quite sensitive to oestrogenic compounds.

16.3.3   Receptor interactions

The study of nuclear and cytoplasmic hormone receptors (oestradiol and progesterone receptors are especially important) in target tissues is a rapidly developing field with important toxicological applications. Chemicals may compete for these receptors, alter their conformation, induce qualitative changes in their cellular content, or uncouple them from intercellular events.

The oestrogen receptor may play a role in the toxicity of many environmental agents. Metabolites of DDT, DMBA, PCBs, and similar aromatic foreign chemicals, have been reported to bind to the cytoplasmic receptors for oestrogen (Dixon and Hall, 1982). Thus, interactions between xenobiotics and cellular receptors for endogenous hormones can result in inadvertent hormonal response (agonist) or can depress normal hormonal balance (antagonist). In either case, abnormal quantitative responses by reproductive tissues can result.

A sensitive and reproducible method for *in vitro* oestrogen receptor analysis involves the use of toxicants to compete with labelled oestradiol in binding to uterine cytoplasmic oestrogen receptors (Clark *et al.*, 1979; Katzenellenbogen *et al.*,

1980; Kupfer and Bulger, 1980). This test involves the addition of various concentrations of the toxicant to uterine cytosol fractions in the presence of labelled oestradiol. If the toxicant is oestrogenic, it will compete with oestradiol for binding to receptor sites, and a classic competitive inhibition curve can be obtained. From this curve, a relative binding affinity can be calculated that reflects the agonistic or antagonistic activity of the toxicant. Such estimates of oestrogenic activity can be used to extrapolate oestrogenic activity in humans. The test is simple and requires little expense.

16.4 INTERFERENCE WITH HYPOTHALAMIC–PITUITARY FUNCTION

The gametogenic and secretory functions of the gonads are dependent upon the secretion of gonadotropins (FSH, LH) and prolactin from the anterior pituitary gland which, in turn, is controlled by the hypothalamus through gonadotropin-releasing hormones. The sex hormones feed back through the hypothalamus to inhibit gonadotropin secretion by controlling releasing factors. FSH stimulates follicular development in the ovary and spermatogenesis in the testis. LH, referred to as interstitial-cell-stimulating hormone (ICSH) in the male, causes luteinization of the ovary and stimulates androgen production by testicular Leydig cells. Prolactin is involved in the initiation and maintenance of lactation in women. In rodents, prolactin maintains the corpus luteum; it is not lutetotropic in women (Thomas and Bell, 1982).

A toxicant can adversely affect reproduction by altering the rate of secretion of one or more hormones that are synthesized and released by the hypothalamus and anterior pituitary gland. Some chemicals (for example, reserpine) act on endogenous catecholamines which, secondarily, influence the ability of the sympathetic nervous system to stimulate gonadotropin release (Coppola *et al.*, 1966; Currie *et al.*, 1969). Others, like phenothiazine derivatives, suppress the hypothalamus and bring about a decrease in gonadotropin levels by suppressing the synthesis and/or release of gonadotropin-releasing factor (Jarvik, 1965). Substances that have oestrogenic activity or act as dopamine antagonists can stimulate the secretion of prolactin and, as a consequence of the hyperprolactinaemia, gonadotropin secretion becomes suppressed.

In vitro model systems are needed for the assessment of toxicants that influence these processes. Currently, little is known about such model systems but their value for predicting toxicity is potentially great. Listed below are a few *in vitro* model systems (ORNL, 1982) which can be used to assess the effects of toxicants on the secretion of gonadotropins by pituitary cells.

16.4.1 Release of hormones from pituitary cells

The ability for a test substance to stimulate the release of gonadotropins from pituitary cells can be measured, using pituitary cells cultured in monolayers from oestrogen–progesterone primed female rats. The gonadotropin-releasing standard should be synthetic gonadotropin-releasing hormone (GnRH). After three to five days in culture, the cells can be incubated in the presence of luteinizing hormone-releasing hormone (LHRH) or the test substance. The response parameter (production of LH, for example) can be measured in the culture medium by a radio-immunoassay (RIA) (Monroe *et al.*, 1968; Millar and Aehnelt, 1977). Using this system, a bioassay can be performed to evaluate the gonadotropin-releasing activity of the test substance and its relative potency in terms of LHRH.

Anterior pituitary tissue from female rats castrated four to six weeks before testing can be used to assay a substance for inhibition of gonadotropin release. For a reference standard, 17β-oestradiol could be used to suppress the release of LH in the culture medium.

The potential of a test substance to stimulate the release of prolactin can be measured in monolayer cultures of anterior pituitary cells obtained from young or mature female rats. The reference standard for the release of prolactin could be haloperidol. After three to five days in culture, the reference standard or the test substance is introduced and prolactin release measured by RIA. RIAs for prolactin have been developed for several species (Hwang *et al.*, 1971; Neill and Reichert, 1971; Clemons and Nicoll, 1977), and for *in vitro* bioassays (Frantz and Turkington, 1972).

To test a substance for inhibition of prolactin release, anterior pituitary tissue from oestrogenized female rats can be used under *in vitro* conditions. For a reference standard, bromoergocriptine could be used. Anterior pituitary tissue can be incubated in the presence of various concentrations of bromoergocriptine or the test substance to establish a dose–response curve. Then a bioassay can be conducted, where the concentration of prolactin in the culture medium is the responsive variable.

At present, there are no suitable model systems for assessment of agents which alter the secretion of GnRH, or the secretion of dopamine and norepinephrine by hypothalamic neurons.

16.4.2 Indirect *in vivo* assays

Levels of pituitary gonadotropins can be assessed indirectly (for example, in the female, measurement of testosterone or the histological assessment of spermatogenesis). Short-term *in vivo* methods for the bioassay of FSH and LH are available. These tests measure a quantitative response of a target organ under stimulation by the hormone or test chemical (Steelman and Pohley, 1953; Parlow, 1961). However, the bioassays of gonadotropins have been largely abandoned due to their lack of sensitivity. The sensitivity of RIAs offers substantial advantages over bioassays, even though cross-reactivity between the gonadotropins and other hormones may weaken the correlation between biological and immunological activities.

16.5   EFFECTS ON FERTILIZATION

Many of the toxic influences on germ cells of both sexes are manifested in reduced rates of conception. There is increasing evidence from animal studies that certain chemicals can inhibit the fertilizing ability of sperm without marked effects on any of the common semen parameters (Tsunoda and Chang, 1976a,b).

The phenomenon of fertilization can be arbitrarily divided into four phases: capacitation; penetration of the egg by the sperm; activation of the egg; and the union of egg and sperm pronuclei. *In vitro* fertilization methods allow the identification of chemicals which alter the fertilization process.

16.5.1   *In vitro* heterologous fertilization tests

In vitro heterologous fertilization tests are the only means available for assessing the fertilizing capacity of human sperm. Human *in vitro* fertilization cannot itself be used as a test, therefore, substitutes are used for the human ovum. These include the zona-free hamster ova (Yanagimachi *et al.*, 1976) and the zona pellucida of stored human follicular oocytes (Yanagimachi *et al.*, 1979).

The heterologous *in vitro* fertilization technique involves a series of steps (Dixon and Hall, 1982). After performing standard semen analysis, the sperm is capacitated. Zona-free hamster ova are added to control and experimental sperm and three hours later fertilizing capacity is assayed (for the sperm binding to the ovum; decondensed sperm head; and/or the presence of the pronucleus with the corresponding sperm tail in the ovum's cytoplasm). Further normal development, such as genetic union of the cells, does not occur under these artificial conditions. A consistent failure of human sperm to penetrate more than 10 per cent of zona-free hamster eggs is considered to reflect an abnormality of the physiological events associated with fertilization (that is, sperm capacitation or the acrosome reaction).

16.5.2   *In vitro* homologous fertilization tests

Effects of chemicals on further fertilization events, for example, activation of the egg and the union of egg and sperm nuclei, can be assessed by homologous *in vitro* fertilization tests utilizing laboratory animals. Sperm penetration of the ovum, cortical reaction, decondensation of sperm nucleus, release of second polar body, appearance of male and female pronuclei, and cleavage of the early embryo are all directly analogous in laboratory animals and man. *In vitro* fertilization can also be coupled with pre-implantation embryo culture, transfer of blastocysts to pseudopregnant recipients, and evaluation of pregnancy outcome to identify critical early developmental targets of environmental chemicals. Male and female gametes can be exposed to environmental agents either *in vitro* or *in vivo* and then be used for *in vitro* fertilization. The zygote is subsequently cultured and the early embryo transferred to a pseudopregnant recipient. Using this approach, the following parameters can be monitored: *in vitro* fertilizing capacity; 4- and 8-cell stage formation; morula and blastocyst development; implantation success, pregnancy rate, and malformations. Thus, chemical effects on the sperm and ova, early development, pre-implantation and post-implantation embryos, and birth defects can be studied.

16.6 SYSTEMS USED AS PRE-SCREENS FOR REPRODUCTIVE AND DEVELOPMENTAL DYSFUNCTION

Various developmental systems (cell and organ cultures, whole-embryo cultures, and whole-animals) have been used as supplements to standard teratology bio-assays. These systems have been used for the elucidation of basic mechanisms involved in abnormal development and for the ranking of chemicals for further standard teratogenesis testing. The latter is especially important, since the number of chemical agents introduced into the environment continues to increase. Rejection of an agent on the basis of a pre-screen test would avoid the implementation of costly and time consuming standard tests.

A simpler system is preferable to the whole organism only if the underlying toxic mechanism is largely understood, occurs universally, and can be completely mimicked. In the short-term tests used in mutagenicity studies, these prerequisites seem to have been fulfilled to some extent, but even there, no single test system has been found to be fully adequate. The situation for prenatal toxicity is more complex than for mutagenicity, since numerous mechanisms are known to result in abnormal development. Thus, no one test system is likely to identify all the abnormal reactions that can occur. Short-term test methods and their applicability have been reviewed by Neubert (1983) and Shepard *et al.* (1983).

An outline of the array of developmental systems now in use is provided in Table 16.1. Those systems which have been more extensively studied and/or utilized as tools of basic research or proposed for pre-screens will be highlighted below.

16.6.1 Mammalian *in vivo* tests

A simple and inexpensive test has been developed which utilizes the tendency of fetal toxicity to manifest itself as reduced perinatal growth and/or increased peri-natal death (due to either *in utero* resorptions or postnatal maternal cannibalism) (Chernoff and Kavlock, 1982). The protocol for this test involves treating the pregnant mammal during the period of organogenesis and allowing the dams to give birth. The litters are examined, counted and weighed at birth. Postnatal growth and viability have been closely correlated with effects seen after the far more laborious standard teratology bioassay (Brown and Fabro, 1981; Doe *et al.*, 1983). This *in vivo* assay maintains the feto–maternal–placental unit and can be utilized with any

Table 16.1   Short-term tests for detecting effects on fetal development

System	Period of development covered	Developmental process studied and endpoint	Reference
I. *Mammalian (In vivo)*	Organogenesis	Perinatal growth and viability	Chernoff and Kavlock (1982); Doe *et al.* (1983)
II. *Mammalian (whole-embryo culture)*			
Mammalian embryos (including human)	Pre-implantation	Fertilization, cleavage, and blastocyst formation	Brinster (1970); Spielmann and Eibs (1978); Hsu (1980)
Rodent embryos	Post-implantation organogenesis	Organogenesis over 2 (or 3) days	New (1966a, b); Cockcroft and Coppola (1977); Shepard *et al.* (1969); Chatot *et al.* (1980); Klee-Trieschmann and Neubert (1981); Sadler and Warner (1984); Priscott *et al.* (1984)
III. *Organ culture*			
Limb buds (avian, rodent)	Late organogenesis	Morphogenesis, cartilage formation, muscle formation	Kochhar (1975); Neubert *et al.* (1974); Neubert and Bluth (1981)
Human digits		Pharmacological effects and growth	Rajan (1969); Rajan *et al.* (1980)
Palatal shelves	Organogenesis	Epithelial fusion and cell death, palate closure	Lahti and Saxén (1967); Saxén (1973); Pratt (1938)
Lens	Organogenesis	Lens differentiation, histogenesis, and protein production	Karkinen-Jaaskelainen *et al.* (1975)
Sex organs	Late organogenesis	Gonodal and organ development, germ cell maturation, accessory sex gland histogenesis	Jost and Bergerard (1949); Josso (1974); Lasnitzki and Mizuno (1981)

Kidney	Late organogenesis	Nephrogenesis, histogenesis	Crocker (1973); Saxén and Ekblom (1981)
Thyroid	Late organogenesis	Thyroid histogenesis functional development	Shepard (1974)
IV. *Tissue culture*			
Lung	Organogenesis	Pattern formation, cell recognition, and adhesion	Merker *et al.* (1981)
Skeletal muscle	Organogenesis	Myogenesis, cell fusion, and histogenesis	Holtzer *et al.* (1958)
Teratocarcinoma	Organogenesis	Histogenesis	Stevens (1967)
Human embryonic cells	Organogenesis	Growth of palatal and mesenchymal cells	Pratt (1983); Pratt *et al.* (1982); Wilk *et al.* (1980)
Neural cells	Organogenesis	Histogenesis	Flint (1983); Flint *et al.* (1984)
V. *Sub-mammalian systems*			
Chick embryo *(in ovo)*	Entire	Whole development	Jelinek (1982); Jelinek and Peterka (1981); Jelinek and Rychter (1979)
Amphibian embryos	Entire	Whole development	Schultz *et al.* (1982)
Fish embryos	Entire	Whole development	Streisinger (1975)
Hydra attenuata	Adult and embryonic	Aggregation and movement, regeneration of damaged and dissociated adults	Johnson (1980); Johnson *et al.* (1982)
Sea urchins	Cleavage	Cell replication and contacts	Costello *et al.* (1957); Hagstrom and Lonning (1973)
Drosophila spp.	Embryogenesis	Embryogenesis	Buzin and Bournias-Vardiabasis (1984)

applicable route of exposure. It has an additional advantage over standard tests in that it can enable investigators to identify postnatal function deficits that may not be apparent in prenatal morphological end-points.

16.6.2   Mammalian embryo cultures

It is now possible to culture mammalian embryos from the one- or two-cell stage to the blastocyst stage. In general, pre-implantation embryos cannot be cultured beyond stages corresponding to implantation or early post-implantation. Hsu (1979) has developed a system in which it is possible to study mammalian development *in vitro* from the pre-implantation phase to the late embryonic stages. However, the success rate of this model has not yet exceeded 10 per cent. Rat embryos (8.5–10.5 day-old) can be cultured over a 48-hour period, and embryonic stages corresponding to about 35-somites can be reached (Fantel, 1982; Sadler *et al.*, 1982).

Some studies have been conducted on mouse (Davis *et al.*, 1981) and hamster embryos (Givelber and Di Paolo, 1968). Rat embryos have been cultured traditionally in a medium containing rat serum, but some investigators have successfully grown them in human serum (Chatot *et al.*, 1980; Klein *et al.*, 1980), dialysed serum (Gunberg, 1976), and in a chemically-defined, serum-free medium (Klee-Trieschmann and Neubert, 1981).

Popov *et al.* (1981), Fantel *et al.* (1979), and others, have used a liver S9 microsomal system added to the culture to activate cyclophosphamide. Oglesby *et al.* (1984) have described an embryo culture system in which rat embryos are grown in the presence of hepatocytes of alternative species by allowing hepatic metabolites of one species to affect development of the other. Only gross morphological evaluations have been performed in most of this study. A morphological scoring system (Brown and Fabro, 1981) may be useful for evaluation but, for more detailed analysis, histological examination is essential (Herken and Anschuetz, 1981).

The applicability of the whole-embryo technique as a routine method is limited because it is expensive, too sensitive to disturbances, often of unknown origin, and prone to abnormal development even under normal conditions. Furthrmore, a maximum culture period of 48 hours is too short compared with the entire period of organogenesis.

The ultimate utility of mammalian embryo culture may lie in the ability to subject laboratory animal embryos to human tissue metabolites where appropriate heterologous systems are developed. Testing of compounds that are insoluble or soluble in toxic solvents is difficult and false positives are common with surface-active compounds.

16.6.3   Chick embryos *in ovo* used as pre-screens

Chemicals have frequently been tested in chick embryos at all stages of development by administration into fertile eggs (Fisher and Schoenwolf, 1983). This approach has not always provided results comparable with those obtained in mammalian systems. Moreover, it is doubtful whether the form and concentration of a chemical, when it reaches the embryo, can be known. A standard window technique for delivering the chemical to the chick embryo has been developed for embryotoxicity and teratogenicity studies in which better control of experimental conditions is possible (Jelinek and Peterka, 1981). The test substance is administered in a single application to the subgerminal portion of the yolk of the embryo on day 2, and intra-amniotically on days 3 or 4. The number of dead, malformed and growth-retarded embryos are counted on day 8 of incubation, when the study is terminated. The method is inexpensive and requires a moderate degree of skill. One of the major problems centres on the fact that the greatly reduced metabolic activity and difference in biochemical composition of the avian egg compared with a mammalian embryo can make the form and concentration of the xenobiotic very different.

16.6.4   Vertebrate embryo cultures

Test systems utilizing the embryos of amphibia and fish have been proposed for teratology screens (Dumont *et al.*, 1983; Streisinger, 1975). These tests are difficult to perform with water-insoluble compounds. Their potential use as screens remains unknown.

16.6.5   Invertebrates used as pre-screens

A number of invertebrates have been proposed as potential teratology pre-screens. These include *Drosophila* (Schuler *et al.*, 1982); *Planaria* (Best and Morita, 1982); and *Hydra* (Johnson, 1980; Johnson *et al.*, 1982). The respective end-points are developmental throughout entire metamorphosis; regeneration; and reassociation of disassociated adult cells. Should these systems be validated, they could be useful for rapid and inexpensive screening of large numbers of chemicals. However, the phylogenetic distance from humans may limit their usefulness for extrapolation.

16.6.6   Organ cultures

Two approaches to organ culture have been used: (a) the fetal organ is maintained on a filter or other support, and differentiates at the culture medium–gas interface (Trowell, 1961; and (b) the fetal organ is submerged in the culture medium and rotated to facilitate gas exchange and diffusion.

The Trowell technique is used for the culture of limb buds from rat (Shepard and Bass, 1970) or mouse (Aydelotte and Kochhar, 1972) embryos. It can also be used for limb buds from embryos of other species, for example, rabbit, chick, or ferret (Lessmollmann *et al.*, 1976; Beck and Gulamhusein, 1980), in a serum-containing medium or a chemically-defined medium. Growth of limb buds in culture is retarded compared with *in vivo* development, but morphological differentiation of the cartilaginous bone anlagen and muscle can be observed. The extent of the morphogenetic differentiation of the cartilaginous bone anlagen depends largely on the stage of development at which the cultures are initiated.

The submerged culture system has also been used successfully for the study of limb bud differentiation *in vitro* (Neubert and Barrach, 1977; Blankenburg *et al.*, 1981). Abnormal development has been induced *in vitro* by adding various teratogens to the culture medium (Welsch *et al.*, 1978; Stahlmann *et al.*, 1981).

It has been possible to quantify the extent of differentiation achieved in nculture and to establish dose–response relationships for abnormal development using the organ culture system. Biochemical variables, such as levels of DNA, RNA, protein, collagen, etc., can be measured (Neubert *et al.*, 1974); or a score system may be used for morphogenetic differentiation (Neubert *et al.*, 1977a,b; 1978).

Growth and differentiation of the palatal shelves have been achieved in organ culture. This system has been used extensively to study cleft palate-inducing agents (Lahti and Saxen, 1967; Pratt, 1983).

Lens development can be followed using human embryonic material. The induction of abnormal development by rubella virus can be mimicked *in vitro*. Cataract formation was observed by Karkinen-Jaaskelainen *et al.* (1975).

Organ culture techniques have been developed for the study of explanted mouse or human embryonic kidney (Crocker,1973; Saxén and Ekblom, 1981). This system may prove useful for investigating the normal mechanism of renal development and also for testing suspected nephrotoxic agents. The expense and time involved are both fairly high since the end-points require histological analysis.

Organ culture of embryonic gonads together with accessory ducts has contributed to the understanding of how hormones and some hormone inhibitors modify sexual development.

16.6.7   Tissue culture systems

Primary cultures from various embryonic tissues have been used in developmental studies, including the chick neural crest (Greenberg, 1982), heart mesenchymal cells, and skeletal muscle cells (Holtzer *et al.*, 1958). However, it must be remembered that some cells may change their characteristics in culture. Pratt *et al.* (1982) have used an established cell line from the human embryonic palatal mesenchyme (HEPM) to study the biochemical basis for the way in which glucocorticoids inhibit palatal mesenchymal cell growth and cause cleft palate in the rodent.

It seems possible that, in some instances, primary cell cultures of embryonic or fetal cells, including those from human embryos or fetuses, can be used for studies on the drug-metabolizing capacity of cells during prenatal, and especially perinatal, development (Nau *et al.*, 1977; Egger *et al.*, 1978; Liddiard *et al.*, 1978; Merker *et al.*, 1981; Kremers *et al.*, 1981).

16.6.8　Studies with non-embryonic tissues

There are a number of non-embryonic tissue systems which can be used to study mechanisms of embryotoxic effects. Basic processes, such as cell–cell interactions, cell migrations, differentiation processes, proliferation processes, and cell death, can be used as end-points, as these are involved in embryonic development. Systems used include the investigation of aggregation phenomena with mammalian cells (Moscona and Moscona, 1952), cell–cell interactions as studied by the attachment of cells to lectin-coated surfaces (Braun *et al.*, 1982), and the inhibition of mammalian cell growth (Freese, 1982). The use of teratocarcinoma cells, which are pluripotent cells capable of many types of embryonic differentiation, might also be considered (Stevens, 1967; Graham, 1977; Martin, 1978).

REFERENCES

Armstrong, D.T. and Dorrington, J.H. (1977). Estrogen biosynthesis in the ovaries and testes. *Adv. Sex Horm. Res.*, **3**, 217–58.

Aydelotte, M.B. and Kochhar, D.M. (1972). Development of mouse limb buds in organ culture: Chondrogenesis in the presence of a proline analog, L-azetidine-2-carboxylic acid. *Dev. Biol.*, **28**, 191–201.

Beck, F. and Gulamhusein, A.P. (1980). The contrast between mouse and ferret limb buds in culture—possible advantages of comparing results from a limb culture system with whole embryo explanation. In: Merker, H.-J., Nau, H. and Neubert, D. (Eds), *Teratology of the Limbs*, Berlin, Walter de Gruyter, pp. 117–27.

Best, J.B. and Morita, N. (1982). Planarians as a model system for *in vitro* teratogenesis studies. *Teratog., Carinog. and Mutag.*, **2**, 277–91.

Blankenburg, G., Bluth, U. and Neubert, D. (1981). On the significance of ascorbate and of cysteine on differentiation of limb buds in organ culture. In: Neubert, D. and Merker, H.-J. (Eds), *Culture Techniques. Applicability for Studies on Prenatal Differentiation and Toxicity*, Berlin, Walter de Gruyter, pp. 197–206.

Braun, A.G., Nichinson, B.B. and Horowicz, P.B. (1982). Inhibition of tumour cell attachment to concanavalin A-coated surfaces as an assay for teratogenic agents: approaches to validation. *Teratog., Carcinog. and Mutag.*, **21**, 343–54.

Brinster, R.L. (1970). *In vitro* cultivation of mammalian ova. In: Raspe, G. (Ed.), *Advances in Biosciences*, volume 4, Oxford, Pergamon Press, pp. 199–233.

Brown, N.A. and Fabro, S. (1981). Quantitation of rat embryonic development *in vitro*: a morphological scoring system. *Teratology*, **214**, 65–78.

Butcher, R.L., Collins, W.E. and Fugo, N.W. (1974). Plasma concentration of LH, FSH, prolactin, progesterone and estradiol-17 beta throughout the 4-day estrous cycle of the rat. *Endocrinology*, **94**, 1704–8.

Buzin, C.H. and Bournias-Vardiabasis, N. (1984). Teratogens induce a subset of small heat shock proteins in *Drosphila* primary embryonic cell cultures. *Proc. Natl. Acad. Sci., USA*, **81**, 4075–9.

Chatot, C.L., Klein, N.W., Piatek, J. and Pierro, L.J. (1980). Successful culture of rat embryos on human serum: Use in the detection of teratogens. *Science*, **207**, 1471–3.

Chernoff, N. and Kavlock, R.J. (1982). An *in vivo* teratology screen utilizing pregnant mice. *J. Toxicol. Environ. Hlth.*, **10**, 541–50.

Clark, J.H. and McCormack, S.A. (1980). The effect of clonid and other triphenylethylene derivatives during pregnancy and the neonatal period. *J. Steroid Biochem.*, **12**, 47–53.

Clark, J.H., Peck, E.J. Jr., Hardin, J.W. and Eriksson, H. (1978). The biology and pharmacology of estrogen receptor binding: relationship to uterine growth. *Recept. Horm. Action,* **2**, 1–31.

Clark, J.H., Hardin, J.W., Eriksson, H., Upchurch, S. and Peck, E.J. Jr. (1979). Hertogeneity of estrogen-binding sites in the rat uterus. *Ontog. Recept. Reprod. Horm. Action,* **1**, 65–77.

Clemons, G.K. and Nicoll, C.S. (1977). Development and preliminary application of a homologous radioimmunoassay for bullfrog prolactin. *Gen. Comp. Endocrinol.,* **32**, 531–5.

Cockcroft, D.L. and Coppola, P.T. (1977). Teratogenic effects of excess glucose in head-fold rat embryos in culture. *Teratology,* **16**, 141–6.

Coppola, J.A., Leonardi, R.G. and Lippman, W. (1966). Ovulatory failure in rats after treatment with brain norepinephrine depletors. *Endocrinology,* **78**, 225–8.

Costello, D.P., Davidson, M.E., Eggers, A., Fox, M.H. and Henley, C. (1957). Methods for obtaining and handling marine eggs or embryos. Woods Hole Marine Biolo. Lab., Woods Hole, Massachusetts.

Crocker, J.F.S. (1973). Human embryonic kidneys in organ cultures: Abnormalities of development induced by decreased potassium. *Science,* **181**, 1178–9.

Currie, G.N., Black, D.L., Armstrong, D.T. and Greep, R.O. (1969). Blockade of ovulation in the rabbit with catecholaminies and sympathomimetics. *Proc. Soc. Exp. Biol.,* **130**, 598–602.

Davis, L.A., Sadler, T.W. and Langman, J. (1981). *In vitro* development of the heart under influence of retinoic acid. In: Neubert D. and Merker, H.-J. (Eds), *Culture Techniques. Applicability for Studies on Prenatal Differentiation and Toxicity,* Berlin, Walter de Gruyter, pp. 101–15.

Dixon R.L. and Hall, J.L. (1982). Reproductive Toxicology. In: Hayes, A.W. (Ed.), *Principles and Methods of Toxicology,* New York, Raven Press, pp. 107–39.

Dixon, R.L. and Lee, I.P. (1980a). Pharmacokinetic and adaptation factors in testicular toxicity. *Fed. Proc.,* **39**, 66–72.

Dixon, R.L. and Lee, I.P. (1980b). Metabolism of benzo(a)pyrene isolated perfused testis and testicular homogenate. *Life Sci.,* **27**, 2439–44.

Doe, J.E., Samuels, D.M., Tinston, D.J. and Wickramaratne, G.A. de Silva (1983). Comparative aspects of the reproductive toxicology by inhalation in rats of ethylene glycol monomethyl ether and propylene glycol monomethyl ether. *Toxicol. Appl. Pharmacol.,* **69**, 43–7.

Dumont, J.N., Schultz, T.W., Buchanan, M.V. and Kao, G.L. (1983). Frog embryo teratogenesis assay: *Xenopus* (FETAX)—A short-term assay applicable to complex environmental mixtures. In: Waters, M.D., Sandhu, S.S., Lewtas, J., Claxton, L., Chernoff, N. and Nesnow, S. (Eds), *Short-term Bioassays in the Analysis of Complex Environmental Mixtures III,* New York, Plenum Press, pp. 393–406.

Egger, H.J., Wittfoht, W. and Nau, H. (1978). Identification of diphenyl-hydantoin and its metabolites, including the dihydrodiol and the catechols in maternal plasma, placenta and fetal tissues of man. In: Neubert, D., Merker, H.-J., Nau, H. and Langman, J. (Eds), *Role of Pharmacokinetics in Prenatal and Perinatal Toxicology,* Stuttgart, Georg Thieme, pp. 483–97.

Eliasson, R. (1978). Semen analysis. *Environ. Health Perspect.,* **24**, 81–5.

Fantel, A.G. (1982). Culture of whole rodent embryos in teratogen screening. *Teratog., Carcinog., and Mutag.,* **2**, 231–42.

Fantel, A.G., Greenaway, J.C., Juchau, M.R. and Shepard, T.H. (1979). Teratogenic bioactivation of cyclophosphamide *in vitro. Life Sci.,* **25**, 67–72.

Fisher, M. and Schoenwolf, G.C. (1983). The use of early chick embryos in experimental embryology and teratology: improvements in standard procedures. *Teratology,* **27**, 65–72.

Flint, O.P. (1983). A micromass culture method for rat embryonic neural cells. *J. Cell Sci.,* **61**, 24–62.

Flint, O.P., Orton, T.C. and Ferguson, R.A. (1984). Differentiation of rat embryo cells in culture: response following acute maternal exposure to teratogens and non-teratogens. *J. Appl. Toxicol.*, **4**, 109–16.

Frantz, W. and Turkington, W. (1972). Formation of biologically active ^{125}I-prolactin by enzymatic radioiodination. *Endocrinology*, **91**, 1545–8.

Freese, E. (1982). Use of cultured cells in the identification of potential teratogens. *Teratog., Carinog., and Mutag.*, **2**, 355–60.

Furuyama, S., Mayes, D.M. and Nugent, C.A. (1970). A radioimmunoassay for plasma testosterone. *Steroids*, **16**, 415–28.

Gellert, R.J., Heinrichs, W.L. and Swerdloff, R.S. (1972). DDT homologs. Estrogen-like effects on the vagina, uterus and pituitary of the rat. *Endocrinology*, **91**, 1095–100.

Givelber, H.M. and Di Paolo, J.A. (1968). Growth of explanted eight-day hamster embryos in circulating medium. *Nature (Lond.)*, **220**, 1131–2.

Graham, C.F. (1977). Teratocarcinoma cells and normal mouse embryogenesis. In: Sherman, M.J. (Ed.), *Concepts in Mammalian Embryogenesis*, Cambridge, Massachusetts, MIT Press, pp. 315–95.

Greenberg, J.H. (1982). Detection of teratogens by differentiating embryonic neural crest cells in cultures; evaluation as a screening system. *Teratog., Carcinog. and Mutag.*, **2**, 319–23.

Gunberg, D.L. (1976). *In vitro* development of post-implantation rat embryos cultured on dialyzed rat serum. *Teratology*, **14**, 65–9.

Gunn, S.A. and Gould, T.C. (1956). The relative importance of androgen and estrogen in the selective uptake of Zn^{65} by the dorsolateral prostate of the rat. *Endocrinology*, **58**, 443–52.

Hagstrom, B.E. and Lonning, S. (1973). The sea urchin egg as a testing object in toxicology. *Acta Pharmacol. Toxicol.*, **32** (Suppl. 1), 3–49.

Haney, A.F. and Schomberg, D.W. (1978). Steroidal modulation of progesterone secretion by granulosa cells from large porcine follicles: a role for androgens and estrogens in controlling steroidogenesis. *Biol. Reprod.*, **19**, 242–8/

Herken, R. and Anschuetz, M. (1981). Differentiation of embryonic tissues in whole-embryo cultures as compared to the development *in vivo*. In: Neubert, D. and Merker, H.-J. (Eds), *Culture Techniques. Applicability for Studies on Prenatal Differentiation and Toxicity*, Berlin, Walter de Gruyter, pp. 19–35.

Holtzer, H., Abbot, J. and Lash, J. (1958). On the formation of multinucleated myotubes. *Anat. Rec.*, **131**, 567–8.

Hsu, Y.C. (1979). *In vitro* development of indivdiually cultured whole mouse embryos from blastocyst to early somite stage. *Dev. Biol.*, **68**, 453–61.

Hsu, Y.C. (1980). Embryo growth and differentiation factors in embryonic sera of mammals. *Dev. Biol.*, **76**, 465–74.

Humphrey, G.F. and Mann, J. (1949). Studies on the metabolism of semen: 5. Citric acid in semen. *Biochem. J.*, **44**, 97–105.

Hwang, P., Guyda, H. and Friesen, H. (1971). A radioimmunoassay for human prolactin. *Proc. Nat. Acad. Sci. USA*, **68**, 1902–6.

Jarvik, M.E. (1965). Drugs used in the treatment of psychiatric disorders. In: Goodman, L.S. and Gilman, A. (Eds), *The Pharmacological Basis of Therapeutics*. Macmillan, New York, pp. 159–80.

Jelinek, R. (1982). Use of chick embryo in screening for embryotoxicity. *Teratog., Carcinog. and Mutag.*, **2**, 255–62.

Jelinek, R. and Peterka, M. (1981). Morphogenetic systems and *in vitro* techniques in teratology. In: Neubert, D. and Merker, H.-J. (Eds), *Culture Techniques. Applicability for Studies on Prenatal Differention and Toxicity*, Berlin, Walter de Gruyter, pp. 553–7.

Jelinek, R. and Rychter, Z. (1979). Morphogentic systems and the central phenomenon of teratology. In: Persand, T.-V.N. (Ed.), *New Trends in Experimental Teratology*, Lancaster, M & P Press, pp. 41–62.

Johnson, E.M. (1980). A subvertebrate system for rapid determination of potential teratogenic hazards. *J. Environ. Pathol. Toxicol.*, **4**, 153–6.

Johnson, E.M., Gorman, R.M., Gabel, B.E.G. and George, M.E. (1982). The *Hydra attenuata* system for detection of teratogenic hazards. *Teratog., Carcinog. and Mutag.*, **2**, 263–76.

Josso, N. (1974). Effect of PGA2 and PGB on the rat foetal mullerian duct '*in vitro*': absence of relationship to testicular anti-mullerian hormone. *Biomedicine*, **21**, 225–9.

Jost, A. and Bergerard, Y. (1949). Culture *in vitro* d'ebauches du tractus genital du foetus de rat. *C.R. Soc. Biol.*, **143**, 608–9.

Karkinen-Jaaskelainen, M., Saxén, L., Vaheri, A. and Leinikki, P. (1975). Rubella cataract *in vitro*: sensitive period of the developing human lens. *J. Exper. Med.*, **141**, 1238–48.

Katzenellenbogen, J.A., Katzenellenbogen, B.S., Tatee, T., Robertson, D.W. and Landvatter, S.W. (1980). The chemistry of estrogens and antiestrogens: Relationships between structure, receptor binding and biological activity. In: McLachlan, J.A. (Ed.),. *Estrogens in the Environment*, New York, Elsevier/North-Holland, pp. 33–51.

Kinouchi, T., Pages, L. and Horton, R. (1973). A specific radioimmunoassay for testosterone in peripheral plasma. *J. Lab. Clin. Med.*, **82**, 309–16.

Klee-Trieschmann, V. and Neubert, D. (1981). Preliminary communication on the feasibility of culturing whole embryos in a chemically-defined medium. In: Neubert, D. and Merker, H.-J. (Eds), *Culture Techniques. Applicability for Studies on Prenatal Differentiation and Toxicity*, Berlin, Walter de Gruyter, pp. 97–100.

Klein, N.W., Vogler, M.A., Chatot, C.L. and Pierro, L.J. (1980). The use of cultured rat embryos to evaluate the teratogenic activity of serum: Cadmium and cyclophosphamide. *Teratology*, **21**, 199–208.

Kochhar, D.M. (1975). Assessment of teratogenic responses to cultured post-implantation mouse embryos: Effects of hydroxyurea. In: Neubert, D. and Merker, H.-J. (Eds), *New Approaches in the Evaluation of Abnormal Embryonic Development*, Stuttgart, Georg Thieme, pp. 250–77.

Korenman, S.G. (1969). Comparative binding affinity of estrogens and its relation to estrogenic potency. *Steroids*, **13**, 163–77.

Kremers, P., Goujon, F. De Graeve, J., Van Cantford, J. and Gielen, J.E. (1981). Multiplicity of cytochrome p-450 in primary fetal hepatocytes in culture. *Eur. J. Biochem.*, **115**, 67–72.

Kupfer, D. and Bulger, W.H. (1980). Estrogenic properties of DDT and its analogs. In: McLachlan, J.A. (Ed.), *Estrogens in the Environment*, Elsevier/North-Holland, New York, pp. 239–62.

Kurilo, L.F., Korogodina, Y.V. and Ignat'eva, E.L. (1983). Effect of thiophosphamide on the differentiation of the germ cell population in female CBA, 101/H and AKR mice. *Biull. Eksp. Biol. Med.*, **95**, 110–13 (in Russian).

Lahti, A. and Saxén, L. (1976). Effect of hydrocortisone on the closure of palatal shelves *in vivo* and *in vitro*. *Nature (Lond.)*, **216**, 1217–18.

Lasnitzki, I. and Mizuno, T. (1981). Interaction of epithelium and mesenchyme in the induction of fetal rat and mouse prostate glands by androgens in organ culture. In: Neubert, D. and Merker, H.-J. (Eds), *Culture Techniques. Applicability for Studies on Prenatal Differentiation and Toxicity*, Berlin, Walter de Gruyter, pp. 359–69.

Lee, I.P. and Dixon, R.L. (1972). Effects of vincristine on spermatogenesis studied by velocity sedimentation cell separation technique and serial mating. *J. Pharmacol. Exp. Therap.*, **181**, 192–9.

Lee, I.P. and Dixon, R.L. (1973). Effects of cadmium on spermatogenesis studied by velocity sedimentation cell separation and serial mating. *J. Pharmacol. Exp. Ther.*, **187**, 641–52.

Lee, I.P. and Dixon, R.L. (1978). Factors influencing reproduction and genetic toxic effects on male gonads. *Environ. Health Persp.,* **24**, 117–27.

Lessmollmann, U., Hinz, N. and Neubert, D. (1976). *In vitro* system for toxicological studies on the development of mammalian limb buds in a chemically-defined medium. *Arch. Toxicol.,* **36**, 169–76.

Liddiard, C., Brnedel, K. and Nau, H. (1978). Drug metabolism in cultures of isolated hepatocytes of the human fetus, the newborn pig and the adult rat. In: Neubert, D., Merker, H.-J., Nau, H. and Langman, J. (Eds), *Role of Pharmacokinetics in Prenatal and Perinatal Toxicology,* Stuttgart, Georg Thieme, pp. 91–108.

Martin, G.R. (1978). Advantages and limitations of teratocarcinoma stem cells as models of development. In: Hohnsonn, M.M. (Ed.), *Development in Mammals,* New York, Elsevier/North-Holland, pp. 225–61.

Mather, J.P., Zhuang, L.-Z., Perez-Infante, V. and Phillips, D. (1982). Culture of testicular cells in hormone-supplemented serum-free medium. In: Bardin, C.W. and Sherins, R.J. (Eds), *The Cell Biology of the Testis,* volume 383, New York, New York, New York Academy of Sciences, pp. 44–84.

Mattison D.R. (1979). Difference in sensitivity of rat and mouse primiordial oocytes to destruction by polycyclic aromatic hydrocarbons. *Chem. Biol. Interact.,* **28**, 133–7.

McNatty, K.P., Makris, A., Degrazia, C., Osanthanondh, R. and Ryan, K.J. (1979). The production of progesterone, androgens and estrogens by granulsoa cells, thecal tissue, and stromal tissue from human ovaries *in vitro. J. Clin. Endocrinol. Metab.,* **49**, 687.

Merker, H.-J., Zimmermann, B. and Riso, J. (1981). The embryonic lung as *in vitro* model for testing teratogenic substances. In: Neubert, D. and Merker, H.-J. (Eds), *Culture Techniques. Applicability for Studies on Prenatal Differentiation and Toxicity,* Berlin, Walter de Gruyter, pp. 301–17.

Millar, R.P. and Aehnelt, C. (1977). Application of ovine luteinizing hormone (LH) radioimmunoassay in the quantitation of LH in different mammalian species. *Endocrinology,* **101**, 760–68.

Monroe, S.E., Parlow, A.F. and Midgley, A.R. Jr. (1968). Radioimmunoassay for rat luteinizing hormone. *Endocrinology,* **83**, 1004–12.

Moscona, A. and Moscona, H. (1952). The dissociation and aggregation of cells from organ rudiments of the early chick embryo. *J. Anat.,* **86**, 287–301.

Mukhtar, H., Lee, I.P., Foureman, G.L. and Bend, J.R. (1978). Epoxide metabolizing enzyme activities in rat testes: postnatal development and relative activity in interstitial and spermatogenic cell compartments. *Chem. Biol. Inter.,* **22**, 152–65.

Nau, H., Liddiard, C., Brendel, K., Wittfoht, W. and Lance, J. (1977). Benzodiazepine metabolism studies in organ and isolated cell cultures of human fetal liver by a gas chromatography mass spectrometer computer system. In: Eggstein, M. and Liebich, H.M. (Eds), *Mass Spectrometry and Combined Techniques in Medicine, Clinical Chemistry and Clinical Biochemistry,* Tübingen, Tübingen University Press, pp. 346–58.

Neal, P. and Baker, T.G. (1974). Response of mouse ovaries *in vivo* and in organ culture to pregnant mare's serum gonadotropin and human chorionic gonadotropin. II. Effect of different doses of hormones. *J. Reprod. Fetil.,* **37**, 399–404.

Neill, J.D. and Reichert, L.E. Jr. (1971). Development of a radioimmunoassay for rat prolactin and evaluation of NIND rat prolactin radioimmunoassay. *Endocrinology,* **88**, 548–55.

Neubert, D. (1983). (Can mutagenicity tests or other *in vitro* methods replace carcinogenicity or other long-term *in vivo* studies?) In: Grosdanoff, P., Schneiders, B. and Uberla, K. (Eds), *Arzneim. Sicher.,* **1**, 83–8 (in German).

Neubert, D. and Barrach, H.J. (1977). Techniques applicable to study morphogenetic differentiation of limb buds in organ cultures. In: Neubert, D., Merker, H.-J. and Kwasigroch, T.E.

(Eds), *Methods in Prenatal Toxciology Evaluation of Embryotoxic Effects in Experimental Animals*, Stuttgart,Georg Thieme, pp. 241–51.

Neubert, D. and Bluth, U. (1981). Feasibility of storing embryonic tissues for subsequent use in organ culture. In: Neubert, D. and Merker, H.-J. (Eds), *Culture Techniques. Applicability for Studies on Prenatal Differentiation and Toxicity*, Berlin, Walter de Gruyter, pp. 171–3.

Neubert, D., Merker, H.-J. and Tapken, S. (1974). Comparative studies on the prenatal development of mouse extremities *in vivo* and in organ culture. *Naunyn-Schmiedeberg's Arch. Pharmacol.*, **286**, 250–70.

Neubert, D., Lessmollmann, U., Hinz, N., Dillmann, I. and Fuchs, G. (1977a). Interference of 6-mercaptopurine riboside, 6-methylmercaptopurine riboside and azathioprine with the morphogenetic differentiation of mouse extremities *in vivo* and organ culture. *Naunyn-Schmiedeberg's Arch. Pharmacol.*, **298**, 93–105.

Neubert, D., Merker, H.-J. and Kwasigroch, T.E. (Eds) (1977b). *Methods in Prenatal Toxicology. Evaluation of Embryotoxic Effects in Experimental Animals*, Stuttgart, Georg Thieme.

Neubert, D., Tapken, S. and Baumann, I. (1978). Influence of potential thalidomide metabolites and hydrolysis products on limb development in organ culture and on the activity of proline hydroxylase. Further data on our hypothesis on the thalidomide embryopathy. In: Neubert, D., Merker, H.-J., Nau, H. and Langman, J. (Eds), *Role of Pharmacokinetics in Prenatal and Perinatal Toxicology*, Stuttgart, Georg Thieme, pp. 359–82.

New, D.A.T. (1966a). Development of rat embryos cultured in blood sera. *J. Reprod. Fertil.,* **12**, 509–24.

New, D.A.T. (1966b). *The Culture of Vertebrate Embryos,* New York, Logos Press-Academic Press, 345 p.

Oak Ridge National Laboratory (ORNL) (1982). *Assessment of Risks to Human Reproduction and Development of the Human Conceptus from Exposure to Environmental Substances.* Proceedings of US EPA sponsored conferences: October 1–3, 1980, Atlanta, Georgia, and December 7–10, 1980, St. Louis, Missouri. Oak Ridge National Laboratory, Oak Ridge, Tennessee, 158 p.

Oglesby, L.A., Ebron, M.T., Carver, B. and Kavlock, R.J. (1984). An *in vitro* system for the co-cultivation of hepatocytes and rat embryos (Abstract). *Teratology,* **29**, 49A.

Parlow, A.F. (1961). Bioassay of pituitary luteinizing hormone by depletion of ovarian ascorbic acid. In: Albert, A. (Ed.), *Human Pituitary Gonadotropins*, Charles Thomas, Springfield, Illinois, 300 p.

Pedersen, T. and Peters, H. (1968). Proposal for a classification of oocytes and follicles in the mouse ovary. *J. Reprod. Fertil.,* **17**, 555–7.

Popov, V.B., Vaisman, B.L. and Puchkov, V.F. (1981). (Embryotoxic action of cyclophosphamide after biotransformation *in vitro* on development of rat embryos) *Buill. Eksp. Biol. Med.,* **91**, 613–15 (in Russian with English abstract).

Pratt, R.M. (1983). Mechanisms of chemically-induced cleft palate. *Trends Pharmacol. Sci.,* **4**, 160–2.

Pratt, R.M., Grove, R.I. and Willis, W.D. (1982). Prescreening for environmental teratogens using cultured mesenchymal cells from the human embryonic palate. *Teratog., Carcinog. and Mutag.,* **2**, 313–18.

Priscott, P.K., Yeoh, G.C.T. and Oliver, I.T. (1984). The culture of 12- and 13-day rat embryos using continuous and non-continuous gassing of rotating bottles. *J. Exp. Zool.,* **30**, 247–53.

Rajan, K.T. (1969). The cultivation *in vitro* of post fetal mammalian cartilage and its repsonse to hypervitaminosis A. *Exp. Cell. Res.,* **55**, 419–23.

Rajan, K.T., Merker, H.-J. and Wilkins, M. (1980). Observations on human digits *'in vitro'* and its possible role in evaluating teratogens. In: Merker, H.-J., Nau, H. and Neubert, D. (Eds), *Teratology of the Limbs,* Berlin, Walter de Gruyter, pp. 307–24.

Sadler, T.W., Horton, W.E. and Warner, C.W. (1982). Whole embryo culture: a screening technique for teratogens. *Teratog., Carcinog. and Mutag.*, **2**, 243–54.

Sadler, T.W. and Warner, C.W. (1984). Use of whole embryo culture for evaluating toxicity and teratogenicity. *Pharmacol. Rev.*, **36** (Suppl. 2), 145s–150s.

Saxén, L. (1973). Effects of hydrocortisone on the development *in vitro* of secondary palate in two inbred strains of mice. *Arch. Oral. Biol.*, **18**, 1469–79.

Saxén, L. and Ekblom, P. (1981). The developing kidney as a model system for normal and impaired organogenesis. In: Neubert, D. and Merker, H.-J. (Eds), *Culture Techniques. Applicability for Studies on Prenatal Differentiation and Toxocity*, Berlin, Walter de Gruyter, pp. 291–300.

Schuler, R.L., Hardin, B.D. and Niemeier, R.W. (1982). *Drosophila* as a tool for the rapid assessment of chemicals for teratogenicity. *Teratog., Carcinog. and Mutag.*, **2**, 293–302.

Schultz, T.W., Dumont, J.N., Clark, B.R. and Buchanan, N.V. (1982). Embryotoxic and teratogenic effects of aqueous extracts of tar from coal gasification electrostatic precipitators. *Teratog., Carcinog. and Mutag.*, **2**, 1–11.

Shepard, T.H. (1974). Onset of function in the human fetal thyroid: biochemical and radio-autographic studies from organ culture. *J. Clin. Endocrinol.*, **27**, 945–58.

Shepard, T.H. and Bass, G.L. (1970). Organ culture of limb buds from riboflavin-deficient and normal rat embryos in normal and riboflavin-deficient media. *Teratology*, **3**, 163–8.

Shepard, T.H., Tanimura, T. and Robkin,M. (1969). *In vitro* study of rat embryos. I. Effects of decreased oxygen on embryonic heart rate. *Teratology*, **2**, 107–10.

Shepard, T.H., Fantel, A.G., Mirkes, P.E., Greenaway, J.C., Faustman-Watts, E., Campbell, M. and Juchau, M.R. (1983). Teratology testing: I. Development and status of short-term prescreens. II. Biotransformation of teratogens as studied in whole embryo culture. *Prog. Clin. Biol. Res.*, **135**, 147–64.

Spielmann, H. and Eibs, H.-G. (1978). Recent progress in teratology: a survey of methods for the study of drug actions during the pre-implantation period. *Arzneim.-Forsch.*, **28**, 1733–42.

Stahlmann, R., Bluth, U. and Neubert, E. (1981). Effects of some 'indirectly' alkylating agents on differentiation of limb buds in organ culture. In: Neubert, D. and Merker, H.-J. (Eds), *Culture Techniques. Applicability for Studies on Prenatal Differentiation and Toxicity*, Berlin, Walter de Gruyter, pp. 207–21

Steelman, S.L. and Pohley, F.M. (1953). Assay of the FSH based on the augmentation with human chorionic gonadotropin. *Endocrinology*, **53**, 604–16.

Stevens, L.C. (1967). The biology of teratomas. *Adv. Morphog.*, **6**, 1–31.

Streisinger, G. (1975). Invited discussion. On the possible use of zebra fish for the screening of teratogens. In: Shepard, T.H., Miller, J.R. and Marois, M. (Eds), *Methods for Detection of Environmental Agents that Produce Congenital Deffects*, Amsterdam, North-Holland, pp. 59–64.

Thomas, J.A., and Bell, J.U. (1982). Endocrine toxicology. In: Hayes, A.W. (Ed.) *Principles and Methods of Toxicology*, Raven Press, New York, pp. 487–507.

Thomas, J.A., Mawhinney, M. and Mason, W. (1968). Sex accessory fructose: an evaluation of biochemical technique. *Proc. Soc. Exp. Biol. Med.*, **127**, 930–37.

Trowell, O.A. (1961). Problems in the maintenance of mature organs *in vitro*. In: *La Culture Organotypique*, Paris, Editions du Centre National de la Recherche Scientifique, pp. 237–49.

Tsunoda, Y. and Chang, M.C. (1976a). Fertilizing ability *in vivo* and *in vitro* of spermatozoa of rats and mice treated with alpha-chlorohydrin. *J. Reprod. Ferti.*, **46**, 401–6.

Tsunoda, Y. and Chang, M.C. (1976b). The fertilizing capacity of spermatozoa from rats and mice treated with CL-88,236 and AY-22,342 as examined both in vivo and in vitro. *Biol. Reprod.*, **14**, 202–11.

Vouk, V.B. and Sheehan, P.J. (Eds) (1983). *Methods for Assessing the Effects of Chemicals on Reproductive Functions*, SCOPE 20, John Wiley & Sons, Chichester, 541 p.

Welsch, F., Baumann, I. and Neubert, D. (1978). Effects of methyl-parathion and methyl-paraoxon on morphogenetic differentiation of mouse limb buds in organ culture. In: Neubert, D., Merker, H.-J., Nau, H. and Langman, J. (Eds), *Role of Pharmacokinetics in Prenatal and Perinatal Toxicology*, Stuttgart, Georg Thieme, pp. 351–8.

Wilk, A.L., Greenberg, J.H., Horigan, E.A., Pratt, R.M. and Martin, G.R. (1980). Detection of teratogenic compounds using differentiating embryonic cells in culture. *In Vitro*, **16**, 269–76.

World Health Organization (1984). *Principles for Evaluating Health Risks to Progency Associated with Exposure to Chemicals during Pregnancy*, Environmental Health Criteria 30, Geneva, Switzerland, 177 p.

Yanagimachi, R., Yanagimachi, H. and Rogers, B.J. (1976). The use of zona-free animal ova as a test system for the assessment of the fertilizing capacity of human spermatozoa. *Biol. Reprod.*, **15**, 471–76.

Yanagimachi, R., Lopata, A., Odom, C.B., Bronson, R.A., Mahi, C.A. and Nicolson, G.L. (1979). Retention of biologic characteristics of zona pellucida in highly concentrated salt solution: the use of salt-stored eggs for assessing the fertilizing capacity of spermatozoa. *Fertil. Steril.*, **31**, 562–74.

Zarrow, M.X., Yochim, J.M. and McCarthy, J.L. (1964). *Experimental Endocrinology, A Source Book of Basic Techniques*, Academic Press, New York, pp. 129–140.

CHAPTER 17

Toxicological versus Ecotoxicological Testing

GUIDO PERSOONE AND JAMES GILLETT

17.1 ANALOGIES AND DIFFERENCES BETWEEN TOXICOLOGY AND ECOTOXICOLOGY

Evolution has gradually brought one species, namely man, above other living creatures on Earth (at least as far as intelligence is concerned). It is logical and justified, therefore, that concerns about the negative effects of man-made chemicals on humans still rank much higher than ecotoxicological considerations in hazard assessment. In contrast to toxicology, which focuses on the protection of the human species (considered by themselves to be the most important creatures on Earth), ecotoxicology concerns the protection and well-being of several millions of species scattered over a variety of terrestrial and aquatic habitats, and of the biological communities and their encompassing ecosystems and processes. Thus, ecotoxicology also indirectly addresses the well-being and ultimately the survival of mankind since noxious chemicals can degrade ecosystems to the extent that the environment may no longer fulfil basic human needs.

We recognize the universality of living processes since we recognize that all life forms have certain basic features in common. However, we are faced with a very wide variety of types and forms of life. Experience has shown that, in general, the greater the differences in form and function, the greater the differences in response to foreign chemicals. These differences are the basis for selective toxicity and are brought about by differences in (i) the mode of uptake of chemicals, (ii) rates of chemical penetration, metabolism, and excretion, (iii) chemical reaction at the toxic site and the mechanism of that reaction, and (iv) the specific habitats of the biota that determine the potential for exposure to chemicals. These same features are important in human toxicology in determining the risk to specific segments of society but the range of responses is obviously much greater in ecotoxicology.

Human toxicological research is, by definition, restricted to the species level and most of our interest is directed at the individual. However, much information is extrapolated from research with animals as well as human epidemiology data. Ecotoxicology, by contrast, encompasses the species and infra-species levels, as well as the impacts on the structure and function of biota at supra-organismal levels (i.e. populations, communities and ecosystems), all of which may be subject to an infinite variety of environmental variables and interactions.

Whereas the loss of individual human lives is of great concern, the disappearance of a few individuals in a population of plants or animals is usually not considered to be serious as long as the proper functioning of the population, communities or ecosystems remains unaffected. Ecotoxicology, therefore, focuses attention on processes and interrelationships of structure and function in populations, communities and ecosystems.

Cairns (1980) emphasized that although natural ecosystems may have so much functional redundancy that the disappearance of certain species does not necessarily lead to impairment of function, it is possible to impair ecosystem function without actually killing organisms.

17.2   EXPOSURE ASSESSMENT VERSUS EFFECTS (HAZARD) ASSESSMENT

Determination of the 'hazard' which a particular chemical may represent for man and other biota is usually approached by relating the magnitude (concentration), frequency and duration of exposure to the magnitude, extent and duration of toxic effects which the xenobiotics have on the living creatures.

Exposure, on the other hand, is determined by a variety of factors including the distribution or partitioning of the chemical between environmental media (such as soil, sediment, water and air), the transformation or degradation of the chemical, and the movement of media containing these agents. Ascertaining these factors is 'exposure assessment' which dictates the magnitude of the potential hazardous effects.

Once the hazard assessment has qualitatively identified the nature of adverse effects and a quantitative dose–response relationship has been defined, it is possible to assess the risk to components, processes and individuals within the system. The most important feature of risk assessment, as emphasized in all recent reviews on the subject, is the determination (or estimation) of the extent to which concentrations of a given chemical released into the environment (i.e. exposure) overlap in time and space with those that are toxic (i.e. hazardous) to selected organisms, populations and ecosystems. Currently, both exposure and the effects of xenobiotics in the natural environment can only be estimated approximately and in a very crude way because of the infinite number of variables involved. The variables arise from the complex biological structure of ecosystems and the numerous interrelationships between their components, and the multivariant pathways of distribution of chemicals in the environment.

17.3   TERRESTRIAL VERSUS AQUATIC ENVIRONMENTS

Ecologically, the terrestrial environments, in many aspects, are similar to aquatic environments since the living components of both are structured in the same way.

Plant and animal species are grouped in populations which, in turn, are well-organized into biological communities. Both types of ecosystems fulfil the same basic functions; namely, primary (photosynthetic) production, consumption and growth as secondary productivity, and degradation and nutrient cycling as major links throughout several types of food chains.

Even though a considerable part of the species which populate terrestrial and aquatic ecosystems are very closely related phylogenetically, the approach to studying impacts of chemicals is, nevertheless, very different for these two environments. This results from the quite different modes of exposure of biota to chemicals in the two types of ecosystems.

In terrestrial ecosystems, exposure to pollutants present in the air seems only to directly affect the plant kingdom; animals are indeed mainly contaminated by uptake of toxicants via the food chain. In the aquatic ecosystem, the pelagic fauna and flora are in continuous contact with chemicals dissolved or suspended in the water column; food chain uptake appears to be very secondary or at least much slower than that from direct contamination. Suspended solids in aquatic environments have about as much contribution to aquatic species as does dust to terrestrial species. In both types of ecosystems, however, the biota living in the soil/sediments can be intoxicated by contact exposure and ingestion of contaminated particles. This more intense contact provides mobility to these deposited chemicals as they enter food webs and disturbed materials re-equilibrate with the water column.

The quantities of chemical substances that can be carried by each of the media (air, water or soil) are not comparable. Moreover, their dynamics, bioavailability and ultimate fate in each medium can be radically different. As a result, experimental approaches to determine the potential effects of pollutants are quite different for terrestrial and aquatic organisms and will be treated separately elsewhere in this volume.

17.4 THE NECESSITY FOR AND DIFFICULTY OF TESTING AT DIFFERENT LEVELS OF BIOLOGICAL ORGANIZATION

In 1983, Cairns addressed the question, 'Are single species toxicity tests alone adequate for estimating environmental hazard?' He noted that 'at each succeeding level of biological organization, new properties appear that would not have been evident even by the most intense and careful examination of lower levels of organization'. Cairns correctly concluded that, to date, 'no scientifically justifiable evidence exists to indicate that degree of reliability with which one may use single species tests to predict responses to higher levels of biological organization'.

Until a few years ago, bioassays on non-human target organisms were restricted almost exclusively to laboratory tests on selected test species (of even age or size) exposed for fixed periods of time to constant concentrations of a toxicant in a predetermined set of physiochemical conditions. The major reason for this is that ecotoxicology, historically, started as an offspring of human toxicology. Originally, the interest was in toxicity ranking of chemicals for a very limited number of test species which were of direct economic or aesthetic interest to man. Standardization of assay conditions provided support for litigation in the control of aquatic pollution (Mount and Gillett, 1982) and in pesticide regulation (Tucker and Crabtree, 1970). Interestingly, these tests had little in common with the reality of impacts on populations and communities which receive stochastic exposure to multiple toxicants under varying physiochemical conditions without reference to species, age or size, or other factors.

The growing concern about pollution in the 1960s, fortunately paralled by a rapid development of ecology, made mankind aware of the need for analysis of the potential impact of chemicals on natural environments at the ecosystem level rather than at the single species level. All the interacting biological components of the systems at risk are exposed, either simultaneously or successively, to varying concentrations of xenobiotics for different periods of time under site-specific, but also variable, environmental conditions. Thus, both direct and indirect effects were expected and confirmed.

Extensive research during the last decade has shown that the 'ecosystem approach' to hazard assessment is very difficult to apply in practice. The difficulty arises from the number of variables involved in multispecies testing either in the laboratory (microcosm or mesocosm) or under actual environmental conditions (field studies). This is a major obstacle to the repeatability of the tests and, as a result, to their predictive potential.

From the practical point of view, there is an undeniable inverse relationship between 'ecological realism' on one hand, and simplicity of testing on the other, as illustrated in Figure 17.1. This inverse relationship sustains the dictum that an understanding of toxic mechanisms is achieved by progressing downward in complexity (i.e. from the organism to the physiologic level, to the organ and finally to the molecular level), whereas the outcome of the toxicologic event can only be fully understood by progressing upward to the more complex system. Enzyme inhibition is only of significance if it causes organ and physiologic systems to fail in ways that make the organism less capable of functioning within the community. The allegory, 'for want of a nail . . . the kingdom was lost', illustrates the vital concept of a critical pathway for a constituent of a system to result in an adverse effect; not every lost nail results in kingdoms falling.

This concept is particularly relevant in the context of this review. It is possible to focus on mechanisms in a single organism while understanding the functional relationships of many component systems of higher biological complexity. For example, a set of separate *in vitro* tests may establish that the chemical penetrates the organism, survives in its various systems, and inhibits a key enzyme. If we know that the enzyme is found in specific organs with functional connections to adverse outcomes, we do not need to test each individual organism to predict that adverse effect. In the human species, an acetylcholinesterase inhibitor effectively deprives the heart of enervation, depriving the brain of oxygen and resulting in death. In other

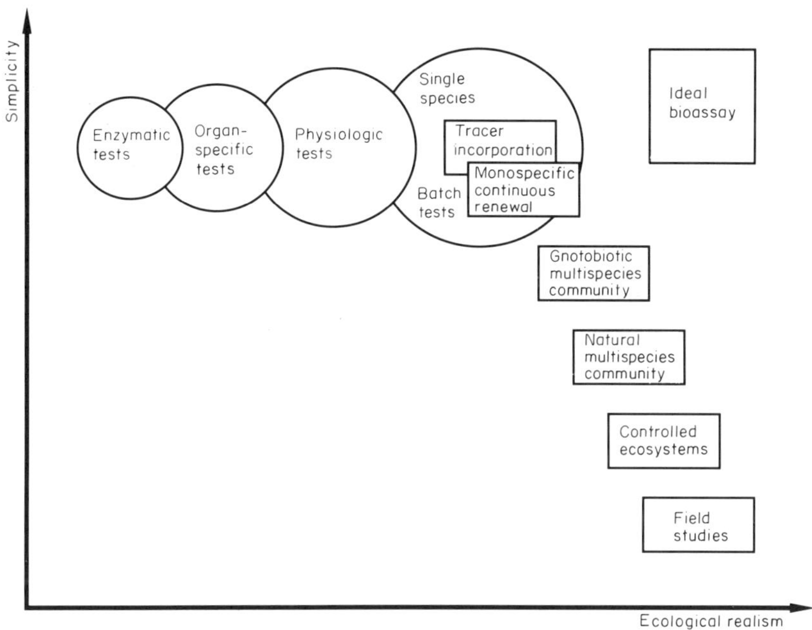

Figure 17.1   Schematic presentation of the inverse relationship between simplicity and ecological realism in test systems of increasing complexity (modified from Calamari *et al.*, 1985).

species, the same enzyme system may have different mechanistic connections, the organs may be more or less redundant and important to organismic vitality, and the individual may have only an infinitesimal role in the population, community or ecosystem. Thus, our testing at lower levels helps us to understand the selective nature of toxicity, the comparative aspects of physiology, and perhaps even something about functional relationships within populations and higher systems. However, the same kind of testing tells us little about the actual outcome; our knowledge of the ecological relationships is so incomplete that any conclusions drawn in this respect may be little more than speculation.

A decade or more ago, compensation for ignorance was achieved by use of safety factors or application factors (Mount and Gillett, 1982). Pragmatically, standards set using such arbitrary factors as 100 or 1000 were effective in reducing pollution and restoring biologic 'livability' to the environment. We do not yet know whether this approach was economically invalid (over-regulation) or ecologically inappropriate (e.g. undiscovered loss of species due to inappropriate standards).

During the decades of the 1960s and 1970s, species- and habitat-specific effects were discovered which revolutionized thinking about environmental problems. Direct toxicity of pesticides to song birds and fish was among the first environmental watersheds crossed, but that was soon overshadowed by the chronic lethal toxicity to robins feeding on contaminated earthworms, which in turn was surpassed by concern about non-lethal, chronic toxicity of pesticides and other toxic substances to birds and fish as seen in reproductive and behavioural effects. These served as warnings to man of potential dangers to his own well-being and illustrated ecological connections previously ignored in anthropocentric haste.

A crude but effective multispecies system was devised by Metcalfe *et al.* (1971)—a 'farm pond' model ecosystem or microcosm—to demonstrate these connections. Although this particular test system has been labelled an 'ecological junk heap', had it been employed before the chlorinated hydrocarbon insecticides were introduced, DDT would never have been used on such a spatial and mass scale over most of the globe. At about the same time, various other systems were excised from fields and ponds to examine, among other things, ecosystem response to stress and radioactive fallout. Together, these sets of tests stimulated multispecies testing and microcosm technology as a legitimate approach to evaluation of higher biologic functions and outcomes.

17.5   SINGLE SPECIES TESTS

Although experience with multispecies testing is being gained rapidly, standardized protocols for multispecies tests are only just becoming available. Because reliable, well-tested and/or cost-effective experimental ecosystem level tests which can be used on a routine basis have been lacking, ecotoxicologic testing to support all national and international hazard assessments of chemicals is still based entirely on single species tests, mostly in a tiered approach.

In principle, the candidate species should be representative of the various biota of natural ecosystems, have a comparable sensitivity, possess the functional community connections, and be sufficiently comprehensive or inclusive to be representative of all critical parts of natural ecosystems. Unfortunately, we are far from achieving this goal. Only a few species have been or can be maintained in the laboratory. Buikema and Benfield (1979) point out that the lack of ecological information needed to establish laboratory populations is a serious handicap to increasing the variety of potential candidate species for ecotoxicological testing. Animal species most widely used for testing in the USA include five mammals, five birds, seven fish, two terrestrial insects, nine aquatic arthropods and one mollusc (Kenaga, 1978).

Most tests so far have been carried out on fish, not only because this group is considered to be the best understood for the aquatic environment, but also (and perhaps mainly) because of its direct interest to man (Cairns, 1982). Also, it appears that many of the species routinely used for toxicity testing are, among their fellows in the natural environment, those with the lowest ecological needs and the largest tolerances regarding many environmental variables (euryspecies); this implicitly makes them the easiest to maintain and handle in the laboratory.

It should be emphasized that the methodology and standardization of testing procedures, even for those of a routine nature, is often very poor. Maki (1983) indicates that although few intercalibration exercises have been carried out, most have been a complete failure either because the experimental protocols have been inadequate or because of the failure to understand some of the basic ecological requirements of the test species. For the aquatic environment, only three tests have successfully passed a 'round robin' inter-laboratory comparison; these are the

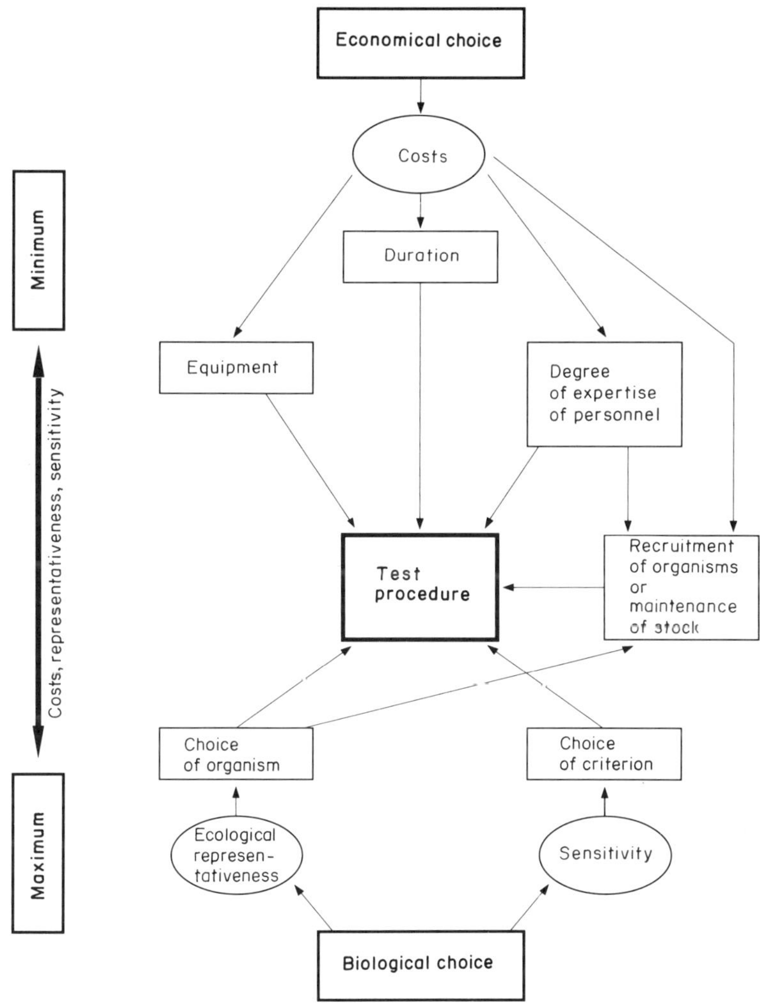

Figure 17.2   Interrelationships of the basic factors determining the choice of bioassay test methods (from Persoone, 1980).

Daphnia magna and the *Brachydanio rerio* short-term bioassays for the freshwater environment (Cabridenc, 1979a,b) and the *Artemia salina* short-term test for the marine environment (Vanhaecke and Persoone, 1982).

The 'ecological realism–simplicity' inverse relationship for the ecosystem approach is, unfortunately, also valid at the single species level. Persoone (1980) clearly demonstrated the paradox between the biological and the economical approach in selecting species and setting up protocols for toxicity tests (Figure 17.2). The biological approach (which is the logical one, of course) aims at the maximim ecological representativeness and sensitivity of the tests. The selection of representative test species (difficult to maintain and handle) and sensitive criteria (growth or reproduction) automatically leads to complicated test methods and long-term experiments which are expensive.

The economical approach, which is the only realistic one for routine testing of a large number of chemicals, is based on simple, short-term tests with limited numbers of species which are easy to culture and on criteria which are simple to assess (e.g. lethality). As noted earlier, this testing strategy, while having merit in terms of economy and expedience, is lacking in terms of representativeness, completeness and sensitivity.

Macek *et al.* (1978), who reviewed the types of aquatic toxicity tests that provide useful data for estimating or predicting the toxicity of chemicals to aquatic organisms, worked out a very informative matrix based on six evaluation criteria (ecological significance, scientific and legal defensibility, availability of routine methods, predictive utility, general applicability and simplicity, and costs); this is reproduced in Table 17.1. Lethality, despite its apparent crudeness, is the most useful of all endpoints considered, both in a single species as well as multispecies tests.

17.6   NECESSITY OF EXPOSURE EVALUATION

In order to make the best use of single species tests in predicting how a particular chemical may influence biota under natural environmental conditions, the inherent toxicity of the particular xenobiotics (determined experimentally) should be related to the quantity of the chemical that will reach the organism under the prevailing conditions of exposure. In recent hazard assessment projects (e.g. OECD, 1982), exposure is determined as 'predicted environmental distribution' (PED) and 'predicted environmental concentration' (PEC). The PED is based on a number of physicochemical characteristics (such as water solubility, vapour pressure, relative molecular mass, soil adsorption coefficient and octanol–water partition coefficient). This gives an estimate of the distribution of the chemical within the environmental compartments of air, water, soil/sediment, and biota. The complementary PEC aims at quantitative prediction of the real concentrations of the chemical likely to be achieved within distinct parts of the ecosystem.

The PED is based on a limited number of parameters. It is usually simple to determine. The PEC is much more difficult to estimate since it requires information

Table 17.1   Consensus evaluation of the relative utility of simple and complex toxicity tests used in assessing the risk associated with the occurrence of chemicals in aquatic environments (from Macek *et al.*, 1978)

Test	Ecological significance	Scientific and legal defensibility	Availability or routine methods	Predictive utility	General applicability	Simplicity and cost	Present relative utility
Simple systems							
Acute lethality	33	36	35	22	24	26	100
Embryo/larval	33	30	23	20	25	14	82
Reproduction	36	30	21	27	24	8	82
Residue accumulation	27	32	22	24	17	14	77
Algal assay	30	23	26	18	14	20	74
Organoleptic	14	25	25	27	13	15	67
Structure/activity	18	21	23	17	16	22	66
Behavioural	21	13	10	9	16	9	44
Histological	10	10	20	10	13	10	41
Physiological and biochemical	12	10	13	8	19	8	40
In vitro	4	5	9	4	11	11	25
Complex systems							
Field	34	24	18	21	21	3	69
Diversity	26	19	25	15	20	10	65
Benthic	21	18	12	18	17	12	56
Microcosm	19	10	15	14	17	9	48

on volumes of production, discharge patterns and detailed knowledge of receiving waters (flows, characteristics, locations, etc.).

17.7 'SHORT-TERM' ECOTOXICOLOGIC ASSAYS

We desire to protect species which will never be tested because they are endangered (e.g. ospreys), physically difficult if not impossible to culture (blue whales, redwood trees), or simply not known. Such an organism might be a 'keystone species' on which ecosystem function depends (e.g. a detritivore that facilitates nutrient cycling in a pond or forest, or a top-level predator structuring the ecosystem by its prey selection). Even to identify such an organism may require years of field and laboratory study. Rarely do toxicity studies provide an opportunity to evaluate impacts on these organisms and the systems they support, because to do so leads to experiments in 'biogeochemical time'.

The short-term view of man in ecological and biogeochemical studies is at the heart of ecotoxicology. Failure to take a long view of the outcomes of anthropogenic inputs into the environment results in problems being discovered after they have progressed to near eco-catastrophe. Global pollution by acid precipitation and stratospheric modification are often cited as examples of such phenomena for which both preventative and mitigative responses are quite difficult. Synthetic organic chemicals, such as DDT, PCBs and phthalate esters, are now widely distributed in the environment. These chemicals have accumulated and biomagnified in some ecosystems, and may gradually change the species composition of an ecosystem. Strenuous efforts have restored species of fish or birds to some such habitats, but others still suffer from the impacts of chemicals long after they have been 'regulated' or 'banned'.

Hence, ecotoxicologic assays not only require multispecies forms and interactions, but they also require multiseasonal studies of succession, adaptation and other interactions. In theory, one can select species with short reproduction and life cycles, such as *Daphnia magna* L. (generation time of days) or *Arabidopsis* spp. (seed-to-seed time of about 30 days). However, that simply begs the question 'Are the critical species affected long-lived or do they have multi-seasonal requirements for critical functions?'. The period during which multi-species test systems and microcosms can be maintained in a suitable operational state is often far short of desirable. How then might 'short-term' assays for ecotoxicologic effects be developed? There are few courses from which to choose; ignore long-term (multiseasonal or multi-generational) phenomenan; ignore multi-species interactions; ignore cryptic species and processes; or assume that broad safety factors (100 or 1000) are adequate. Pragmatically, as noted earlier, the application of safety factors has served well for a time, but as economic issues intruded into environmental protection in the wake of a global energy crisis and slump in both industrial and developing nations, the question of over-regulation is not a rhetorical one.

Unpublished studies by Mount and his co-workers, and similar analyses by others using large databases, have revealed some features of comparative toxicity that provide cautious encouragement for the possibilities of ecotoxicologic testing within a shorter timeframe. For example, it is possible to test 'clusters' of organisms and extrapolate to a value of a theoretical LCO (the lethality to the zeroth organism) (Gillett, unpublished). This 'cluster' is a set of species (e.g. rainbow trout, *D. magna*, and bluegill, or white rat, bobwhite quail, and housefly) for which commensurate doses (mg/kg) or exposures (mg/m^3) are available and for which there is some understanding of the relationship of toxic response to the class of chemical involved in the test. Thus, for heavy metals, a sensitive micro-organism (such as *E.coli*) could be included. If phytotoxicity is expected or a concern, an alga might be used.

The spread of LD50 or LC50 data from the cluster is used to estimate selective toxicity, while the mean value estimates its qualitative nature (i.e. very highly toxic, moderately toxic, etc.). Provisional analysis of a large database from the US Department of the Interior, Fish and Wildlife Service reveals that there is greater variation between, say, rainbow trout under a variety of test conditions (temperature, age or size, hardness, salinity, pH, etc.) than there is among all fish tested (Johnson and Finley, 1980). Thus, one suspects that any laboratory test is not likely to reveal specific sensitivities, but simply ranks chemicals among species qualitatively. About as much information is gathered from the test cluster (designed to provide taxonomic spread in response) as from more extended testing. However, when selectivity is high (wide range in response) or a pollutant is suspected to affect several media, then the use of a larger cluster (5–8 species) is advisable.

A second approach assumes that chronic lethality occurs at about an order to magnitude lower in exposure than acute toxicity. Non-lethal but serious effects on reproduction and behaviour may be two orders of magnitude lower than lethality or morbidity. Without a sound understanding of chemical ecology and the behavioural relationships, one can never be sure that disruption will not occur as a direct or indirect result of the chemical in the environment. However, in practice, the use of this estimated chronic value (1/10 of the lowest LC50) does protect many species. However, we are never confident about how many species are protected or of their functional importance.

Multi-species and microcosm studies provide a short-cut to investigating these functional relationships, even though these tests frequently require weeks to months for completion and analysis. Once preliminary single species tests and physiochemical data have provided estimates of chronic exposure and chronic response, the model ecosystem can be used to confirm the activity of a candidate chemical or mixture or to demonstrate its probable safety, at least under the conditions of the test. We do not know with what certainty one can extrapolate from a given test set (species, habitat conditions) to others. Therefore, systems most likely to be exposed and/or anticipated to be sensitive to a particular class of chemical should be tested first.

Attention must be paid both to broad functions (primary production, nutrient cycling, etc.) and species composition. For example, Harte *et al.* (1980) found that their lotic microcosm tracked primary production and nitrogen cycling in the source reservoir — even beyond the time when a sensitive diatom was eliminated (due to a deficiency in silicon) and replaced by a blue-green alga. The presence of the undesirable organism (*Anabaena* sp.) would not have been found by simple functional analysis.

This review began by emphasizing that the objectives in ecotoxicology differ markedly from those in human toxicology. We have attempted to demonstrate concerns about approaches to testing which depend on biological simplification for quick answers. At the same time, the complexity of the systems and the species which form them demand greater attention that can only be given to them if we can find economical, accurate and simple means of determining their responses to concentrations of potential toxicants.

REFERENCES

Buikema, A.L. Jr., and Benfield, E.F. (1979). Use of macroinvertebrate life history information in toxicity tests. *J. Fish. Res. Bd. Can.*, **36**, 321–8.

Cabridenc, R. (1979a). Inter-laboratory ring test concerning the study of ecotoxicity of a chemical substance with respect to Daphnia. Commission of the European Communities. *Study D.8368*, 18 p.

Cabridenc, R. (1979b). Inter-laboratory ring test concerning the study of the ecotoxicity of a chemical substance with respect to the fish. Commission of the European Communities. *Study D.8368*, 18 p.

Cairns, J. Jr. (1980). Beyond single species toxicity testing. *Mar. Environ. Res.*, **3**, 157–9.

Cairns, J. Jr. (1982). Predictive and reactive systems for aquatic ecosystem quality control. In: *Scientific Basis of Water-Resource Management*, Geophysics Study Committee, National Research Council, National Academy Press, Washington, D.C., pp. 72–84.

Cairns, J. Jr. (1983). Are single species toxicity tests alone adequate for estimating environmental hazard? *Hydrobiologia*, **100**, 47–57.

Calamari, D., Chiaudani, G., and Vighi, M. (1985). Methods for measuring the effects of chemicals on aquatic plants. In: Vouk, B., Butler, G.C., Hoel, D.G., and Peakall, D.B. (Eds), *Methods for Estimating Risk of Chemical Injury: Human and Non-Human Biota and Ecosystems*, SCOPE 26, John Wiley & Sons, New York, pp. 549–71.

Harte, J., Levy, D., Rees, J., and Saagebarth, E. (1980). Making microcosms an effective assessment tool. In: Giesy, J. (Ed.), *Microcosms in Ecological Research*, DOE Symposium No. 52, US Technical Information Service, Springfield, VA, pp. 105–7.

Johnson, W.W., and Finley, M.T. (1980). *Handbook of Acute Toxicity of Chemicals to Fish and Aquatic Invertebrates*, Resource Publication Series, No. 37, US Fish and Wildlife Service, Washington, D.C., 98 p.

Kenaga, E.E. (1978). Test organisms and methods useful for early assessment of acute toxicity of chemicals. *Environ. Sci. Tech.*, **12**, 1322–8.

Macek, K., Birge, W., Mayer. F.L., Buikema, A.OL. Jr., and Maki, A.W. (1978). Discussion Session Synopsis. In: Cairns, J. Jr., Dickson, K.L., and Maki, A.W. (Eds), *Estimating the Hazard of Chemical Substances to Aquatic Life*, ASTM, Special Technical Publication 657, American Society for Testing and Materials, Philadelphia, pp. 27–32.

Maki, A. (1983). Exotoxicology—critical needs and credibility. *Environ. Toxicol. Chem.*, **2**, 259–60.

Metcalfe, R.L., Sangha, G.K., and Kapoor, I.P. (1971). Model ecosystem for the evaluation of pesticide degradability and ecological magnification. *Environ. Sci. Technol.,* **5**, 709–13.
Mount, D.I., and Gillett, J.W. (1982). Progress in research on ecotoxicology. In: Mason, W.T. (Ed.), *Research on Fish and Wildlife Habitat,* EPA-600/8-82-022, US Environmental Protection Agency, Washington, D.C., pp. 143–64.
OECD (1982). *Guidelines for Ecotoxicologic Testing of Chemicals,* Organization for Economic Cooperation and Development, Paris.
Persoone, G. (1980). Standardization of aquatic bioassays: comprises between biological and economical criteria. In: Klaverkamp, J.F., Leonhard, S.L., and Marshall, K.E. (Eds), *Proceedings of the 6th Annual Aquatic Toxicity Workshop,* Winnipeg, Canada, Can. Tech. Rep. Fish. Aquat. Sci., pp. 111–22.
Tucker, R.K., and Crabtree, D.G. (1970). *Handbook of Toxicity of Pesticides to Wildlife,* Resource Publication Series No. 84, US Fish and Wildlife Service, Washington, D.C., 131 p.
Vanhaecke, P., and Persoone, G. (1982). Report on an intercalibration exercise on a short-term standard toxicity test with *Artemia nauplii.* In: Leclerc, H., and Dive, D. (Eds), *Les tests de toxicité aigue en milieu aquatique,* volume 106, Editions INSERM, pp. 359–76.

Short-term Toxicity Tests for Non-genotoxic Effects
Edited by P. Bourdeau *et al.*
© 1990 SCOPE. Published by John Wiley & Sons Ltd.

CHAPTER 18

Possibilities and Limitations of Predictions from Short-term Tests in the Aquatic Environment

GUIDO PERSOONE, DAVID CALAMARI AND PETER WELLS

18.1 INTRODUCTION

In the previous chapter (Persoone and Gillett, Chapter 17, this volume) attention has been drawn to the large number of biological and physicochemical variables which determine the structure and functioning of ecosystems. The variety and the interrelationship of these factors present difficulties for the precise determination of the hazard which chemicals may pose for the natural environment and its biota.

Because of the complexity of the ecosystems involved, one would be inclined to believe that short-term aquatic toxicity tests cannot have any predictive value. However, in this chapter, it will be shown that tests of short duration (a few days up to one month) can be useful in many instances for predicting effects of chemicals on aquatic biota.

18.2 PREDICTION OF ACUTE POISONING IN THE FIELD

Data on lethal concentrations of chemicals in short-term tests are well-suited to predict mortalities in the field. In one of many examples of 'field validation' of lethal concentrations determined in laboratory experiments, Hasselrot (1965) studied the high mortality in caged yearling salmon and adult minnows in a polluted river in Sweden; mean and maximum concentrations of zinc of 0.15–0.28 and 0.25–0.95 mg/litre respectively, in a water with hardness between 21 and 48 mg CaCO/litre were found. The conclusion of this author that the zinc was the main factor responsible for the fish kills was validated by, and could have been predicted from, data published by Lloyd (1960, 1961) which indicated that short-term fish LC50s (4–10 days) are situated between 0.5 and 1.0 mg Zn/litre in waters of similar hardness. Calamari and Marchetti (1974) confirmed laboratory data on the toxicity of copper and ammonia by keeping rainbow trout in cages in Lake Orta (Italy) where the concentrations of these two chemicals varied during the seasons from 0.006 to 0.066 mg Cu/litre and from 5.8 to 7.2 mg N/litre (NH_3 plus NH_4^+). The field results correlated well with the acute toxicity values obtained experimentally.

An extensive review on the toxicity of mixtures prepared by the Working Party on Water Quality Criteria for European Fresh Water Fish (EIFAC/FAO, 1980) includes a number of cases in which the toxicity of mixtures could have been predicted on the basis of simple addition of the proportional contribution of each toxicant. In particular, laboratory data on the joint effect of different chemicals on fish gave an observed median value of 0.95 of that predicted, while the corresponding value for sewage effluents, river waters and a few industrial wastes, based on the toxicity sum of their constituents, was 0.85. Mixtures which contain pesticides were slightly (1.3 times) more toxic than predicted.

18.3   PREDICTION OF TOXICITY IN DIFFERENT PHYSICOCHEMICAL CONDITIONS

When data on the toxicity in two or more different physicochemical conditions are available, interpolations can be made and have proven of practical value. A classical example is the variation in the toxicity of metals in relation to water hardness in which there is a linear relationship, the slope of which is a function of the metal (USEPA, 1980; Sprague, 1985). Several other parameters such as oxygen concentration, temperature and chelating substances, in combination with various kinds of pollutants, are referred to in the series of EIFAC reviews defining water quality criteria (Alabaster and Lloyd, 1982). These relationships have practical utility in the prevention of massive fish kills; these could often be avoided by preventing discharges of effluents contaminated to levels which, according to laboratory data, are lethal for biota.

18.4   PREDICTION OF TOXICOLOGICAL RELATIONSHIPS AMONG DIFFERENT SPECIES

Detailed toxicological relationships among species have been defined in recent years for several types of chemicals. Kenaga (1978) collected acute toxicity data on 75 insecticides and herbicides for eight animal organisms commonly used as test-species in environmental hazard assessment. These species belonged to two phyla, five classes and eight families. The correlations of the acute toxicity between the organisms and the chemicals showed useful predictive values for closely related species within classes. However, useful predictive correlations were not observed between or within phyla, or between terrestrial and aquatic organisms. From this study, Kenaga concluded that, among the species studied, the most useful organisms for an early indication of toxicity in the aquatic environment seem to be a fish and a crustacean. Suter *et al.* (1983) used the database of the Columbia National Fisheries Research Laboratory in the USA to compare 96 h LC50 values for 28 fish species from 17 genera, 10 families and 6 orders submitted to 271 toxicants. This author found that there is an increasing sensitivity relationship for the pesticides when correlations are made at the order, family, genus and species level.

More recently, Blanck (1984) and Blanck *et al.* (1984) correlated the acute sensitivities of several species of aquatic organisms to chemicals ('non-pesticide organics', pesticides and metals) using polynomial regression analysis. He demonstrated that all of the species analysed—algae, invertebrates and fish (freshwater and marine) had a similar toxicity response to non-pesticide organics. When averaged into three categories, i.e., closely-related species (fish versus fish), more distantly-related species (fish versus invertebrates), and most distantly-related species (fish versus algae), the average correlation indices are 0.82, 0.80 and 0.70 respectively. These findings corroborate the results of many others who also demonstrated that certain sensitivity correlations are possible between related species. However, since different types of toxicants have different modes of action, no 'general' toxiological relationship exists which is applicable to all categories of chemicals and for all species.

It should be emphasized, therefore, that the original concept of 'very sensitive' species which are, at the same time,'good representatives' for specific groups of organisms or for specific trophic levels, makes sense only when correlated with well-defined categories of chemicals.

Kenaga (1982a) demonstrated that although certain species are frequently very sensitive or very resistant overall, there are also many exceptions to this general rule. As a result, any particular species can, in principle, never represent any other for establishing the sensitivity of the latter to a variety of different chemicals. However, when toxicity data from a variety of test-species, preferably of remote phylogenic relationship, are considered together, an 'overall' range of sensitivities will be obtained which is reasonably representative for aquatic biota in general.

Kenaga (1982a) noted that the problem still to be resolved is to know how many species and what types of species need to be tested to adequately represent the whole range. Sloof *et al.* (1983) and Sloof and Canton (1983) tried to find out how the three organisms recommended by the OECD and the EEC for the first steps in testing chemicals (alga–Daphnia–fish acute toxicity) cover the sensitivity range of other aquatic biota. For 25 to 30 per cent of the chemicals used in their study, a difference exceeding one order of magnitude between the results obtained with the three candidate species and an extended set of test organisms belonging to various groups of aquatic biota was observed.

In considering toxicological relationships between species, it is clear that attention should also be paid to salinity, i.e., whether toxicity results from freshwater biota can be used to predict toxicity in marine species and vice versa. Samoiloff and Wells (1984), reviewing some of the literature on the subject, showed that the differences in toxicity caused by different salinities are usually small (with some exceptions that may be due to osmoregulation). However, one should not overlook basic physicochemical differences between freshwater and seawater which may

affect the form and availability of many pollutants; the degree of exposure of the
biota to toxicants can be very different in these two environments and should, of
course, be taken into consideration.

18.5   PREDICTIVE VALUE OF ACUTE TOXICITY DATA FOR CHRONIC TOXICITY

In ecotoxicology, the concentration of a chemical considered 'safe' for the environment is usually derived from the no observed effect level (NOEL) determined in
chronic, life cycle, or reproduction tests.

In order to decrease the time, the effort, and the costs required to conduct chronic
tests, scientists have been endeavouring to extrapolate safe levels from short-term
acute (lethal) tests. Figure 18.1 shows how extrapolation of non-toxic levels from
lethal concentrations is both species- and toxicant-dependent due to differences in
the shape of the toxicity curve as well as in the distances between specific points of
effect (threshold, intoxication, mortality). There is no overall constant ratio between
acute and chronic toxicity levels because both the effect (lethal versus sublethal) and
the time of exposure are different.

In a detailed comparative study of acute and chronic toxicity data of 84 chemicals
tested on eleven species of aquatic animals, Kenaga (1982a,b) found that the
ACR—the acute to chronic toxicity ratio—ranged from 1 to 18 000. This study,
however, also revealed that 86 per cent of the ACR values were below 100, that the
ACRs for the crustacean *Daphnia magna* and the fish *Pimephales promelas* are
similar in most cases for a given chemical, and that ACR values for most chemicals

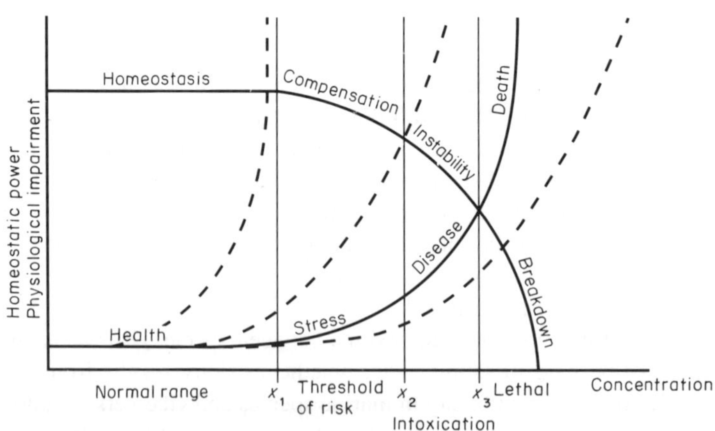

Figure 18.1   Diagram of effects of a chemical, at increasing concentrations on the physiological processes of an organism. Different chemicals have different toxicity curves, with
different threshold concentrations for different effects (X_1, X_2, X_3).

are within one order of magnitude between species. Moreover, it appeared that chemicals with large ACR values also have 'unusual' specific modes of toxic action. This is the case of metals and pesticides, which are chemicals that have received very much attention in comparison to industrial organic compounds. Since for 93 per cent of the chemicals in the latter category, the ACR values are below 25, Kenaga considers that one may use application factors based on an ACR of 25 or less to predict the chronic toxicity of industrial organic chemicals from acute toxicities.

Sloof *et al.* (1983) and Sloof and Canton (1983) compared the acute and chronic toxicity to daphnids and fish for 126 data pairs taken from the literature; a very high degree of correlation ($r = 0.88$) was found. These authors also confirmed Kenaga's findings that the differences between acute and chronic levels were less than a factor of 100.

18.6   TESTS WITH DEVELOPMENTAL STAGES OF FISH FOR PREDICTING LONG-TERM TOXICITY

Fish are exposed to the toxicants throughout their life cycle and effects are measured on survival, growth and reproduction. The early life stages of fish have long been recognized as very sensitive biological material (Marchetti, 1965). Mount and Stephan (1967) described a life-cycle fish toxicity test which involves all developmental stages. For several years, life-cycle toxicity tests have provided the best data for the establishment of water quality criteria. However, the cost, the time involved and, not least, the continuous risk of biological (infection, diseases) or technological (mechanical failures) problems are very high; moreover, experience has demonstrated that certain life stages are more sensitive than others.

Reviewing the existing data, McKim (1977) demonstrated that the sensitivities of embryo-larval and early juvenile stages are, in most cases, comparable with those of full life-cycle tests within a factor of two. Therefore, tests of a few days or a few weeks duration (depending on the type of fish) could be a good substitute for life-cycle tests with a much longer duration. In the same context, Calamari and Marchetti (1978) reviewed the experiments performed at the Water Research Institute in Italy on early life stages of fish and emphasized the relevance of studies on developmental and young stages of *Salmo gairdneri* for the establishment of water quality criteria for fisheries.

18.7   PREDICTIONS BASED ON THE SHAPE OF TOXICITY CURVES

Toxicity curves in aquatic toxicology are drawn by plotting the logarithms of the median lethal exposure time (log LT50) against the logarithms of the concentration (log C) of toxicant to improve data interpretation. As the time of exposure is part of the stimulus, more information is obtained from such graphs than from classical curves expressed as 'percentage of effect versus concentration' for a fixed time.

Wuhrmann and Woker (1948) considered such curves as equilateral hyperboles and modified the classical equation in:

$$\log (T-Ta) + n \log (C+Ca) = \log K$$

in which T and C are time and concentration respectively and Ta and Ca the asymptotic values for time and concentration.

This equation theoretically expresses thresholds at which, for an infinite time of exposure, no additional effects are observed or for which, at an infinite concentration, the minimum time to obtain the effect has already been reached. Although experience has revealed many exceptions, this concept of a threshold of toxicity has remained in practical use. Sprague (1969) termed this the 'incipient lethal level' in his review on aquatic toxicity and he considered the threshold concept as a key factor in ecotoxicological effect assessment. Sprague defined the asymptotic concentration as 'that level of the environmental entity beyond which 50% of the population cannot live for an indefinite time'.

The classical toxicity curve (LT50–C) provides an overall impression of what is happening in the test. A steep vertical asymptote, for example, indicates that acute mortality has stopped, whereas the absence of an asymptote, e.g., after 96 hours, indicates that acute morality is probably still occurring in the experimental population. Idealized examples of such toxicity curves are shown in Figure 18.2.

Where a tiered testing approach is adopted, analysis of the shape of the log LT50s may, according to Lloyd (1979) be very helpful in determining if further testing is

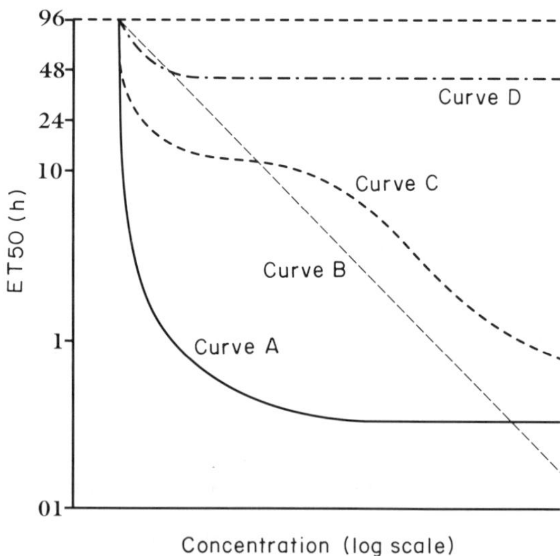

Figure 18.2   Types of toxicity curves found in practice for aquatic organisms exposed to toxic substances. Concentrations are plotted as the multiple of the 96-h LC50 (from Lloyd, 1981).

needed. The importance of this fact has been acknowledged by the International Standardization Organization (ISO, 1978) and by the OECD (1981) both of which propose that reports on fish toxicity tests should include the concentration response curve in addition to the 96-hour LC50. Lloyd (1979) even suggests the use (if necessary) of different application factors.

18.8 PREDICTIONS ON THE BASIS OF CHEMICAL STRUCTURE

The correlation of molecular structure with biological activity is an important aspect of ecotoxicology because of its predictive potential.

Although more and more papers are now published on the subject, the potential of the Hansch equation (1973) has, to date, not yet been fully exploited in aquatic toxicology. The equation:

$$\log \frac{1}{EC50} \; a \log P + b \, (\log P2) + cpKa + dEs + e$$

relates biological effects, with lipophilic properties, and electronic and steric characteristics. Theoretically, the Hansch equation allows one to predict the effects of certain molecules without testing. This possibility is currently under study by the OECD within the framework of setting principles for the establishment of a priority list of chemicals for testing. For the thousands of chemicals on the market, ecotoxicological information is indeed, in many cases, scarce or even totally lacking.

The value and the limitations of the QSAR (Quantitative Structure Activity Relationship) have been determined in experimental work. Published works include those of Veith *et al.* (1983) on narcotic chemicals, of Konemann (1981) on fifty substances commonly found as industrial pollutants, of Calamari *et al.* (1980, 1983) on several amines and chlorobenzenes, and of McLeese *et al.* (1979) on phenols, anilines and other aromatic compounds. All of these authors agree on the usefulness and applicability of QSARs in short-term aquatic toxicology, as do Veith *et al.* (1980) and Konemann and Calamari (1983) in two reviews. More explicitly, it is the opinion of the latter two authors that:

(1) QSARs have been developed for several classes of chemicals; within these classes, good estimates of the toxicity of chemicals can be predicted solely on the basis of their chemical relationship.
(2) Most QSARs have been calculated for a small number of chemicals. Expert judgement is necessary to set the limits to the validity of QSARs as well as reliable confidential limits to the predicted effect values.
(3) When correctly applied, QSARs can be useful in the selection of priority chemicals even where no experimental data are available.
(4) Toxicity data calculated from QSARs are rough estimates and should not be used as a substitute for experimental data.

18.9 PREDICTION OF BIOCONCENTRATION FACTORS

Neely *et al.* (1974) demonstrated that a good linear relationship exists between the bioconcentration of several organic chemicals in trout muscle and the n-octanol–water partition coefficient of these substances. In the same paper, the bioconcentration factor (BCF) was defined as the ratio of the concentration of the chemical substance in the fish muscle (measured at equilibrium) and the contaminated water in which the fish were kept. Several other workers subsequently confirmed this finding. Veith *et al.* (1979), in particular, comparing actual measurements in short-term tests with estimated BCF, found the following equation for 55 chemicals analysed:

$$\log \mathrm{BCF} = 0.85 \log P - 0.70.$$

This formula allows one to calculate the potential for bioaccumulation of a molecule simply on the basis of physicochemical parameters. The relationship has been confirmed in many field studies although it is not applicable where biomagnification through the food chain plays an important role. Moreover, it has been demonstrated that the BCF cannot be estimated by this method in early life stages of fish because of the very high contents in lipids of the latter; for example, Galassi *et al.* (1982) showed that the amount of paradichlorobenzene accumulated by fish larvae was one order of magnitude higher than in adults.

18.10 USE OF TOXICOKINETICS FOR PREDICTIVE PURPOSES

Good results have been obtained in a limited number of cases using toxicokinetic models to predict the accumulation of chemicals in biota based on short-term exposures (Galassi *et al.*, 1982; Galassi and Calamari, 1983). This was demonstrated, for example, in the case of 1,2,3- and 1,2,4-trichlorobenzenes for which 48-hour tests proved to be an adequate substitute for longer exposures using flow-through techniques. This new approach has significant possibilities considering the effort required and the problems inherent in the proper maintenance of early life stages of fish in the laboratory and in conducting toxicity tests with embryo-larval organisms.

18.11 RELEVANCE OF SHORT-TERM TESTS FOR THE DEFINITION OF WATER QUALITY CRITERIA

The data obtained in short-term tests are an essential component of the information necessary to establish water quality criteria. Gross effects can be reliably predicted based upon acute toxicity tests. However, short-term tests may be inadequate in the prediction of more subtle effects, especially those relating to environmental situations of greater complexity.

This was illustrated in the work of Hansen and Garton (1982) on the possibility of using standard toxicity tests to predict the effects of the insecticide Diflubenzuron on laboratory stream communities. Effects such as direct lethality to the biota of the ecosystem analysed could be clearly predicted but indirect effects due to altered interspecies interactions could be predicted only with 'a priori' knowledge of the trophic dynamics of the system.

Field validation of toxicological data is strongly recommended although it is rarely performed; most of the water quality criteria proposed by various organizations have never been verified in this way. Nevertheless, it is encouraging to note that in the few cases that validation has been attempted, the results were reassuring. Geckler *et al.* (1976), in a three-year study on a natural stream, found that copper already produced an effect at half of the concentration predicted from laboratory data. The effects which were noted were, however, only of a functional type since they consisted of a mass migration of animals from the test area in an avoidance reaction to the poison.

An extensive study on fish and fisheries in an area with a number of lakes polluted by copper and zinc was performed in Norway (EIFAC/FAO, 1977). In Lake Ringvatnet and Lake Hostovatnet, where there was a good fishery, the sum of the concentrations of copper and zinc slightly exceeded the water quality criteria proposed by EIFAC/FAO (Alabaster and Lloyd, 1982); in Lake Bjorra, where copper and zinc concentrations were much higher than EIFAC standards, all fish had disappeared. Van Loon and Beamish (1977) did not find any fish in Ross Lake with a high level of copper and zinc; they noted a slight decrease of the fish population in Hamell Lake where, during limited periods of the year, the sum of the metal concentrations exceeded the 95 percentile of water quality criteria formulated by EIFAC, while the 50 percentile of the sum of the two metals was 0.5. In Lake Cliff, on the contrary, where copper and zinc concentrations were lower, fish populations were flourishing. Such studies are an indirect confirmation of the utility of short-term laboratory tests, the results of which were used to establish the relevant water quality criteria.

18.12   CONCLUSIONS

There are numerous interactions between biota, and between biota and their surroundings; the complexity of these interactions make it theoretically impossible to predict the hazard which chemicals may represent for ecosystems by the use of tests on individual component parts of the system, e.g., single species. In consequence, greater attention has been directed during the last decade to multiple species and microcosm–mesocosm tests in the laboratory as well as in the field (Smies, 1983).

Multispecies tests are mostly long-term assays (several months up to years) and usually quite expensive. Due to the large number of variables involved, standardization of experimental microecosystems is, unfortunately, virtually impossible in either the field or in the laboratory. As a result, they suffer from an intrinsic lack of reproducibility which, in turn, makes them unsuitable for predicting effects in any other 'field situation' by extrapolation. Although ecological knowledge on the factors which rule structure and function of natural ecosystems is rapidly expanding, there is no multispecies toxicity protocol available which could be generally applied for predictive hazard assessment. According to Smies (1983), experimental micro-ecosystem assays are, however, becoming increasingly popular and have already proved valuable in the validation of bench tests for the assessment of real world hazards. Rodgers *et al.* (1983) demonstrated the potential of microcosms for the verification of theoretical models based on the distribution and fate of chemicals which, as indicated earlier, are of utmost importance for a correct exposure assessment.

Despite these limitations, it appears, in practice, that single species tests are extremely useful and are the major and only reliable means of estimating probable damage from anthropogenic stress at the present time (Cairns, 1983). Short-term bioassay data are an 'early warning' in predicting acute poisoning in the field; they can be used to predict the toxicities of mixtures and they can also serve to prognose effects in various physicochemical conditions.

Interesting extrapolations of predictive value can be made with acute toxicity curves; this can help in deciding if further testing for particular chemicals is needed.

REFERENCES

Alabaster, J..S., and Lloyd, R. (1982). *Water Quality Criteria for Freshwater Fish*, Second Edition, Butterworths, London.

Blanck, H. (1984). Species dependent variation among aquatic organisms in their sensitivity to chemicals. *Ecol. Bulletin,* **36**, 107–19.

Blanck, H., Wallin, G., and Wangberg, S.A. (1984). Species-dependent variation in algal sensitivity to chemical compounds. *Ecotoxicol. Environ. Safety,* **8**, 339–51.

Calamari, D., and Marchetti, R. (1974). Predicted and observed acute toxicity of copper and ammonia to rainbow trout (*Salmo gairdneri* Rich.). *Prog. Water Technol.,* **7**, 569–77.

Calamari, D., and Marchetti, R. (1978). Relevance of studies on developmental and young stages of *Salmo gairdneri* in establishing water quality criteria for fisheries. Berichte 10/78 Umweltbundesamt, 201–10, Berlin.

Calamari, D., Da Gasso, R., Galassi, S., Provini, A., and Vighi, M. (1980). Biodegeneration and toxicity of selected amines on aquatic organisms. *Chemosphere,* **9**, 753–62.

Calamari, D., Galassi, S., Setti, F., and Vighi, M. (1983). Toxicity of selected chlorobenzenes to aquatic organisms. *Chemosphere,* **12**, 253–62.

Cairns, J. Jr. (1983). Are single species toxicity tests alone adequate for estimating environ-mental hazard? *Hydrobiologia,* **100**, 47–57.

EIFAC/FAO (1977). Report on the effects of zinc and copper pollution on the salmonid fisheries in a river and lake system in central Norway. *EIFAC Tech. Pap.,* **29**, 34 p.

EIFAC/FAO (1980). Report on combined effects on freshwater fish and other aquatic life of mixtures of toxicants in water. *EIFAC Tech. Paper.,* **37**, 49 p.

Galassi, S., and Calamari, D. (1983). Toxicokinetics of 1,2,3 and 1,2,4 tichlorobenzenes in early life stages of *Salmo gairdneri Chemosphere,* **12**, 1599–603.

Galassi, S., Calamari, D., and Setti, F. (1982). Uptake and release of p-dichlorobenzene in early life stages of *Salmo gairdneri. Ecotoxicol. Environ. Safety,* **6**, 439–47.

Geckler, J.R., Horming, W.B. Neiheisel, T.M., Pickering, Q.H., and Robinson, E.L. (1976). Validity of laboratory tests for predicting copper toxicity in streams. Environmental Protection Agency, EPA-600/3-76-116, Washington, D.C.

Hansch, C. (1973). Quantitative approaches to pharmacological structure–activity relationships. In: Cavallito, C.J. (Ed.), *Structure Activity Relationships*, volume 1, Pergamon Press, Oxford, pp. 75–165.

Hansen, S.R., and Garton, R.R. (1982). Ability of standard toxicity tests to predict the effects of the insecticide diflurobenzuron on laboratory stream communities. *Can. J. Fish. Aquat. Sci.*, **39**, 1273–88.

Hasselrot, T.B. (1965). A study of remaining water pollution from a metal mine with caged fish as indicators. *Vattenhygien*, **21**, 11–16.

International Standards Organization (1978). Recommended changes to the ISO proposed flow-through test procedure ISO/TC 147/SC5 WG 3 DOC 18. Document presented to ISO Meeting, Ottawa, Canada, May 1978.

Kenaga, E.E. (1978). Test organisms and methods useful for early assessment of acute toxicity of chemicals. *Environ. Sci. Tech.*, **12**(12), 1322–9.

Kenaga, E.E. (1982a). Predictability of chronic toxicity from acute toxicity of chemicals in fish and aquatic invertebrates. *Environ. Toxicol. Chem.*, **14**, 347–58.

Kenaga, E.E. (1982b). Review: the use of environmental toxicology and chemistry data in hazard assessment: progress, needs, challenges, *Environ. Toxicol. Chem,.* **1**(1), 69–80.

Konemann, H. (1981). QSARs in fish toxicity studies, part 1: relationship for 50 industrial pollutants. *Toxicology*, **19**, 209–21.

Konemann, H., and Calamari, D. (1983). QSARs in aquatic toxicology. OECD Existing Chemicals Programme, 2nd Meeting, November 1983, Berlin.

Lloyd, R. (1960). The toxicity of zinc sulphate to rainbow trout. *Ann Appl. Biol.*, **48**, 84–94.

Lloyd, R. (1961). The toxicity of mixtures of zinc and copper sulphates to trout (*Salmo gairdneri* Rich.) *Ann. Appl. Biol.*, **49**, 535–8.

Lloyd, R. (1979). The use of the concentration–response relationship in assessing acute fish toxicity data. In: Dickson, K.L., Maki, A.W., and Cairns, J. Jr. (Eds), *Analyzing the Hazard Evaluation Process*, Water Quality Section, American Fisheries Society. Washington, D.C.

Lloyd, R. (1981). The role of acute toxicity tests with aquatic animals in chemical registration and notification schemes. In: Stokes, P.M. (Ed.), *Ecotoxicology and the Aquatic Environment*, Pergamon Press, Oxford, pp. 5–8.

Marchetti, R. (1965). The toxicity of nonylphenol ethoxylate to the development stages of the rainbow trout: *Salmo gairdneri* Rich. *J. Appl. Biol.*, **55**, 425–30.

McKim, J.M. (1977). Evaluation of tests with early life stages of fish for predicting long-term toxicity. *J. Fish. Res. Bd. Can.*, **34**, 1148–54.

McLeese, R.W., Zitko, V., Sergeant, D.B., Burridge, L., and Metcalfe, C.D. (1979). Structure–lethality relationship for phenols, anilines and other aromatic compounds in shrimps and clams. *Chemosphere*, **8**, 53–60.

Mount, D.I., and Stephan, C.E. (1967). A method for establishing acceptable toxicant limits for fish—malathion and the butoxyethanol ester of 2,4-D. *Trans. Am. Fish. Soc.*, **96**, 185–93.

Neely, B.W., Brauson, D.R., and Blau, G.E. (1974). Partition coefficient to measure bioconcentration potential of organic chemicals in fish. *Environ. Sci. Tech.*, **8**, 1113–15.

Organizatiron for Economic Cooperation and Development (OECD) (1981). *Guidelines for Testing of Chemicals*, OECD, Paris.

Rodgers, J.H. Jr., Dickson, K.L., Saleh, F.Y., and Staples, C.A. (1983). Use of microcosms to study transport, transformation and fate of organics in aquatic systems. *Environ. Toxicol. Chem.*, **2**(2), 155–67.

Samoiloff, M.R., and Wells, P.G. (1984). Future trends in marine ecotoxicology. In: Persooone, G., Jaspers, E., and Claus, C. (Eds), *Ecotoxicology Testing for the Marine Environment*, volume 1, State Univ. Ghent, and Inst. Mar. Scient. Res., Bredene, Belgium, pp. 733–50.

Sloof, W., and Canton, J.H. (1983). Comparison of the susceptibility of 11 fresh-water species to 8 chemical compounds. 2. (semi) chronic toxicity tests. *Aquat. Toxicol.*, **4**(3), 271–82.

Sloof, W., Canton, J.H., and Hermens, J.L.M. (1983). Comparison of the susceptibility of 22 freshwater species to 15 chemical compounds. 1. (sub)acute toxicity tests. *Aquat. Toxicol.*, **4**, 113–28.

Smies, M. (1983). On the relevance of microecosystems for risk assessment: some considerations for environmental toxicology. *Ecotoxicol. Environ. Safety*, **7**, 355–65.

Sprague, J.B. (1969). Measurement of pollutant toxicity to fish. 1. Bioassay methods for acute toxicity. *Wat. Res.*, **3**, 793–821.

Sprague, J.B. (1985). Factors that modify toxicity. In: Rand, G.M., and Petrocelli, S.R. (Eds), *Fundamentals of Aquatic Toxicology*, Chapter 6, Hemisphere Publishing Corp., Washington, D.C., pp. 124–63.

Suter, G.W. III, Vaughan, D.S., and Gardner, R.H. (1983). Risk assessment by analysis of extrapolation error: a demonstration for effect of pollutants on fish. *Environ. Toxicol. Chem.*, **2**(3), 369–78.

U.S. Environmental Protection Agency (EPA) (1980). Ambient water quality criteria for lead. EPA 440/5-80-057, Washington, D.C.

Van Loon, J.C., and Beamish, R.J. (1977). Heavy-metal contamination by atmospheric fallout of several Flin Flon area lakes and the relation to fish populations. *J. Fish. Res. Bd. Can.*, **34**, 899–906.

Veith, G.D., Call, D.J., and Brooke, L.T. (1983). Structure-toxicity relationships for the fathead minnow, *Pimephales promelas:* narcotic industrial chemicals. *Can. J. Fish. Aquatic. Sci.*, **40**, 743–8.

Veith, G.D., DeFoe, D.L., and Bergstedt, B.V. (1979). Measuring and estimating the bioconcentration factor of chemicals in fish. *J. Fish. Res. Bd. Can.*, **36**, 1040–48.

Veith, G.D. Macek, K.J., Petrocelli, S.R., and Carroll, J. (1980). An evaluation of using partition coefficients and water solubility to estimate bioconcentration factors for organic chemicals in fish. In: Eaton, J.G., Parish, P.R., and Hendricks, A.C. (Eds), *Aquatic Toxicology*, ASTM STP 707, ASTM, Philadelphia, PA, pp. 116–29.

Wuhrmann, K., and Woker, H. (1948). Beitrage zur Toxikologie der Fische. II. Experimentelle Untersuchungen uber die Ammoniak und Blausaurevergiftung. *Schweiz. Z. Hydrol.*, **11**, 210–44.

CHAPTER 19

Possibilities and Limitations of Short-term Tests for Ecotoxicologic Effects: Terrestrial Approaches

JAMES W. GILLETT

19.1 INTRODUCTION

This chapter attempts to set forth the problems of evaluation and assessment of impacts of organic chemicals in the terrestrial environment. It is very difficult to distinguish between and separate terrestrial and aquatic systems over concerns about chemical pollution. Land use patterns determine much of water quality. At the interfaces between terrestrial and aquatic environments (wetlands, stream- and lake-side, beaches), there are many cross-inputs. Some species (invertebrates and amphibians) spend parts of their lives in one and then another habitat. Some, apparently terrestrial, species may associate almost exlcusively with the aquatic environment. The osprey, for example, only touches land in the form of its nest and perch, feeding exclusively on fish. Is it an aquatic or terrestrial species?

19.2 PAST AND PRESENT APPROACHES TO TERRESTRIAL ECOTOXICOLOGY

19.2.1 Animals

19.2.1.1 General considerations

Terrestrial toxicologic investigations have mainly focused on health effects in mammalian species as models of potential impact on human health. However, the responses of white rats to acute oral, chronic dietary, and lifetime dietary exposures provide basic mammalian toxicological data not only on mortality and pathology, but also on growth, reproduction, gross organ toxicity, and functional impairment (e.g. neurotoxicity). Since these same concerns pertain to wild terrestrial mammals as well as humans, then rat toxicity studies (and surrogate *in vitro* tests) also serve terrestrial ecotoxicology.

Most single species toxicity testing has been conducted with insects (to screen the effectiveness of products against injurious (pest) or beneficial insects) and rodents (mainly rats, mice and guinea-pigs and undertaken for human health and safety reasons). Other species have received much less attention. Interest in impacts on avifauna, spurred by Rachel Carson's *Silent Spring* (1962), led to extensive testing of chemicals in birds (Tucker and Crabtree, 1970). However, the ecotoxicologic problems that became evident (Pimentel, 1971) involved sparse species at the top of the food chain, and the extensive testing which took place on birds such as chickens, quail and pheasant (all gallinaceous species and grain eaters) did not result in the same effects that were being observed in predators such as eagles, hawks, owls, ospreys and pelagic sea birds (which suffered from egg-shell thinning and reproductive failure).

Substantial efforts by the US Fish and Wildlife Service and other research organizations around the world have developed laboratory-reared species for such tests (e.g. the sparrowhawk (kestrel) and barn owl). Routine testing of pesticides, however, continues to involve bobwhite quail, pheasants and mallard ducks, selected to represent indigenous species at risk of exposure. Protocols in use for the evaluation of pesticides call for acute, subchronic, and field pen testing for mortality and effects on reproduction and behaviour. However, factors such as impact of migration and cross-exposure to the same or other pesticides in global transits are not readily tested.

Acute tests (of species) are usually performed as rangefinding tests to ascertain levels to use in chronic exposures. Chronic or iterative exposures in turn are used not only for determining mortality but also to obtain information about toxic effects on specific physiological functions, some examples of which are shown in Table 19.1. These examples demonstrate effects that have been found to be useful in analysing or predicting outcomes of the use of pesticides and other toxic substances in natural environments. They can be critical for one or more species, but may be irrelevant in terms of human toxicity. On the other hand, alternative animal models can provide better prediction of adverse human impacts on specific physiological functions than many traditional laboratory species (such as the rat). Examples of these alternative animal models are given in Table 19.2.

Single species toxicity tests serve only as a measure of impact on individual members of an ecosystem. Of greater importance are measures of irremedial or irreversible loss of species or function due to chronic or iterative exposure to a toxicant (Cairns *et al.*, 1981). Neuhold and Ruggerio (1976) noted at least five types of serious adverse effects for which ecotoxicologic concerns are high:

   (i)   loss of primary productivity;
  (ii)   loss of secondary productivity, growth and reproduction;
 (iii) disturbance in material and nutrient cycling;
 (iv) altered ecosystem structure, diversity and complexity; and
  (v)   loss of endangered species or their habitats.

Table 19.1   Tests with end-points other than mortality for the measurement of toxicity in terrestrial environments

Species	Test
Avian	
Chicken, quail, pheasant, grouse, sparrowhawk, mallard, barn owl	Reproduction—egg-shell thinning
Herring gull	Salt gland
Doves, finches	Reproductive behaviour
Amphibian	
Frogs, toads	Morphogenesis
Arthropods	
Honeybees	Communication, other behaviours
Crickets	Calling behaviour
Various spp.	Metamorphosis
Spiders	Web-spinning
Protista	
Bactteria	Nitrogen-fixation, ammonification, sulphate reduction, cellulytic decomposition
Fungi	Decomposition process

Table 19.2   Animal models used to predict toxic effects on human health

Species	Test
Chicken, cat	Delayed type neurotoxicity
Armadillo	Genotoxicity (quadruplicate birth)
Various rodents, poultry	Nutritional effects of toxicant
Rats, mice	Genotoxicity (cancer, reproduction)
Monkeys	Behavioural toxicology
Swine	Cardiovascular and gastrointestinal effects

19.2.1.2   Bioaccumulation

Studies with birds and field studies were among the first activities that revealed the significance of food chain uptake and magnification of chemicals, both of which continue to be a strong focus of ecotoxicologic testing. Uptake by all routes (bioaccumulation) and the transfer of that accumulated chemical between species (biomagnification) are often confused. In terrestrial species, bioaccumulation is dependent on many factors, including:

(1) exposure rate or concentration (Kenaga, 1972),
(2) properties of the chemical determining its stability, ability to pass through membranes, and extent of retention in tissues (Hansch, 1980); and
(3) pharmacodynamics of the chemical in the organism, in turn governed by physiological and biochemical factors such as blood flow and tissue- or organ-specific degradation or binding (Lindstrom *et al.*, 1974; Bungay *et al.*, 1980).

The physicochemical properties of a chemical are adequate to indicate *potential* bioaccumulation. The ability to predict bioaccumulation (Kenaga, 1980) partly depends on the octanol–water partition coefficient (K_{ow} or P), which may be measured, or may be predicted from the chemical structure of the toxicant (Leo *et al.*, 1971). The extent of bioaccumulation is proportional to P for values of P between 10^3 and 10^6. However, if the value of log P exceeds 6 (i.e. P exceeds 10^6), bioaccumulation may be substantially less than predicted. Nevertheless, suspected bioaccumulation is readily diagnosed from structure, providing that covalent reaction in biota is not in question.

This latter exception is demonstrated with the example of methyl mercury. As a fungicide, methyl mercury had been tested in various formulations without notable problems being apparent. Based on its relatively high water solubility and low log P, it had not been suspected of bioaccumulation. Shortly thereafter, it was recognized that mobilization of mercury from sediments (in the form of methyl mercury) was the cause of Minimata disease, and environmental surveys revealed heavy residues of mercury in many game birds suspected of having fed on fungicide-dressed seeds. Further investigation showed that the methyl mercury, accumulated by covalent reaction with protein sulphydryl groups, was chronically neurotoxic, although not especially lethal in acute doses. Thus, animals are capable of developing heavier total mercury loadings from methyl mercury than inorganic forms (Gillett, unpublished observations).

With some notable exceptions, biodegradability may also decrease with increasing log P. One such exception are the easily photolysed and hydrolysed pyrethroid chemicals which are not bioaccumulated in spite of high values of Log P. This covariant relationship is also affected by species-specific enzyme nature and amount, so that full predictability for all species is unattainable.

19.2.2 Plants

Most of the concern for toxicity to plants has been for indirect or non-target phytotoxic effects of chemicals such as insecticides, and concern is generally low unless crop productivity is significantly decreased. Testing of plant responses has focused largely on germination and early seedling growth, by means of field observation of effects. Various efforts to improve the seed germination-early seedling growth assays have been successful, but practically no effort has been made to standardize the several methods in use.

Relatively little testing of lower plants, other than algae, has taken place, since these tend to be of neither economic importance nor pest species. Because of emphasis on crop and pest species (largely rooted, higher plants) in agriculture, relatively little information on non-agricultural species and on later life stages, interspecies interactions, succession and community structure is available.

One exception is the body of information developed around the sensitivity of lichens (fungal–algal associations) to air pollutants (Duffus, 1980). The distribution of lichens between and within communities has served as a convenient index of air pollution. However, laboratory testing has not been widely employed, in part due to technical difficulties.

Much of the phytotoxicology centres around interference with photosynthesis, both because of the primary energetic considerations and because of the uniqueness of this system in plants. Many herbicides (Audus, 1964) depend on inhibition of one or more reactions of the photosynthetic cycle for their effectiveness. Tschan *et al.* (1975) developed an especially sensitive test for photosynthetic inhibitors, using light emission by a marine bacterium activated by the oxygen generated by photosynthesis. Any toxicant affecting reduction of water to oxygen or decreasing algal photosynthetic and oxidative efficiency leads to lower light emissions. Although theoretically operable for general metabolic toxicants (interfering with any oxygen-producing or oxygen-utilizing reactions), the Tschan test appears most sensitive to photosynthetic inhibitors. Improvements and modifications have been made, but the test still requires elaborate and expensive equipment without offering any better insight into ecotoxicologic problems.

Seed germination tests only examine a brief part of a plant's life cycle. Usually, the test provides an opportunity to examine early effects on morphology, susceptibility to pathogens and growth of root and hypocotyl. However, these observations are not always made or evaluated. Plant sensitivity to the action of chemical agents at later stages of its life cycle can be determined through field observation or greenhouse tests. The reproductive process (flowering, pollination, fruit formation and development), maturation, and senescence may also be affected by synthetic organic chemicals.

Attempts to establish a plant life cycle test using *Arabidopsis* spp. are underway (Tingey, personal communication). This small member of the wort family has a seed-to-seed time of around 30 days permitting it to be studied in botany classes. Its biology is thus well known, but its sensitivity to toxicants and the degree to which it may represent other, longer-lived species are in question. Furthermore, the mechanical difficulties in handling the very small seeds present a particular problem.

19.2.3 Microcosms

Given the status of single species testing, it is hardly surprising that multi-species tests of ecological effects, although considered most important, are just being developed and have only a small database to support their interpretation and use

(Cairns *et al.*, 1981). The laboratory model ecosystem or microcosm represents the highest order of testing outside of the field. A variety of terrestrial, aquatic and mixed media systems have been developed and applied to the evaluation of various synthetic chemicals, mostly pesticides. The technology has been reviewed extensively (Gillett and Witt, 1979; Giesy, 1980; Hammonds, 1981; Van Voris *et al.*, 1983a).

The microcosm is inherently safer and more easily manipulated than field sites, provides detail unattainable in the field, and is not subject to the vicissitudes of weather and geologic cataclysm. It permits rigorous testing of hypotheses developed from the laboratory (chemical or single species toxicity tests). While combining good features of both laboratory and field tests, microcosms have a variety of shortcomings including: never fully representing all ecological processes; being difficult to make self-sustaining with adequate complexity; and being fraught with methodologic difficulties. In a number of cases, the microcosm has been demonstrated as useful in assessing effects on primary productivity (Cole *et al.*, 1976; Van Voris *et al.*, 1983b), growth and reproduction (Gillett *et al.*, 1983a), nutrient cycling (Van Voris *et al.*, 1980), and interspecies interaction (Gillett *et al.*, 1983a). Because these are meaningful ecotoxicologic end-points, they suggest that further development will be worthwhile.

19.3 FUTURE TRENDS FOR SHORT-TERM TESTING IN TERRESTRIAL ECOTOXICOLOGY

19.3.1 General considerations

The trend towards the increasing use of short-term tests (especially *in vitro* tests) could result in a situation where the results of tests on whole animals (now used to support ecotoxicologic assessments as well as to assess the safety for human beings), might not be available. There is a significant implication in this since much as the single species test fails to provide integration of effects for the ecosystem (Cairns *et al.*, 1981; Levin and Kimball, 1983), so the short-term *in vitro* test fails to provide integration of effects at the organism level. For example, *in vitro* test systems such as perfused rat liver or hepatocytes may reveal much about the effects of a chemical on liver but other important effects (e.g. behaviour, feeding efficiency, etc.) may not be evidenced.

The challenge, then, is to establish a testing system which minimizes testing resources, adverse environmental impact (caused by the test itself), and excessive use of laboratory test species while gaining better information capable of ecological integration. The sheer complexity of this task suggests that a variety of approaches will have to be combined.

19.3.2   Structure–activity relationships

For new chemicals (and inadequately tested older chemicals), much can be gained by analysis of known structure–activity relationships (SAR). Even when there are few or no data available from toxicity tests, it is possible to express the nature and extent of concerns for a chemical from simple relationships (Gillett, 1983) in order to develop testable hypotheses which must then be investigated by means of additional testing. Many physicochemical characteristics of a specific chemical can be predicted from consideration of its structure or from other measured physicochemical properties (Lyman *et al.*, 1982). These estimated values can be employed in mathematical models (Neely, 1980) to estimate potential exposures. As part of a screening system, the estimation of physicochemical properties has already contributed much to simplifying assessment and testing. Unfortunately, as with all simplifications, much has been done without adequate background documentation.

Presently, SAR are based on statistical analysis of empirical data. For example, extensive investigation of bioaccumulation has provided substantial support for the use of SAR in predicting bioaccumulation potential. For interpolations, these SAR are quite accurate (error factors of only 2 or 10); however, extrapolation is less certain.

Acute toxicity for a given chemical in the laboratory rat can be predicted with some confidence if the acute toxicities of other members of the same class of compound are already known. However, chronic toxicity (where lethality is not the end-point) is much harder to predict. Numerous databases contain much information which would help bolster SAR efforts, but no suitable means of bringing together these data from around the world has been developed. Furthermore, there are questions about the quality of such data which have usually been generated over a decade or more.

The USEPA has instigated comprehensive acute and chronic toxicity databases for wildlife (TERRATOX) and plants (PHYTOX) to accompany the aquatic database AQUIRE and the chemical properties databases CHEMFATE, DATALOG and BIOLOG in the master program SPHERE (Miles *et al.*, 1983). Based on material in peer-reviewed, open literature and further screened for quality, these systems will be heavily employed in evaluation of new chemicals under the Toxic Substances Control Act and other legislation. Use of sophisticated computerized structural connectivity indices (UNICORN) will further enhance data accessibility. The LOG P DATABASE™ (Technical Database Services, Inc.) contains measured and evaluated partitioning data on over 5000 chemicals. Other commercial endeavours are largely oriented toward human health.

Subsequently, it may be possible to estimate unmeasured values through a number of multivariant analyses and other statistical techniques. Hudson *et al.* (1979) showed that acute (single dose) and subchronic (5-day dietary exposure plus 3-day feed-off) toxicity of chemicals to birds could be estimated from rat data within one order of magnitude. The degree to which such computerized SAR devices will substitute for actual testing will depend on the acceptability of this degree of error.

Although there are many relationships identified for SAR at the enzymatic level and a number at the species level, no such relationships have been developed for functions at levels of biological organization above the organism. The Pre-Biologic Screen (Gillett, 1983) uses a combination of log P (octanol–water partition coefficient), log (Henry's law constant), and log (biodegradation half-life) to pose testable hypotheses about a chemical in regard to ecotoxicologic concerns (bioaccumulation and chronic action; multi-species/multi-media involvement; chronic action in the water column, including leaching and plant uptake; and indirect effects due to atmospheric action). Concerns are ranked as high, moderate, and low (or negligible). While providing a useful means of ranking chemicals in relation to potential adverse effects, these methods do not constitute a guarantee of actual effects or serve as a surrogate for actual data.

It must be emphasized that testing is only one of the links in a complete assessment (Goss and Wyzga, 1982). Unnecessary testing has costs to the regulatory agency, the public and, of course, the manufacturer. Devising unambiguous criteria is an important objective so that much thinking has gone into the interpretation of schemes employing various SAR screens. Even so, for non-mammalian species, we are still very far away from predicting end-points other than death or genotoxic responses.

19.3.3   Generalized toxicity tests

The initial hope that these tests might serve as surrogates for predicting effects on higher organisms has not been borne out in several investigations. In the past two decades, several microbial tests have been proposed as means of estimating toxicity of individual chemicals, complex effluents and other mixtures. The Microtox™ test (Beckman Instruments, Inc., 1980) employs a marine bioluminescent bacteria which releases light through normal metabolism; toxic chemicals reduce luminescence (Dutka and Kwan, 1981). The Tschan test (described earlier) assesses phytotoxic chemicals acting through inhibition of the Hill reaction in photosynthesis. Respiratory inhibition (Liu, 1981; Bauer *et al.*, 1981) is more readily measured at a lower cost and without elaborate equipment (Gillett *et al.*, 1983b). Analyses of respiratory inhibition have shown (Dutka and Kwan, 1981; Gillett *et al.*, 1983b) that measurements were primarily affected by the size of the active microbial population rather than by inhibition of enzymes. Mixed population sources of organisms cultured under equivalent conditions were not statistically different, but selected species (pure cultures) might be more or less sensitive (Bauer *et al.*, 1981).

Now the question changes from, 'Are such generalized assays applicable to higher species, levels of biological organization, etc.?' to 'Are such *in vitro* tests applicable to even the tested species in the field?' Various *in vitro* studies have not yielded responses relevant to field results. The *in vitro* tests were either too sensitive or exposure was radically different in the field. In a microcosm study of 3,4-dichlorophenol (to which the bacteria of soil and sewage sludge were expected to be 'naive'), the *in vitro* EC50 was 10 to 20 mg/litre for pure and mixed cultures from a variety of sources (Gillett *et al.*, 1983b). However, soil respiration was uninhibited by 1000 p.p.m. (mg/kg dry soil) (Gillet *et al.*, unpublished results). The test chemical appeared to be both adsorbed and tightly bound to the soil in an unextractable form. The unextractable portion increased in proportion and extent as the proportion of organic matter increased between soil series, but also declined with time, releasing free (extractable) 3,4-DCP.

Thus, our inability to describe the chemodynamics of chemicals in sufficient detail, as to ascertain the specifics of exposure, limits laboratory-to-field extrapolation and the applicability of generalized toxicity assays. Much more work is needed to validate the capacity of all these toxicity tests to predict potential effects under field conditions.

Use of other species in generalized assays has not produced acceptable methods either. *Daphnia* spp., houseflies, earthworms (especially *Eisenia foetida*), honeybees and other invertebrates can be assayed accurately, reproducibly, and sensitively for numerous chemicals. On the other hand, each species or group is insensitive to certain classes of chemicals. Therefore, the effects noted in one species are not necessarily applicable or able to be extrapolated to other species. Lack of detailed research at higher levels of biological organization over a sufficient range of chemical classes, exposure scenarios, etc., precludes the general use of single species tests as indicators of ecotoxicologic concerns.

19.3.4   Microcosm studies

Microcosm tests are the principal alternative to single species tests for ecotoxicologic effects. These are expected to gain in value and significance as they are widely applied to environmental problems (Gillett and Witt, 1979). Initially, this type of study suffered from relatively high capital and operating costs and from heavy requirements for professional expertise. Recent efforts to develop standardized protocols have resulted in evidence that simple microcosms are cost-effective means of examining complex situations. Improvements in multi-seasonal operation of terrestrial systems indicate the ability to shorten the testing period. However, these same studies have not provided support for the earlier idea of microcosms as broad screening tools.

Further development of microcosm screening assays is likely to occur. Very small soil core microcosms (10 cm in diameter and 10 cm deep) (Draggan, 1976) are too highly variable (Gile *et al.*, 1979) for much use in terrestrial tests, but the soil litter microcosm (Lighthart *et al.*, 1982) of approximately 100 g of soil in a glass canning jar, and larger soil cores (with or without intact plant communities) of 15 cm diameter and 60 cm depth (Van Voris *et al.*, 1984) have suitable sensitivity, low variability and cost for some screening and confirmation uses.

Microcosms for agroecosystems can be readily and rationally constructed and operated under conditions that provide for substantial management decision-making power in assessments; however, there is a lack of understanding about the sensitivity and operation of microcosms representing non-agricultural systems. Although many mathematical models of ecosystem function have been constructed, few analyses of sensitivity of processes within systems or between systems have been performed relative to organic chemical insults. In part, this is due to deficiencies in knowledge of ecosystem science as applied to environmental impacts, but also to operational difficulties in developing and maintaining microcosms representing certain system (wetlands, forest systems) or general lack of interest in impacts on certain ecosystems (desert biomes, for example).

19.4 CONCLUSIONS

Terrestrial ecotoxicologic assessments are not likely to be enhanced by short-term *in vitro* toxicity test methods that depend on effects at a lower order of biological integration than currently practised in toxicologic studies. Present methods are already under criticism (Levin and Kimball, 1983) for inadequacies regarding representativeness, completeness, meaningful sensitivity, statistical validity, and quality assurance.

Terrestrial ecotoxicologic assessments currently utilize much information generated in the course of human health assessments, especially mammalian toxicity data. Two other approaches seem useful in enhancing currently available techniques and tests:

(1) The development and improvement of SAR methods, which can shorten and focus testing requirements, obviating all but those needed to confirm or discriminate particular problems. Development to extend those methods from the sub-organismal and organismal levels to higher levels of biological organization is required. As computer-accessible databases are developed and organized, attention to quality assurance of data and other details are suspected to be important.

(2) Microcosm technology, which needs a broader database with more chemical classes and types of observations of higher level functions within the model ecosystems. Validation of the applicability of this technology in particular assessments is needed, as well as further system improvements and broader representation of ecotypes.

Because of the potential cost-effectiveness and incisiveness of microcosm studies, particularly when used in conjunction with SAR techniques to establish testable hypotheses of adverse action, this technology may lead to reduced resource needs and costs, the basic objective of short-term testing.

REFERENCES

Audus, L.J. (1964). *The Physiology and Biochemistry of Herbicides,* Academic Press, New York, NY, 555 p.

Bauer, N.J., Seideler, R.J., and Knittel, M.D. (1981). A simple, rapid test for pollutant effects on microbiota. *Bull. Environ. Contam. Toxicol.,* **27,** 577–82.

Beckman Instruments Inc. (1980). *Microtox™ Assay Interim Manual* N. 11067.9B-9-80.

Bungay, P.M., Dedrick, R.L., and Matthews, H.B. (1980). Pharmacokinetics of environmental contaminants. In: Haque, R. (Ed.), *Dynamics, Exposure and Hazard Assessment of Toxic Chemicals,* Ann Arbor Science Publishers, Ann Arbor, MI, pp. 369–78.

Cairns, J. Jr., Alexander, M., Cummin, K.W., Edmonson, W.T., Goldman, R., Harte, J., Isensee, A.R., Levin, R., McCormick, J.F., Peterle, T.J., and Zar, J.H. (1981). *Testing for Effects of Chemicals on Ecosystems,* National Academy Press, Washington, D.C., 103 p.

Carson, R. (1962). *Silent Spring,* Houghton, Mifflin, Boston, MA, 368 p.

Cole, L.K., Sanborn, J.R., and Metcalf, R.L. (1976). Inhibition of corn growth by aldrin and the insecticide's fate in the soil, air and wildlife of a terrestrial model ecosystem. *Econ. Entomol.,* **5,** 583–9.

Draggan, S. (1976). The microcosm as a research tool for estimation of environmental transport of toxic materials. *Intern. J. Environ. Studies,* **10,** 5–10.

Duffus, J.H. (1980). *Environmental Toxicology,* Edward Arnold Publishers Ltd., London, 164 p.

Dutka, B.J., and Kwan, K.K. (1981). Comparison of three microbial screening tests with the Microtox test. *Bull. Environ. Contam. Toxicol.,* **27,** 755–7.

Giesy, J. (Ed.) (1980). *Microcosms in Ecological Research,* DOE Symposium No. 52, US National Technical Information Service, Springfield, VA, 1008 p.

Gile, J.D., Collins, J.C., and Gillett, J.W. (1979). *The Soil Core Microcosm—A Potential Screening Tool,* EPA 600/3-79-089, US Environmental Protection Agency, Corvallis, OR, 40 p.

Gillett, J.W. (1983). A comprehensive prebiologic screen for ecotoxicologic effects. *Environ. Toxicol. Chem.,* **2,** 463–76.

Gillett, J.W., and Witt, J.M. (1979). *Terrestrial Microcosms,* NSF-RA-790034, National Science Foundation, Washington, D.C., 34 p.

Gillett, J.W., Gile, J.D., and Russell, L.K. (1983a). Predator–prey (vole–cricket) interactions: the effects of wood preservatives. *Environ. Toxicol. Chem.,* **2,** 185–93.

Gillett, J.W., Knittel, M.D., Jolma, E., and Coulombe, R. (1983b). Applicability of microbial toxicity assays to assessment problems. *Environ. Toxicol. Chem.,* **2,** 185–93.

Goss, B.L., and Wyzga, R. (1982). A conceptual framework of ecological risk analysis. Presented at Pacific Div., Amer. Assoc. Adv. Sci., 20 June, 1982.

Hammonds, A. (Ed.) (1981). *Methods for Ecological Toxicology—A Critical Review of Laboratory Multi-Species Tests,* Ann Arbor Science Publishers, Woburn, MA. 310 p.

Hansch, C. (1980). The role of the partition coefficient in environmental toxicity. In: Haque, R. (Ed.), *Dynamics, Exposure and Hazard Assessment of Toxic Chemicals,* Ann Arbor Science Publishers, Ann Arbor, MI, pp. 273–86.

Hudson, R.H., Haegle, M.A., and Tucker, R.K. (1979). Acute oral and percutaneous toxicity of pesticides to mallards: correlations with mammalian toxicity data. *Toxicol. Appl. Pharmacol.,* **47,** 451–60.

Kenaga, E.E. (1972). Guidelines for environmental study of pesticides: Determination of bioconcentration potential. *Residue Rev.,* **44,** 73–114.

Kenaga, E.E. (1980). Correlation of bioconcentration factors of chemicals in aquatic and terrestrial organisms with their physical and chemical properties. *Environ. Sci. Technol.,* **14,** 553–6.

Leo, A., Hansch, C., and Elkins, D. (1971). Partition coefficients and their uses. *Chem. Rev.,* **71**, 525–616.

Levin, S.A., and Kimball, K.D. (Eds) (1983). *New Perspectives in Ecotoxicology,* Ecosystems Research Center, Cornell University, Ithaca, NY, 158 p.

Lighthart, B., Baham, J., and Volk, V.V. (1982). Microbial respiration and chemical speciation in metal-amended soils. *J. Environ. Qual.,* **12**,. 543–8.

Lindstrom, F.T., Gillett, J.W., and Rodecap, S.E. (1974). Distribution of HEOD (dieldrin) in mammals: I. Preliminary model. *Arch. Environ. Contam. Toxicol.,* **2**, 9–42.

Liu, D. (1981). A rapid biochemical test for measuring chemical toxicity. *Bull. Environ. Contam. Toxicol.,* **26**, 145–9.

Lyman, W.J., Reehl, W.F., and Rosenblatt, D.H. (1982). *Handbook of Chemical Property Estimation Methods: Environmental Behavior of Organic Compounds,* McGraw-Hill, New York, NY, 580 p.

Miles, P.C., Auer, F.M., and Hasson, M.A. (1983). New developments of the EPA SPHERE database. Presented at the 4th annual meeting of the Society for Environmental Toxicology and Chemistry, Arlington, VA, Nov. 1983.

Neely, B. (1980). A method for selecting the most appropriate environmental experiments on a new chemical. In: Haque, R. (Ed.), *Dynamics, Exposure and Hazard Assessment of Toxic Chemicals,* Ann Arbor Science Publishers, Ann Arbor, MI, pp. 287–96.

Neuhold, J., and Ruggerio, L. (1976). *Ecosystem Processes and Organic Contaminants,* NSF-RA-760008, National Science Foundation, Washington, D.C., 41 p.

Pimentel, D. (1971). *Ecological Effects of Pesticides on Non-Target Species,* Office of Science and Technology, US Govt. Printing Office, Washington, D.C., 220 p.

Tschan, Y.T., Roseby, J.E., and Funnell, G.R. (1975). Toxicity and persistence of herbicides. *Soil Biol. Biochem.,* **7**, 34–40.

Tucker, R.K., and Crabtree, D.G. (1970). *Handbook of Toxicity of Pesticides to Wildlife,* Resource Publication Series No. 84, US Fish and Wildlife Service, Washington, D.C., 131 p.

Van Voris, P., O'Neill, R.V., Emanuel, W.R., and Shugart, H.H. (1980). Functional complexity and ecosystem stability, *Ecol.,* **6**, 1352–60.

Van Voris, P., Tolle, D.A., Arthur, M.F., Chesson, J., and Brocksen, R.W. (1983a). Terrestrial microcosms: validation, applications and cost-benefit analysis. Presented at 4th annual meeting of the Society of Environmental Toxicology and Chemistry, Arlington, VA, Nov. 1983.

Van Voris, P., Arthur, M.F., and Tolle, D.A. (1983b). *Field and Laboratory Evaluation of Terrestrial Microcosms for Assessing Ecological Effects of Utility Wastes,* Project Report 1224–5, Electric Power Research Institute, Palo Alto, CA, 183 p.

Van Voris, P., Arthur, M.F., and Tolle, D.A. (1984). *Standard Method and Technical Support Document for the Soil Core Microcosm,* Draft document to Office of Toxic Substances, US Environmental Protection Agency, Washington, D.C.

CHAPTER 20

Predicting Safe Levels of Chemicals

I. V. SANOCKIJ

20.1   INTRODUCTION

The capacity of existing toxicological laboratories is insufficient to evaluate the toxicity, hazard and safe (permissible) exposure levels of all known chemicals, or all new chemical compounds before they are introduced to the environment. Therefore, there is a need to develop methods of rapidly predicting safe exposure levels in the absence of extensive toxicological information. In the USSR, a variety of methods have been proposed for the rapid prediction of safe levels of chemicals for human exposure. These have been developed for chemicals or families of chemicals with well-known properties and established toxicities. The effectiveness of each approach has been determined by examining the correlation of the properties under investigation with the existing maximum acceptable concentrations (MACs), established by traditional methods, for the chemicals being considered.

20.2   LIMITATIONS IN EXTRAPOLATING THE RESULTS OF TRADITIONAL TOXICOLOGY TO MAN

Traditional toxicology involves experimentation with laboratory animals (generally mammals) with the aim of extrapolating the results to humans. However, there are a number of factors in this approach which limit the validity of data interpretations and extrapolations.

20.2.1   Variation in toxicity with route of exposure

It is often necessary to extrapolate toxicity data for one route of exposure to establish safe levels for a different route of exposure. This may arise, for example, when attempting to set MACs for chemicals in the air of the occupational environment based on data derived from exposure of animals via the diet. However, the toxicity or hazard of a chemical can be markedly different for different routes of exposure, as demonstrated in Table 20.1.

Table 20.1   Degree of toxicity of substances by ingestion and inhalation

Substance	Ingestion		Inhalation	
	LD50 (mg/kg)	Hazard classification*	LC50 (mg/m^3)	Hazard classification*
m-aminobenztrifluoride	220	III	440	I
Benzyl chloride	1500	III	390	I
Benzyl chloride	1400	III	210	I
Benztrichloride	1300	III	60	I
Bromacetopropylacetate	600	III	149	I
2-Vinylpyridine	420	III	460	I
Dinitril perfluoroglutaric acid	997	III	58	I
Benzidine	327	III	290	I
2-Chloroethanesulphochloride	240	III	250	I

* Harmful substances are classified into the following four classes of hazard: I, extremely hazardous; II, very hazardous; III, moderately hazardous; IV, slightly hazardous.
These hazard classes are defined and described in detail in the State Standard GOST 12.1.007–76 entitled 'System of Occupational Safety Standards. Harmful Substances. Classification and General Safety Requirements'.

20.2.2   Variation with age and size

There is a concern with regard to variation of toxic response with age and size, not only in the laboratory animals upon which tests are conducted, but also with respect to the workforce for which occupational exposure limits are being established.

To some extent, species differences in response to a toxic chemical may be explained by variation in size. Allometric relationships, such as size and age variation in metabolism, can be correlated to inter- and intraspecies differences in responses to toxic chemicals.

With regard to worker protection, MACs are usually established for a healthy, mature, young adult, whereas increasing numbers of adolescents and older persons are making up the workforce. Variations in the responses of these different subpopulations are seldom considered when MACs are being established.

20.2.3   Variations in species sensitivity

Interspecies differences in sensitivity to specific chemicals can be represented by the coefficient of species sensitivity (CSS):

$$CCS = \frac{LD50_{max}}{LD50_{min}}$$

where the $LD50_{max}$ is the LD50 of the most tolerant (i.e. least sensitive) species tested, and the $LD50_{min}$ is the LD50 of the least tolerant (most sensitive) species tested.

Table 20.2 displays CSS values for 52 chemicals tested with four species of laboratory rodents.

Table 20.2   LD50 values for different species under administration into the stomach and the CSS values

No	Substance	Mouse LD50 (mg/kg)	Rat LD50 (mg/kg)	Guinea-pig LD50 (mg/kg)	Rabbit LD50 (mg/kg)	CSS
1	Acetocyanhydrine	2.9	13	9	13	4.4
2	Acetphos	210	45	27	45	7.7
3	Ammonium perchlorate	1 900	4 200	3 310	1 900	2.2
4	Acetonenitrile	48	105	50	19	5.5
5	Butylacetate	7 700	13 100	4 700	3 200	4.0
6	1,4-Butanediol	2 062	1 525	1 200	2 531	2.1
7	1,4-Butinediol	104	104	130	150	1.5
8	Butyphos	179	217	146	242	1.6
9	*N*-Butylpyro-catechol	3 000	4 700	1 400	2 800	3.3
10	Gramoxon	37	188	38.6	49.8	3.2
11	Hydrazine hydrate	83	129	40	55	3.2
12	Hexachlorobutane	2 000	1 413	940	1 071	2.1
13	Hexachloro-butadiene	87	350	90	90	4.0
14	3,4-Dichloroaniline	500–700	500–700	500–700	500–700	1.0
15	2,5-Dichloroaniline	2 500–3 000	2 500–3 000	2 500–3 000	2 500–3 000	1.0
16	Dichlorobutyl-tin	35	112	190	125	5.4
17	DDT	180	400	400	300	2.2
18	α-2,4-Dinitrophenol	46	31	81	30	2.7
19	1,2-Dibrom-3-chloropropane	410	300	210	180	2.2
20	Diethanolamine	3 300	3 460	2 200	2 200	1.5
21	Ammonium dimethyldithio-carbonate	592	1 458	1 680	450	3.7
22	1,2-Dibromoethane	420	117	110	55	7.6
23	Diphenylpropane	2 400	12 000	4 000	4 000	5.0
24	Indalon	11.6	7.4	3.2	5.4	3.6
25	Carbathione	266	700	815	320	3.0
26	Monoethanolamine	1 476	2 050	620	1 000	3.3
27	Monoethanol-ethylenediamide	3 550	3 600	1 500	2 000	2.4

Table 20.2   *(continued)*

28	Methylacetophos	322	380	214	420	1.9
29	Murbetol	50	250	250	200	5.0
30	Melprex	266	1 118	176	535	6.3
31	Nicotine (base)	24	50	220	30	9.1
32	*n*-Nitrotoluene	330	2 400	3 600	2 400	10.9
33	Sodium fluoride	80	200	250	100	3.1
34	Parachlorobenzene	3 220	2 512	7 593	2 812	3.0
35	Pentachlorobutane	2 500	2 108	1 410	1 560	1.7
36	Reglone	79.7	281.9	123.6	227.8	3.5
37	Ethyl alcohol	9 488	13 660	1 600	6 300	8.5
38	Carbon disulphide	2 780	3 188	2 125	2 550	1.5
39	Titanium	150	472	100	100	4.7
40	Tetraethyl-tin	40	15	37	7	5.7
41	1,1,1-Trichloroethane	17 200	12 300	9 470	5 660	3.0
42	Phenylhydrazine	175	188	80	80	2.4
43	Triethanolamine	7 750	8 400	5 160	5 300	1.6
44	2-Phenylcyclo-hexenal	5.4	3.5	1.6	2.7	3.3
45	3-Chloro-4-methylcoumarinyl	28	38	57	75	2.6
46	Chlorobenzene	1 445	2 390	5 060	2 250	3.5
47	Chloroindane	1 000	700	1 000	500	2.0
48	Carbon tetrachloride	9 066	6 200	5 760	5 760	1.5
49	Calcium cyanamide	415	513	415	353	1.4
50	Ethyleneglycol	8 348	6 122	8 213	9 000	1.4
51	Epichlorohydrine	194	141	280	345	2.4
52	Ethoxyphos	375	190	300	375	1.9

It has been shown that a threefold difference in LD50 and LC50 is within the normal limits of experimental error and cannot, therefore, serve as a criterion of species differences in sensitivity. This variability, and its significance compared with experimental error, must be considered when extrapolating this data to human beings.

20.2.4   Extrapolation of animal results to man

When differences in species sensitivity are strongly manifested, the extrapolation of test results to humans must be done with caution. Extrapolation is most valid when differences in interspecies sensitivity are small (i.e. CSS≤3). If the CSS value for a substance is less than or equal to 3, then the data suggest that there is a 2:1 probability that the sensitivity of humans to that substance will be in the same range (within error limits; i.e. animal:human $CSS(K_2)$≤3). For 34 substances for which

Table 20.3   LD50 values (mg/kg) and their ratio for different species of laboratory animals and for man

No	Substance	Mouse	Rat	Guinea-pig	Rabbit	Man	$LD50_{max}/LD50_{min}$	$LD50_{min}/LD50_{man}$
1	Barium carbonate	200	125	235	—	12.1	1.9	10.3
2	Barium chloride	350	350	—	170	5.0	2.1	34.0
3	Sodium chloride	—	12 000	—	10 000	4 285	1.2	2.3
4	Mercury dichloride	17.5	80	—	30	4.2	4.6	4.2
5	Zink sulphite	—	2 200	—	2 057	107.1	1.1	19.2
6	Calcium cyanamide	415	513	415	353	642.5	1.4	0.5
7	Cichloremethane	5 600	—	—	1 896	2 385	3.0	0.8
8	Chloroform	1 750	2 180	1 750	—	856.5	1.2	2.0
9	Carbon tetrachloride	9 066	6 200	5 760	5 760	428	1.6	˙13.4
10	Dichlorethane	910	770	—	910	671	1.2	1.1
11	Phenol	—	415	—	510	140	1.2	3.0
12	Methyl alcohol	8 712	12 880	—	9 029	338.5	1.5	25.7
13	Ethyl alcohol	9 488	13 660	2 400	7 900	4 514.2	5.7	0.5
14	Butyl alcohol	2 835	4 360	—	1 750	2 892.8	2.5	0.6
15	Ethyleneglycol	8 348	7 331	8 213	9 000	1 667.5	1.2	4.4
16	Chloralhydrate	—	650	—	1 300	142	2.0	4.6
17	Formaldehyde	—	800	260	—	142	3.1	1.8
18	Paraldehyde	1 790	1 650	—	5 000	1 715	3.0	0.96
19	Malathione (carbophos)	1 187.5	3 000	570	—	17.8	5.3	32.0
20	Octamethyl	22.5	16	—	—	12.5	1.4	1.3
21	Parathione (thiophos)	17	10.5	18.5	50	1.7	4.8	6.2
22	Tricresyl-phosphate	—	—	400	100	7.1	4.0	14.1
23	Chlorophos	377.5	525	—	—	40	1.4	9.4
24	Luminal	325	660	—	150	71	4.4	2.1
25	Barbitol (veronal)	600	200	—	262.5	100	3.0	2.0
26	Mephenizine	150	110	—	50	17.5	3.0	2.8
27	DDT	190	500	400	300	107.1	2.6	1.8
28	Aldrin	20	49	—	—	27.5	2.4	0.7
29	Dieldrin	25	68.5	—	—	27.5	2.7	0.9
30	Salicylic acid	430	900	—	1 100	214	2.3	2.2
31	Aniline	1 075	—	2 500	1 000	285	2.5	3.5
32	Nitrobenzene	—	640	—	660	21.4	1.0	29.9
33	Dinitroorthocresol	47	28	—	—	11.4	1.7	2.4
34	Sodium fluoride	80	200	250	150	87.5	3.1	0.9

Table 20.4 Biological activity (l_i) values of chemical bonds of standardized compounds belonging to different homologous series

Bond	l_i(litres/μmol)	Series
C−H	0.8	Saturated and unsaturated, cyclic and non-cyclic and mixed hydrocarbons
C−H	21 273.9	Saturated aldehydes (joined to the carbonyl group)
C−C	51.4	Saturated non-cyclic hydrocarbons
C−C	173.7	Saturated cyclic hydrocarbons
C=C (conjugated bond)*	242.4	Unsaturated cyclic hydrocarbons
C=C	451.8	Unsaturated non-cyclic hydrocarbons
C=C	1 126.5	Unsubstituted aromatic hydrocarbons
C=C	507.9	Substituted aromatic hydrocarbons with one and two side chains
C=C	7 057.9	Substituted aromatic hydrocarbons with an unsaturated side chain
C≡C	2 097.1	Unsaturated hydrocarbons containing a triple bond
C−N	−6 242.7	Aliphatic nitro compounds (one C−N bond joined to carbon)
C−N	154 446.3	Aliphatic nitro compounds (four C−N bonds joined to carbon) from tetranitromethane
C−N	119 027.8	Cyclic mono-nitro compounds
C−N	27 970.0	Aromatic mono-nitro compounds
C−N	77 851.5	Aromatic di-nitro compounds
C−N	66 442.0	Aromatic tri-nitro compounds
C−N	6 113.5	Aliphatic primary amines
C−N	1 565.7	Aliphatic secondary amines
C−N	3 266.2	Aliphatic tertiary amines
C−N	35 914.6	Aliphatic diamines
C−N	97 551.4	Cyclic amines
C−N	33 302.0	Aromatic amines
C−N	16 680.8	Amides
C−N	4 817.6	Heterocyclic compounds
C=N	9 635.2	Heterocyclic compounds
C≡N	97 856.8	Cyanides
C−O	21 987.7	Non-cyclic oxides
C−O	2 465.7	Heterocyclic oxides
C−O	68.1	Aliphatic ethers
C−O	6 535.3	Esters of saturated alcohols
C−O	10 306.9	Esters of unsaturated alcohols
C=O	213.8	Saturated ketones
C=O	8 753.8	Cyclic saturated ketones
C=O	−12 517.8	Saturated aldehydes (joined to the carbonyl group)

Table 20.4   *(continued)*

O–H	8 507.9	Organic acids
O–H	–21 648.2	Monohydric saturated alcohols
O–H	100 223.6	Unsaturated alcohols
O–H	–5 214.5	Aromatic alcohols
N–H	283.3	Ammonia
N–O	2 230.3	Oxides of nitrogen
N=O	4 460.6	Oxides of nitrogen
N=C	1 644 538.3	Aliphatic isocyanides
N=C	139 778.4	Aromatic isocyanides
N–N	318 864.8	Inorganic amines

* The conjugated bond (C=C) differs from an unconjugated bond in that, in the molecule of the compound, it alternates with (C–C) bonds.

human lethality data was available, it was found that about two thirds of those substances with low interspecies variability (CSS $\leq$3; 26 substances) also had low animal/human variability in toxic response (K_2 $\leq$3; 16 substances) (Table 20.3). The parameter K_2, is calculated as follows:

$$K_2 = \frac{LD50_{min}}{LD50_{man}}$$

where $LD50_{min}$ is the LD50 for the most sensitive (least tolerant) species tested, and the $LD50_{man}$ is the LD50 for man.

Therefore, generally, when CSS is $\leq$3, there is a strong probability (i.e. 2:1) that K_2 will be $\leq$3.

The validity of extrapolation to humans is greater when the threshold of chronic action (Lim_{ch}) is considered instead of the LD50. Therefore, the probability of establishing an adequately safe human exposure level based on animal lim_{ch} data is greater than when using lethal toxicity data.

20.3   METHODS FOR ESTABLISHING SAFE LEVELS OF OCCUPATIONAL EXPOSURE VIA INHALATION

There have been three basic approaches for the rapid determination of safe levels of occupational exposure to chemicals:

(1)   derivation on the basis of molecular structure;
(2)   derivation on the basis of physicochemical properties;
(3)   derivation on the basis of biological activity.

20.3.1 Molecular structure

The derivation of safe exposure levels in air (maximum acceptable concentration (MAC)) on the basis of chemical structure and the biological activity of chemical bonds was proposed by G. N. Zaeva. In this approach, an index of biological activity (l_i) was established for various chemical bonds (Table 20.4). The MAC for a compound could be calculated as follows:

$$MAC = \frac{M(1000)}{\Sigma l_i} \ (mg/m^3)$$

For example, the MAC for valerianic acid would be calculated as:

$$CH_3CH_2CH_2CH_2COOH \qquad Valerianic\ acid$$

$$MAC = \frac{102(1000)}{9(C–H) + 4(C–C) + 1(C = O) + 1(C–O) + 1(O–H)}$$

$$= \frac{102(1000)}{9(0.8) + 4(51.4) + 1(-12517.8) + 1(2197.7) + 1(8507.9)}$$

$$= 5.6\ mg/m^3.$$

The MAC for valerianic acid legislated by the USSR is 5 mg/m^3. MAC values calculated by this approach generally agree with MACs established for saturated organic acids and alcohols of aliphatic series.

20.3.2 Physicochemical properties

Extensive studies have been carried out on the correlation of physicochemical properties of chemicals and their toxicity by E. I. Ljublina and co-workers at the Leningrad Institute of Industrial Hygiene and Occupational Diseases. Their work examined the relationships of various properties (Table 20.5) of chemicals with the two hour LC50, the two-hour NC50 (NC = narcotic concentration) and with C_{lim} (the threshold concentration causing changes in the bending reflex of rabbits after a 40-minute exposure). The physicochemical properties most closely associated with biological activity were molecular weight, density, refractive index and melting point.

A variety of equations were developed for the calculation of an MAC for inhalation exposure based on correlations with physicocheical properties. These equations included the following:

Table 20.5 Physicochemical properties correlated with biological activity

No.	Name	Units
1	Molecular weight	
2	Density	g/cm^3
3	Molar volume	cm^3/mol
4	Refractive index	
5	Molar refraction	cm^3/mol
6	Melting point	°C
7	Boiling point	°C
8	Saturated vapour pressure	mm Hg
9	Equilibrium temperature	°C
10	Rate of change of t_{boil} with pressure	°C/mm Hg
11	Critical density	g/cm^3
12	Critical temperature	°C
13	Critical pressure	atm
14	Latent heat of fusion	kcal/mol
15	Latent heat of vaporization	kcal/mol
16	Heat of combustion	kcal/mol
17	Heat of formation of gas	kcal/mol
18	Helmholtz energy of formation of gas	kcal/mol
19	Logarithm of distribution coefficient (olive oil/water)	
20	Logarithm of distribution coefficient (water/air)	
21	Surface tension	dyne/cm
22	Kinematic viscosity	centistokes
23	Dynamic viscosity	centipoise
24	Solubility	mmol/litre
25	Specific heat capacity	cal/mol °K
26	Specific heat of vapour	cal/mol °K
27	Themal conductivity	cal/cm s °K
28	Atomic polarization	cm^3
29	Electric dipole moment	Debye
30	Dielectric constant	
31	Specific dispersion	cm^3/g
32	Absolute dispersion	
33	Primary ionization potential	electronvolt
34	Entropy of liquid	cal/mol °C
35	Entropy of gas	cal/mol °C

$$\log(\text{MAC}) = 0.4 - 0.01M + \log M \ (\text{mg/m}^3)$$

$$\log(\text{MAC}) = 1.6 - 2.2(p) + \log M \ (\text{mg/m}^3)$$

$$\log(\text{MAC}) = 14.2 - 10(n_{\text{D}}) + \log M \ (\text{mg/m}^3)$$

$$\log(\text{MAC}) = 0.6 - 0.01(t_{\text{boil}}) + \log M \ (\text{mg/m}^3)$$

$$\log(\text{MAC}) = -1.2 - 1.012\,(t_{\text{melt}}) + \log M \ (\text{mg/m}^3)$$

$$\log(\text{MAC}) = 0.48\log(v) - 1.0 + \log M \ (\text{mg/m}^3)$$

where p is the density (g/cm^3), n_D is the refractive index, t_{boil} is the boiling point (°C), t_{melt} is the melting point (°C), and v is the saturated vapour pressure (mm Hg).

Additional equations were developed to more accurately predict MACs for chemicals in homologous series (Table 20.6). However, an intermediate method is still required for the accurate calculation of MACs or other toxicity indices which, although not necessarily all-embracing, would not be limited to particular homologous series.

Table 20.6   Reliability of correlations between the existing maximum allowable concentration (in mmol/m^3) and equations for the calculation of the MAC based on the molecular weight (M), the boiling point (t_{boil}) and the melting point (t_{melt})

Substances	No. of pairs (n)	Correlation coefficient (r)	Probability (p)	Mean deviation (S_{yx})	Equation log MAC =
Hydrocarbons	42	−0.65	<0.001	0.70	0.99–0.012 M
	42	−0.71	<0.001	0.65	0.41–0.006 t_{boil}
	34	−0.62	<0.001	0.73	−0.72–0.007 t_{melt}
Saturated	18	−0.56	<0.02	0.85	1.00–0.015 M
monohydric	17	−0.68	<0.01	0.77	1.41–0.012 t_{boil}
alcohols	10	−0.66	<0.05	0.77	−0.47–0.008 t_{melt}
Nitro compounds	25	−0.72	<0.001	0.71	0.15–0.013 M
without unsaturated	16	−0.70	<0.001	0.69	−0.01–0.008 t_{boil}
bonds in open chains	21	−0.67	<0.001	0.71	−1.67–0.009 t_{melt}
Amines, nitroamines	40	−0.50	=0.001	0.56	−1.04–0.006 M
and other derivatives	31	−0.49	<0.01	0.61	−1.18–0.003 t_{boil}
of amines	27	−0.52	<0.01	0.58	−1.62–0.004 t_{melt}
Chlorinated	35	−0.61	<0.001	0.77	0.12–0.011 M
hydrocarbons	32	−0.51	<0.01	0.83	−0.57–0.007 t_{boil}
	22	−0.65	<0.01	0.58	−1.60–0.009 t_{melt}

20.3.3   Biological activity

K. K. Sidorov proposed a method for deriving MACs based on the threshold of chronic action (lim_{ch}):

$$MAC = \frac{lim_{ch}}{safety\ factor}$$

lim_{ch} is based on a chronic exposure by inhalation for four months (4 hours/day; 5 days a week). Alternatively, lim_{ch} (in units of mg/m^3) can be calculated by one of the following two equations:

$$\log(\text{lim}_{ch}) \ (mg/m^3) = 0.62 \times \log[LC_{50} \ (mg/m^3)] - 1.08;$$
$$\log(\text{lim}_{ch}) \ (mg/m^3) = 0.77 \times \log[\text{lim}_{ac} \ (mg/m^3)] - 1.56.$$

The safety factor is determined from differences in interspecies sensitivity (CSS; see Table 20.7) and the 'degree of cumulative effects' (see Table 20.8) as the product of points attributed to the values for CSS and Z_{biol} or Z_{ch} determined from the toxicity data. For example, the MAC for bromobenzene would be calculated as follows:

Table 20.7   Coefficient of species sensitivity (CSS)

Degree	CSS	Points
Low	<3	2
Moderate	3.1–9	3
High	>9	4

Table 20.8   Degree of cumulative effects

Degree of cumulation	$Z_{biol} = LC50/\text{lim}_{ch}$	$Z_{ch} = \text{lim}_{ac}/\text{lim}_{ch}$	Points
Low	<10	<2.5	2
Moderate	11–100	2.5–4.9	3
High	101–1000	5–10	4
Very high	>1000	>10	5

From experimental data:
LC50 = 21 000 mg/m^3
LD50 = 2700 mg/kg (mouse)
     = 3200 mg/kg (rat)
     = 1500 mg/kg (guinea-pig)
     = 3300 mg/kg (rabbit)

$$\log \text{lim}_{ch} = 0.62 \times \log(21 \ 000) - 1.08$$
$$= 0.62 \times 4.32 - 1.08$$
$$= 1.60$$

$$\text{lim}_{ch} = 40 \ mg/m^3$$

$$Z_{biol} = LC_{50}/\text{lim}_{ch}$$
$$= 21 \ 000/40$$
$$= 525.$$

From Table 20.8, a Z_{biol} value of 525 corresponds to 4 points.
CSS = 3300/1500 = 2.2
From Table 20.7, a CSS value of 2.2 corresponds to 2 points. Finally:

$$MAC = lim_{ch}/safety\ factor$$
$$= 40/(4 \times 2) = 40/8 = 5\ mg/m^3.$$

(The MAC for bromobenzene legislated in the USSR is 3 mg/m^3.)

To derive MACs for substances with irritation effects, two equations were proposed by N. G. Ivanov. These were:

$$log(MAC) = 0.69\ log(lim_{ac(rat)}') - 0.18\ log(lim_{ac(man)}) - 0.7\ log(Z_{ir}) - 0.51\ (r=0.96;$$
$S_{xy} = \pm 0.27$; when correlated with established MAC values)

$$log(MAC) = 0.11\ log(LC50) + 0.65\ log(lim_{ir(rat)}) - 0.72\ log\ (Z_{ir}) - 0.65$$
($r = 0.97$; $S_{zy} = \pm 0.27$; when correlated with established MAC values)

where $Z_{ir} = lim_{ac}/lim_{ir}$. Some values for Z_{ir} are listed in Table 20.9.

Table 20.9 · Limits of acute and irritative action for rats

Substance	lim_{ac} (mg/m^3)	lim_{ir} (mg/m^3)	Z_{ir}
1. Ammonia	462	228	2
2. Nitrogen dioxide	58	20	2.9
3. Bromine	50	10	5
4. 2-Chloroethanesulphchloride	97	12	8
5. Tributyl hydroperoxide	340	180	1.9
6. Phosphorus chloroxide	8	0.8	10
7. Sulphur monochloride	90	8.7	10
8. Bromoacetopropylacetate	13.5	4.3	3.1
9. Acetoperopylacetate	150	470	0.3
10. Glycidole	98	98	1
11. Pyromellite acid dianhydride	70	106	0.66
12. Chlorine	20	10	2
13. Sulphur anhydride	500	80	6.2

Responses considered when identifying an end-point for detection of lim_{ir} include respiration rate, olfactory responses, cellular reactions of the lungs and upper respiratory tract, and vital staining of lung tissue. For lim_{ac}, responses include body temperature, motor activity, muscular strength, orientation and oxygen consumption.

20.4 CONCLUSION

Although significant correlations do exist, on the whole, deriving occupational exposure limits based on chemical structure and physicochemical properties is not sufficiently exact for use with all chemicals. However, the establishment of equations specific to homologous or analogous series of chemicals can significantly increase the validity of calculated MACs.

Deriving MACs based on measures of biological activity appears to be the most valid approach, particularly when thresholds of action (either acute—$\lim_{ac}$—or chronic—$\lim_{ch}$) are used. The widespread use of rapid methods for deriving safe exposure levels is a necessity, but toxicological investigations should continue after an MAC has been established and the MAC should be recalculated as more and better data become available. It is also recommended that rapid methods of evaluating MACs only be used for classes of compounds with well understood properties and which do not have delayed or long-term effects, especially if manifested through limited contact with the substance.

BIBLIOGRAPHY

Bukovsky, M.I., Zhukov, V.I., and Kozhukhova, T.V. (1984). *Maximum Allowable Concentrations and Tentative Safe Exposure Levels of Harmful Substances in the Environmental Media* (Hygienic Standards Officially Approved in the USSR), Centre of International Projects, GKNT, Moscow, United Nations Environment Program, 114 p.

Bustueva, K.A., and Roscin, A.V. (1975). Safe levels of biological exposure to chemicals in the air of industrial premises and in the atmosphere. In: *Methods Used in the USSR for Establishing Biologically Safe Levels of Toxic Substances*, World Health Orgaization, Geneva, pp. 139–47.

Krasovskij, G.N. (1975). Species and sex differences in sensitivity to toxic substances. In: *Methods Used in the USSR for Establishing Biologically Safe Levels of Toxic Substances*, World Health Organization, Geneva, pp. 109–25.

Ljublina, E.I., and Filov, V.A. (1975). Chemical structure, physical and chemical properties and biological activity. In: *Methods Used in the USSR for Establishing Biologically Safe Levels of Toxic Substances*, World Health Organization, Geneva, pp. 19–44.

Santosky, I.V. (1975). Investigation of new substances: permissible limits and threshold of harmful action. In: *Methods Used in the USSR for Establishing Biologically Safe Levels of Toxic Substances*, World Health Organization, Geneva, pp. 9–18.

Sanotsky, I.V., and Ulanova, I.P. (1983). *Hygienic and Toxicological Criteria of Harmfulness in Evaluating Hazards of Chemical Compounds*, Centre of International Projects, GKNT, Moscow, United Nations Environment Program, 296 p.

Sidorenko, G.I., and Pinigin, M.A. (1975). Establishment of safe levels of chemicals in communal hygiene: methodological approaches. In: *Methods Used in the USSR for Establishing Biologically Safe Levels of Toxic Substances,* World Health Organization, Geneva, pp. 126–38.

Ulanova, I.P. (1975). Toxicometry and prophylactic toxicology. In: *Methods Used in the USSR for Establishing Biologically Safe Levels of Toxic Substances*, World Health Organization, Geneva, pp. 45–55.

CHAPTER 21

Computer-aided Chemical Structure-handling techniques in Structure–Activity Relationship Systems

JOSEF FRIEDRICH, WOLFGANG SCHUBERT AND IVAR UGI

2.1 INTRODUCTION

Structure–property correlation uses the occurrence of specific structural features within chemical molecules in statistical analyses. The features are correlated with physicochemical properties or biological activities. Quantitative structure–activity relationships (QSAR) have been predominantly applied to the design of drugs (see Ariens, 1971) and to the understanding of drug disposition (Lien,1981). Recently, considerable effort has been applied to the identification of chemicals with potential anticancer properties (Nasr *et al.*, 1984). The application of QSAR to the design of less toxic molecules has been recently reviewed by Hansch (1985).

21.2 STRUCTURE-HANDLING TECHNIQUES

21.2.1 General considerations

The general approach to structure-handling for SAR studies is depicted in Figure 21.1. Before any retrieval or correlation can be accomplished, the molecule file has to be processed by a feature recognition procedure. Not only structural features (such as the presence or absence of a carbonyl group) may be recognized, but also quantitative values such as topological indices or thermodynamic parameters may be included. The resulting file of structural and quantitative features will be used for further processing in retrieval or correlation.

Property estimation can be achieved by summation of substructures which contribute to a thermochemical or physicochemical property. The Hansch form of linear free energy relationship studies is a special case of the summation procedure (Kim *et al.*, 1979). The Free–Wilson method (Free and Wilson, 1964) works on the assumption that the contribution of a substituent to a given property or activity of a

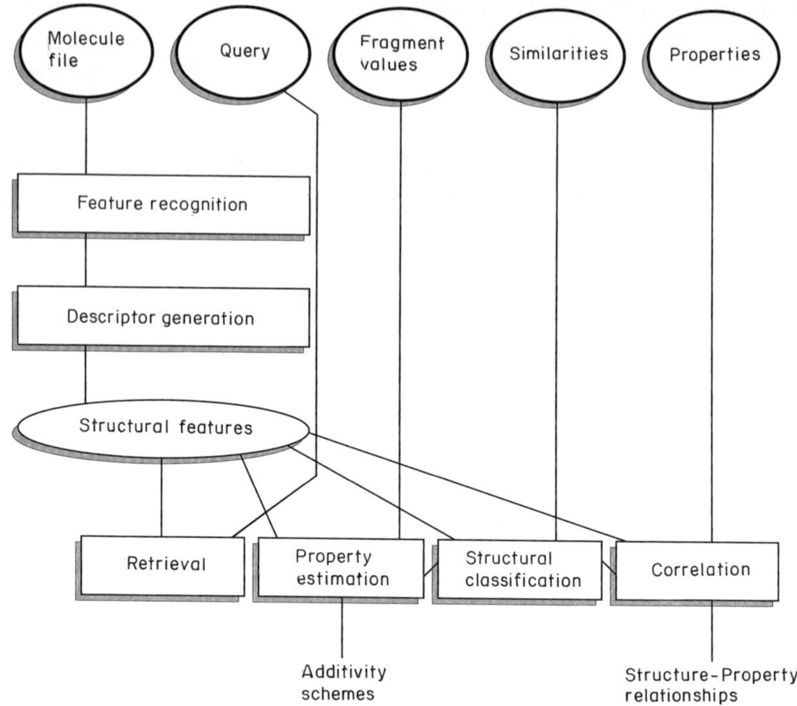

Figure 21.1   General overview of a SAR system.

molecule is independent of the contributions of other substituents at other positions in the molecule. Similarity measures, like the minimum chemical distance (Jochum *et al.*, 1982) may be used to classify structures.

21.2.2 Structural features

The simple types of structural features include basic structural units such as the total number of atoms, bonds, rings, multiple bonds, and particular atoms. Descriptors of this type do not discriminate well except in a molecule data set where all the compounds are very similar. However, in conjunction with additional structural features, they have been used in multiple regression, discriminant analyses and pattern-recognition studies.

A more sophisticated approach to defining structural features is to identify sub-structures or 'fragments' of a whole molecule. These may include, for example, rings or specific functional groups. Such variables have been widely used by manual assignment in linear discriminant analyses. Ring/functionality variables have been derived from Wiswesser line notation (WLN) for structure–toxicity analyses

(Enslein and Craig, 1979). In addition to the fragment itself, the type and relative positions of heteroatoms and substituents in six-membered ring systems were used in regression analysis of physicochemical, thermochemical and biological properties and cluster analyses.

Templates are similar to fragments but represent a 'superstructure' which is superimposed on all molecules of the data set. Free–Wilson analysis falls within this category. The template-fitting process may be done manually or automatically, derived from structures encoded in the form of connection tables.

Paths of atoms and bonds through the molecule have been used, such as a path joining two heteroatoms or chains of four to six specified atoms with bonds specified only as ring or non-ring. The most extreme approach is to take any possible path and build a molecular descriptor on the basis of autocorrelation vectors. For each property, the components of the descriptor consist of all the products of two atoms having different pathlengths between each other (Moreau and Broto, 1980). Such a descriptor has nice mathematical properties but chemical interpretation becomes difficult.

21.2.3 Feature selection

Features such as ring fragments, heteropaths, atom chains or augmented atoms may be valuable in defining pharmacophoric patterns in a single fragment. Selection of such features may be done automatically if the structures are represented by a fragment code such as WLN, or manually. Using an automated approach, the descriptors are fixed and some important substructures may not be detected. Manual selection is more flexible but is subjective and introduces bias.

Algorithmically-drived variable (feature) sets tend to represent the molecule much better than preselected sets do. For property estimation, it is essential to consider the whole molecule, so that the incremental contributions of all structural units are included. However, for correlations with physicochemical properties, a fixed set of features representing only a part of the total structure may be sufficient.

If variables overlap, problems of redundancy may arise. This could mean that some variables correlate strongly. In particular, the mixed-descriptor approach, where structural features and physicochemical parameters together constitute a descriptor, may create problems. Different types of descriptors with different weights may substitute for one another and thus create difficulties in interpretation. These problems might be eliminated by restricting the types of descriptors; by running a step-by-step analysis procedure in order to select a subset of the descriptors or to create new variables by a transformation process.

Often, less complex variables can be more effective for prediction, as demonstrated by Adamson and Bawden (1977). Sometimes, a hierarchy of descriptor types, where a higher descriptor also contains the features of any lower one, may be better (Friedrich and Ugi, 1979, 1980).

21.3 DESIGN OF A STRUCTURE–ACTIVITY CORRELATION SYSTEM

21.3.1 Design features

An ideal QSAR system would be easy to use, have a rapid response time, and would be able to handle large data sets and large molecules. It would also incorporate a procedure for the selection of structural features which is flexible, and applicable to any kind of molecule. The procedure would also create features which do not overlap or intercorrelate, are appropriately distributed through the data set and which are not given too much weight.

The two most important system features, flexible structural features and fast response time, are difficult to incorporate. Therefore, most systems in use are based on fixed feature descriptors (such as WLN) and run as batch programs. To overcome some of these difficulties, we devised an algorithm and implemented the corresponding computer program (Friedrich and Ugi, 1980). The essence of this system is the pregeneration of all conceivable substructures in a hierarchical order (Figure 21.2). Once the complete set of substructures and their interconnections through 'father–son' relations has been established, 'OR', 'AND' and 'NOT' substructure queries are performed on the stored network of substructures without the need to analyse and manipulate graphs or to reproduce structural representations out of other fixed fragment descriptions. For instance, a search for molecules containing a certain substructure (for example, $C = O$) would only lead to computing the corresponding substructure point in the network, entering there, and pursuing the substructure interconnections 'upwards' towards their 'fathers' (i.e. towards the unfragmented molecules of the data set). Following the network in the other direction from a subset of tagged 'active' terminal molecules leads to the substructures which are statistically the most significant for the activity in question; they have the highest ratio of active/inactive embedding molecules.

Thus we deal not only with flexible structural features covering any kind of molecule, we also avoid strong overlap (where one structure contains others) by selecting the most 'active' substructures, which are determined to have no substructures of greater activity in the hierarchy 'above' or 'below'.

It is an important feature of the design of the substructure network that each substructure is generated and stored only once, regardless of the number of molecules or larger substructures in which it occurs. Due to the fact that smaller substructures are more likely to be encountered, the introduction of a new molecule may add only a few larger substructures to the total network. Therefore, the more molecules the data set contains, the more economically the fragmentation process works.

It may happen that the size of some big molecules will lead to a disproportionately large number of large substructures requiring excessive amounts of computer space and computing time. In order to overcome problems created by these large molecules and their large molecular fragments, without relinquishing the speed and generality of the system with respect to the more widely occurring smaller

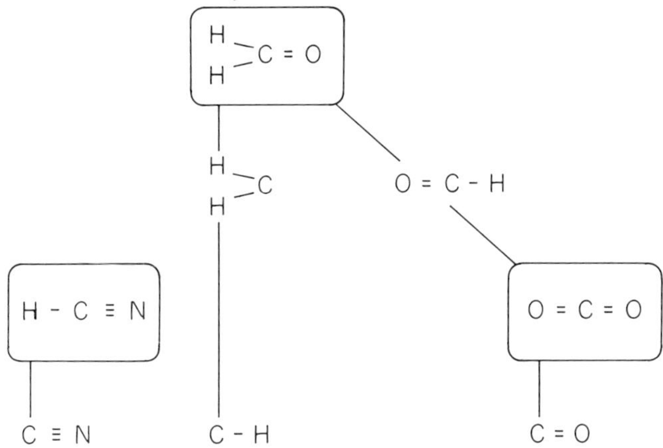

Figure 21.2   Example of a hierarchical approach for handling chemical fragments and substructures in a QSAR system.

substructures, screens of a predetermined size are generated by a fast algorithm. Here the requirements in computer time and space increase only quadratically with the chosen screen size, whereas the full substructure generation would increase with the 3rd power of the molecule's size. These screens overcome the problem of too many large substructures but also prevent the user from introducing any bias into the substructure network if manual screening procedures were used.

21.3.2   System performance

To test this system we investigated the influence of a series of substituted *o*-toluenesulphonylthioureas and *o*-toluencsulphonylureas on the level of blood sugar in rats using the data of Dove and Franke (1979). Our system automatically found the molecular fragments responsible for the effects of concern and determined the probability of incorrectly classifying the fragments. We have also tested the system using Japanese data on the accumulation of about 100 substances in fish. These substances included polychlorinated aromatic compounds, heterocyclics, alcohols and aliphatic compounds. Figure 21.3 represents the preliminary findings of our investigation.

21.4   ACKNOWLEDGEMENTS

Development and design of this computer program was funded mainly by the Commission of the European Communities. Several versions of this program now exist. One operates in Ispra, Center of Euratom and at the University of Copenhagen, Denmark. Another version was given to the Bayer AG, Leverkusen.

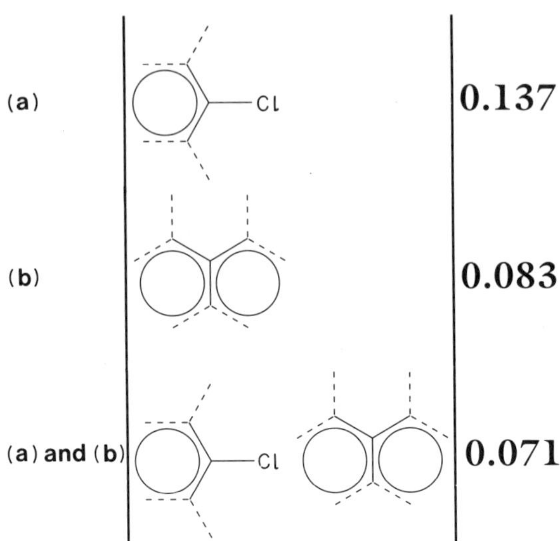

Figure 21.3   Results of a preliminary QSAR analysis of accumulation of chemicals in fish.

The Sumitomo Chemical Company received its version from the literature (i.e. from Friedrich and Ugi, 1980). The program is still under development at the Technical University of Munich.

REFERENCES

Adamson, G.W., and Bawden, D. (1977). A substructural analysis method for structure–activity correlation of heterocyclic compounds using Wiswesser Line Notation. *J. Chem. Inf. Comput. Sci.*, **17**, 164–71.

Ariens, J. (Ed.) (1971). *Drug Design*, Academic Press, New York.

Dove, S., and Franke, R. (1979). Discriminant-analytical investigation on the structure dependence of hyperglycemic and hypoglycemic activity in a series of substituted *o*-toluenesulfonylthioureas and *o*-toluenesulfonylureas. *J. Med. Chem.*, **22**, 90–95.

Enslein, K., and Craig, P.N. (1979). Status report on development of predictive models of toxicological endpoints. Genese Corp., Rochester, NY.

Free, S.M., and Wilson, J.W. (1964). A mathematical contribution to structure–activity studies. *J. Med. Chem.*, **7**, 395–9.

Friedrich, J., and Ugi, I. (1979). Substructure searchng and structure property locating by means of subgraph generation. *Match*, **6**, 201–211.

Friedrich, J., and Ugi, I. (1979). Substructure retrieval and the analysis of structure–activity relations on the basis of complete and ordered set of fragments. *J. Chem. Res.*, microfilm 1301z–80, 1401–97 and 1501–50.

Hansch, C. (1985). The QSAR paradigm in the design of less toxic molecules. *Drug Metab. Rev.*, **15**(7), 1279–94.

Jochum, C., Gasteiger, J., Ugi, I., and Dugundji, J. (1982). The principle of minimal chemical distance and the principle of minimum structure change. *Z. Naturforsch.*, **37b**, 1205–15.

Kim, K.H., Hansch, C., Fukunaga, J.Y., Steller, E.E., Jow, P.T.C., Craig, P.N., and Page, J. (1979). Quantitative structure–activity relationships in 1-aryl-2-(alkylamino)ethanol anti-malerials *J. Med. Chem.*, **22**, 366–91.

Lien, E.J. (1981). Structure–activity relationships and drug disposition. *Ann. Rev. Pharmacol. Toxicol.*, **21**, 31–61.

Moreau, G., and Broto, P. (1980). The autocorrelation of the topological molecular structure: a new molecular descriptor. *Nouveau Journal de Chimie*, **4**, 359–60.

Nasr, M., Paull, K.D., and Narayanan, V.L. (1984). Computer-assisted structure–activity correlations. *Adv. Pharmacol. Chemother.*, **20**, 123–90.